PSYCHOSOCIAL
CARE for People with Diabetes

Deborah Young-Hyman, PhD
Mark Peyrot, PhD

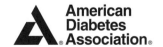
American
Diabetes
Association

Director, Book Publishing, Abe Ogden; *Managing Editor,* Greg Guthrie; *Acquisitions Editor,* Victor Van Beuren; *Production Manager,* Melissa Sprott; *Copyediting,* Cenveo Publisher Services; *Composition,* ADA; *Cover Design,* Koncept, Inc.; *Printer,* Versa Press.

Printed in the United States of America
1 3 5 7 9 10 8 6 4 2

The suggestions and information contained in this publication are generally consistent with the *Clinical Practice Recommendations* and other policies of the American Diabetes Association, but they do not represent the policy or position of the Association or any of its boards or committees. Reasonable steps have been taken to ensure the accuracy of the information presented. However, the American Diabetes Association cannot ensure the safety or efficacy of any product or service described in this publication. Individuals are advised to consult a physician or other appropriate health care professional before undertaking any diet or exercise program or taking any medication referred to in this publication. Professionals must use and apply their own professional judgment, experience, and training and should not rely solely on the information contained in this publication before prescribing any diet, exercise, or medication. The American Diabetes Association—its officers, directors, employees, volunteers, and members—assumes no responsibility or liability for personal or other injury, loss, or damage that may result from the suggestions or information in this publication.

♾ The paper in this publication meets the requirements of the ANSI Standard Z39.48-1992 (permanence of paper).

ADA titles may be purchased for business or promotional use or for special sales. To purchase more than 50 copies of this book at a discount, or for custom editions of this book with your logo, contact the American Diabetes Association at the address below, at booksales@diabetes.org, or by calling 703-299-2046.

American Diabetes Association
1701 North Beauregard Street
Alexandria, Virginia 22311

DOI: 10.2337/9781580404396

Library of Congress Cataloging-in-Publication Data

Young-Hyman, Deborah.
  Psychosocial care for people with diabetes / Deborah Young-Hyman.
      pages cm
  Includes bibliographical references and index.
  ISBN 978-1-58040-439-6 (alk. paper)
  1. Diabetics--Services for--Unites States--Standards. 2. Diabetes--Social aspects. 3. Clinical health psychology--United States. 4. Diabetics--Rehabilitation--Psychological aspects. I. American Diabetes Association. II. Title.
  RA645.D5Y68 2012
  362.1964'62--dc23
                                    2012031896

Contents

Acknowledgments   v
Mark Peyrot
Deborah Young-Hyman

Introduction   vii

I. Behavioral Health

1. Depression and Diabetes   1
Mary de Groot, PhD

2. Eating Disorders and Disordered Eating Behavior   17
Deborah Young-Hyman, PhD, CDE

3. Hypoglycemia   33
Linda Gonder-Frederick, PhD
Daniel J. Cox, PhD, ABPP
Harsimran Singh, PhD
Jaclyn A. Shepard, PsyD

4. Cognitive Difficulties in Children with Type 1 Diabetes   57
Clarissa S. Holmes, PhD

5. Neurocognitive Dysfunction in Adults with Diabetes   69
Christopher M. Ryan, PhD

II. Self-Management

6. Assessment of Diabetes Knowledge, Self-Care Skills,
   and Self-Care Behaviors by Questionnaire   101
Garry Welch, PhD
Softja E. Zagarins, PhD

7. Adherence to Medical Regimens   117

Suzanne Bennett Johnson, PhD

8. Lifestyle Modification: Nutrition   131
   Judith Wylie-Rosett, EdD, RD
   Linda M. Delahanty, MSRD

9. Lifestyle Modification: Exercise   147
   David G. Marrero, PhD
   Paula M. Trief, PhD

III. Implementation of Treatment Technology

10. Subcutaneous Insulin Infusion or Insulin Pump Therapy   159
    Jill Weissberg-Benchell, PhD, CDE

11. Psychosocial Considerations Regarding Adoption
    of Intensive Management   171
    Lori Laffel, MD, MPH

12. Bariatric Surgery   193
    Brooke A. Bailer, PhD
    Thomas A. Wadden, PhD
    Lucy F. Faulconbridge, PhD
    David B. Sarwer, PhD

IV. Life Course Issues

13. Psychosocial Adjustment to Diabetes and
    Critical Periods of Psychological Risk   219
    Richard R. Rubin, PhD
    Mark Peyrot, PhD

14. Special Issues in Children and Adolescents   229
    Tim Wysocki, PhD
    Barbara J. Anderson, PhD

15. Lifespan Development Issues for Adults   251
    Paula M. Trief, PhD

16. Diabetes-Related Functional Impairment and Disability   273
    Felicia Hill-Briggs, PhD

List of Contributors   291

Index   293

Acknowledgments

We would like to thank several people involved in the planning and development of this work who are not named authors. These include current and former American Diabetes Association (ADA) officers and staff, particularly Nathaniel Clark, as well as those behind the scenes who supported revisions to the ADA standards of care to include psychosocial issues and those at the ADA who facilitated the approval and financing of this volume. We also want to acknowledge several behavioral diabetes experts who contributed to this effort, including Robert Anderson, William Polonsky, and Paul Ciechanowski.

We would be remiss in not giving special thanks to Barbara Anderson and Richard Rubin for their tireless and longstanding leadership in the field of behavioral diabetes research and treatment, including editing a key publication in this arena (Anderson 2002). Finally, we offer our sincerest thanks to our editor at ADA, Victor Van Beuren. Without his assistance, encouragement, and support, this volume would never have seen the light of day.

Mark Peyrot
Deborah Young-Hyman
September 1, 2012

BIBLIOGRAPHY

Anderson BJ, Rubin RR: *Practical Psychology for Diabetes Clinicians: How to Deal With the Key Behavioral Issues Faced by Patients and Health Care Teams.* 2nd ed. Alexandria, VA, American Diabetes Association, 2002

Introduction

It is well recognized that diabetes is a chronic illness managed in a collaborative fashion between health care providers, patients, and patients' families; that diabetes and routine diabetes care affect virtually all aspects of the patient's daily life (including his or her emotional life); and that life events, in turn, influence his or her ability to manage diabetes. Diabetes does not *have* psychosocial issues; at a fundamental level diabetes *is* a psychosocial issue, or rather a set of psychosocial issues. Medical management of diabetes is inextricably intertwined with these psychosocial issues, and it can be daunting for the clinician to undertake responsibility for addressing them simultaneously. Yet addressing both sets of issues is imperative if either is to be addressed successfully. Psychosocial issues range widely, including such disparate elements as management of depression and other psychological disorders or conditions; how to work effectively with low literacy patients; helping patients develop effective, long-lasting self-management plans by considering patients' priorities, goals, resources, attitudes, and knowledge about diabetes; and how disease management fits into a patient's or family's lifestyle.

To date there has been little in the way of guidelines to help clinicians address critical psychosocial issues. Although psychosocial issues are included in the American Diabetes Association's annually published *Clinical Practice Recommendations*, they are only briefly mentioned, primarily in terms of their association with medical management. Evaluations are recommended and clinicians are advised to refer their patients to behavioral specialists "as indicated." However, outcomes of diabetes care include patient psychosocial well-being, not just medical outcomes, and the interrelationship between the two makes a resource book essential.

The body of literature on diabetes-related psychosocial issues has become quite substantial. Studies have documented the relationship between diabetes outcomes and psychosocial factors. A multifactorial approach suggests that these relationships are dynamic and reciprocal. *Psychosocial Care for People with Diabetes* presents recommendations for dealing with psychosocial factors as a part of routine care as well as assessment and referral for diabetes-specific psychosocial problems requiring the intervention of specialists. This volume addresses the major psychosocial issues facing the clinician and patient in the context of living with and managing diabetes, including factors such as the life stage of the patient, socio-cultural context and resources (technical, financial, and interpersonal), the patient-provider relationship, and responsibility for implementing diabetes self-management as well as behavior change strategies. Chapters address the specifics of and the interface between components of treatment (such as insulin pump use, continuous glucose monitoring, medical nutrition therapy, and physical activity), patient and provider adherence to recommended care, age-specific life-course issues, psychological adjustment to and sequelae of illness, as well as special population needs. Critical periods for psychological risk are addressed, as well as issue-specific recommendations for assessment and treatment. Clinical recommendations are based on published literature and expert opinion.

This volume is organized into four main sections: Behavioral Health, Self-Management, Implementation of Treatment Technology, and Life Course Issues. While there are many connections and overlaps among the topics covered in these sections, it was necessary to impose a somewhat artificial division of the material into separate sections and chapters. Behavioral Health, covering conditions that are thought of as being the special purview of behavioral specialists, may be a major reason for clinicians to seek guidance from this volume. Similarly, while behaviors through which patients self-manage their diabetes are *the* essential component of diabetes management, it is generally accepted that behavioral specialists have an important role to play in assisting clinicians deal with issues of behavior change and maintenance; thus, a section on Self-Management is included. There is a separate section on Implementation of Treatment Technology, as the focus shifts to considering the role of behavioral and psychosocial factors in the use of technologic aids in diabetes care. Finally, the last section, Life Course Issues, returns to consideration of fundamental life processes in which diabetes and its care are embedded.

Chapters in the section on Behavioral Health include the conditions of depression (Chapter 1) and disordered eating behavior (Chapter 2), which can be considered psychological disorders. Compared to healthy populations, patients with diabetes have been shown to have higher prevalence of these conditions, at both subclinical and diagnostic levels. These symptoms, conditions, or diagnoses (depending on severity) illustrate the interaction between patient adjustment to illness and underlying physiologic processes of the disease(s). Recent research has begun to establish reciprocal relationships between the onset of these disorders and diabetes (see Chapter 1 on depression and Chapter 2 on disordered eating behavior). Thus, attention to the presence of depression and disordered eating behavior is essential to the successful management of the disease. While hypoglycemia is not a purely behavioral health issue, Chapter 3 demonstrates that its occurrence, course, and consequences are inextricably linked to behavior. Severe hypoglycemia and glucose toxicity (hyperglycemia) have been associated with cognitive function in individuals with diabetes across the life span. Chapters 4 and 5 on neurocognitive functioning present what is known regarding glycemia and cognitive function: neurocognitive issues regarding the accomplishment of age-appropriate tasks, brain function and how it relates to cognitive tasks that can be impaired by glycemia, and structural changes in the brain consequent to the disease. A main focus of both neurocognitive chapters regards patients' ability to accomplish self-management behaviors and what steps should be taken when cognitive impairment is suspected.

The next section of this volume, Self-Management, targets knowledge, skills, behaviors, and lifestyle modifications that enable patients to successfully manage the disease. The authors address the interactions among care providers, patients, and the patients' physical, interpersonal, and community environments. Chapter 7 gives a general framework for addressing issues of self-management in the framework of adherence to medical regimen, paying special attention to patient-provider communication. Chapter 6 on assessment/monitoring of the various components of self-management provides a foundation for intervention efforts. Evidence-based studies and theory-based conceptualization demonstrate how access to resources (see Chapter 9 on exercise), responsibility taking (see Chapter 7 on adherence), and structured interventions (see Chapter 8 on nutrition) impact adoption and maintenance of self-care behaviors, thereby improving or inhibiting treatment success. This section underscores the need for multidisciplinary screening and care, and should help the clinician identify appropriate resources for non-medical aspects of care.

The chapters in the Implementation of Treatment Technology section present what is known about prescribing and implementing advances in intensive treatment technologies such as use of insulin pumps (see Chapter 10), aids for improving adherence such as continuous glucose monitoring (CGM) and intensification of regimens (see Chapter 11), and bariatric surgery (see Chapter 12), proven to ameliorate type 2 diabetes in obese individuals. These technologies are relatively new in our treatment armamentarium, and therefore long-term outcome data is not yet available. However, the chapters present recommendations for screening, use, and monitoring of psychosocial issues related to technology implementation. Although these advanced treatment technologies are potentially available to all individuals with diabetes, systematic protocols for screening regarding patient suitability and psychosocial monitoring of their use are not broadly disseminated or standardized. Inclusion of these chapters is meant to facilitate clinicians' choice of psychosocial criteria to consider when implementing intensive treatment regimens, and to suggest psychological processes and developments that need monitoring.

The final section, Life Course Issues, contains chapters that address both the life course of the patient and psychosocial issues inherent in the life course of the disease. With the exception of diabetes remission via bariatric surgery or transplantation (the latter technology still in the experimental stage), the disease is chronic and progressive. Therefore there are predictable times when disease management becomes more difficult, distress can be expected, and more resources are needed (see Chapter 13). It is unclear how often this treatment perspective, anticipatory guidance regarding expected difficulties, is implemented in clinical care. Complicating expected disease progression is the idiosyncratic life course of the individual. Three chapters focus on how care can be enhanced for the specific needs of these populations at particular stages of life: childhood and adolescence (Chapter 14), adulthood (Chapter 15), and when disability occurs—often in later life (Chapter 16). The intersection between the life course of the individual and the progression of the disease becomes of greater concern as more children are diagnosed with type 2 diabetes, and as treatment for all types of diabetes improves so that patients can be expected to live longer with the disease.

It is hoped that these recommendations will serve to inform and influence public policy for guiding diabetes care and research, as well as the reimbursement policies of the various insurers and managed care organizations. In addition to being a clinical resource, the systematic presentation of this body of information should serve to enhance the likelihood that adequate resources are available to respond effectively to the psychosocial needs of patients with diabetes. Recent pharmacologic and technical advances have made available increasingly complex treatment regimens that can improve medical outcomes. In the final analysis, however, adoption of effective treatment is based on the knowledge, beliefs, attitudes, and behaviors of patients, caretakers, and health care providers about how psychosocial barriers can be overcome to improve the health and quality of life of people with diabetes and their families.

Chapter 1
Depression and Diabetes

Mary de Groot, PhD

ASSESSMENT AND DIAGNOSIS OF DEPRESSION

Depression refers to a spectrum of disorders and cluster of symptoms that involve sad or blue mood or anhedonia, neurovegetative symptoms (e.g., changes in appetite, sleep), and cognitive impairments occurring during a discrete period of time. Major depressive disorder (MDD) is defined as a cluster of five or more of the following symptoms occurring two weeks or longer: depressed or sad mood, loss of pleasure or interest in routine activities, changes in weight or appetite, hyper- or hyposomnia, fatigue, psychomotor agitation or retardation, worthlessness or excessive guilt, decreases in concentration, and/or suicidal ideation or attempt (American Psychiatric Association [APA] 2000). Episodes may be recurrent or single events.

Subsyndromal depression or minor depressive disorders include dysthymia (low-grade depression lasting more than half of the time during a two-year period), adjustment disorder with depressed mood (a period of depression lasting no more than 6 months in response to an identifiable psychosocial stressor such as a major life event or medical event), and depressive disorder not otherwise specified (a period of depressive symptoms resulting in impairment in social or occupational functioning that does not meet criteria for other diagnostic categories) (APA 2000).

Diabetes-related distress is distinguished from depression spectrum disorders in that concerns are directly related to diabetes management and/or social support (e.g., interactions with relatives pertaining to self-care behaviors) (Fisher 2007). Distress is specifically associated with the experience of living and managing diabetes. Diabetes-related distress may coincide with or exist separately from depressive symptoms or episodes (Fisher 2007). Although diabetes-related distress is an appropriate target for psychosocial interventions, it is not currently designated as a psychiatric diagnosis.

Analyses of several national surveys have identified demographic and psychosocial correlates of MDD or depressive symptoms in individuals with diabetes that include: female sex, younger age, BMI >30 kg/m^2, high school education, poverty, smoking, treatment with insulin, higher A1C, single marital status, poor health status perception, and increased number of complications (Egede 2003, Jones 2004, Katon 2004b, Nichols 2007). The onset of symptoms may be gradual or correspond closely to an external event that is readily identifiable by the patient.

DIFFERENTIAL DIAGNOSES

The diagnosis of MDD is excluded in the presence of primary psychotic disorders (e.g., schizophrenia, schizoaffective disorder, delusional disorders) or the presence of manic or hypomanic periods resulting in the diagnosis of bipolar disorder I or II, respectively (APA 2000). Anxiety spectrum disorders (e.g., panic disorder, agoraphobia, specific phobia, social phobia, obsessive compulsive disorder, generalized anxiety disorder) may co-occur with the diagnosis of a depression spectrum disorder (APA 2000) (Table 1.1).

Table 1.1. DSM-IV Criteria for a Major Depressive Episode

A. Five or more of the following symptoms have been present during the same 2-week period and represent a change from previous functioning; at least one of the symptoms is either *1*) depressed mood or *2*) loss of interest or pleasure
    1. depressed mood most of the day, nearly every day, as indicated by either subjective reports or observation made by others
    2. markedly diminished interest or pleasure in all, or almost all, activities most of the day, nearly every day (as indicated by either subjective account or observation made by others)
    3. significant weight losses when not dieting or weight gain, or decrease or increase in appetite nearly every day
    4. insomnia or hypersomnia nearly every day
    5. psychomotor agitation or retardation nearly every day (observable by others, not merely subjective feelings of restlessness or being slowed down)
    6. fatigue or loss of energy nearly every day
    7. feelings of worthlessness or excessive or inappropriate guilt (which may be delusional) nearly every day (not merely self-reproach or guilt about being sad)
    8. diminished ability to think or concentrate, or indecisiveness, nearly every day (either by subjective account or as observed by others)
    9. recurrent thoughts of death (not just fear of dying), recurrent suicidal ideation without a specific plan, or a suicide attempt or a specific plan for committing suicide

B. The symptoms do not meet criteria for a Mixed Episode

C. The symptoms cause clinically significant distress or impairment in social, occupational, or other important areas of functioning

D. The symptoms are not due to the direct physiological effects of a substance (e.g., a drug of abuse, a medication) or a general medical condition (e.g., hypothyroidism)

E. The symptoms are not better accounted for by bereavement, i.e., after the loss of a loved one, the symptoms persist for longer than 2 months or are characterized by marked functional impairment, morbid preoccupation with worthlessness, suicidal ideation, psychotic symptoms, or psychomotor retardation.

MEASUREMENT OF DEPRESSION

Depressive symptoms may be adequately measured using self-report symptom inventories such as the Beck Depression Inventory-II (BDI-II) (Beck 1996), the nine-item depression scale of the Patient Health Questionnaire (PHQ-9)

(Kroenke 2001), or the Center for Epidemiologic Studies Depression Scale (CES-D) (Radloff 1977). These measures vary in the number and content of items and may be used selectively for a variety of purposes (e.g., clinical screening, research). All have been developed for the general population (i.e., they are not diabetes specific) and have demonstrated acceptable levels of validity and reliability. For each measure, clinical cutoff scores that correspond to clinically significant and diagnosable depression have been developed and validated in psychiatric samples (Radloff 1977, Beck 1996, Kroenke 2001). The BDI has been specifically validated for use in patients with type 1 diabetes (T1D) and type 2 diabetes (T2D) (Lustman 1997a). It should be noted that the BDI-II and PHQ-9 gather specific information about suicidal ideation and/or intent and plan. These measures should be used in a setting where patient responses can be evaluated by providers immediately following completion and where follow-up evaluation of risk of self-harm and referral are available.

Psychiatric interview protocols available for the assessment of depression range from semi-structured interviews such as the Schedule for Affective Disorders and Schizophrenia-Lifetime Version (SADS-L) and Structured Clinical Interview for the DSM-IV-TR (SCID) (Spitzer 1992, Williams 1992) to structured interviews such as the Composite International Diagnostic Interview (CIDI) (Robins 1988) and the Diagnostic Interview Schedule (DIS) (Helzer 1988) that can be administered and scored through computer interface (Erdman 1992). The DIS has been validated for use in patients with T1D and T2D (Lustman 1986). These interview protocols require expert training in psychopathology and interview assessment. A clinician version of the SCID (Spitzer 1992, Williams 1992) is available; however, these interviews are more commonly used in the context of clinical research protocols.

Two measures have been created to measure diabetes-related distress: the Problem Areas in Diabetes (PAID) and Diabetes Distress Scale (DDS) (Welch 1997, Polonsky 2005, Fisher 2007). These measures show some shared variance with self-report depression questionnaires (Fisher 2007) as well as unique variance (Welch 1997, Hermanns 2006).

PREVALENCE OF COMORBID DEPRESSION AND DIABETES

The majority of studies have examined cross-sectional rates of MDD and/or depressive symptoms in samples diagnosed with T1D and T2D. Meta-analyses of the literature of prevalence rates of depression or depressive symptoms in patients with T1D have shown increased rates of depression in diabetes samples compared with nondiabetic control subjects (21.6 T1D vs. 11.4% nondiabetic) (Anderson 2001, Barnard 2006, Shaban 2006). Similarly, meta-analyses conducted on studies of depression in people with T2D have found increased rates of depression compared with nondiabetic control subjects (27 vs. 17.6%) (Anderson 2001, Ali 2006). Depression assessment methods and thresholds vary considerably in this literature as do rates of MDD and depressive symptoms (e.g., psychiatric interview protocols yield an average rate of depression of 11% compared with 31% in those using self-report questionnaires) (Anderson 2001). Psychiatric interviews provide greater diagnostic precision, and therefore lower prevalence rates, by permitting interviewers to determine the timing, origins, and alternative diagnostic explanations for individual depressive symptoms that may be endorsed by the patient (e.g., expectable bereavement vs. major depressive disorder). These distinctions are not made in self-report measures, so depressive symptoms attributable to any cause may be reported by respondents.

Overall, rates of depression among patients with T1D and T2D are ~2 times greater than those in the general population (Anderson 2001) (see one exception: Pouwer 2003). Women with diabetes are 1.6 times more likely to report depressive symptoms than their male counterparts with diabetes, with one study finding a stronger association among younger women (<40 years) (Anderson 2001, Zhao 2006). Rates of depression among men with T1D have been shown to exceed those in nondiabetic comparison samples (Barnard 2006, Shaban 2006). The majority of studies have been conducted with white, middle-class samples; however, rates of depressive symptoms do not appear to vary considerably across diverse racial, ethnic, or international samples (Gary 2000, Grandinetti 2000, Fisher 2001, Roy 2001, de Groot 2006, Wagner 2006, Asghar 2007, de Groot 2007). Few studies have used well-controlled prospective designs.

Well-controlled prospective longitudinal studies of the psychological characteristics of children and adolescents with T1D have shown mixed findings with regard to elevated rates of comorbid depression. Some studies have observed elevated rates (Kokkonen 1995, Kovacs 1997, Grey 2002), whereas others observed no differences in rates of depression compared to healthy control subjects (Jacobson 1997b). In one study, women with diabetes showed greater risk for depression recurrence than males with diabetes or psychiatric counterparts (Kovacs 1997). In a sample of youth (ages 10–21 years), men with T2D showed greater risk of self-reported depressive symptoms compared with men with T1D (Lawrence 2006). Depressive symptoms appear to increase the risk for worsened glycemic control, earlier-onset diabetic retinopathy, and increased adolescent hospitalizations and emergency department visits (Kovacs 1995, Stewart 2005, Lawrence 2006).

Few studies have examined the naturalistic course of depression in adults with T1D and T2D. Depressive symptoms and affective disorders have been found to be highly persistent (e.g., 73–79% remain depressed) in prospective longitudinal investigations over 1–5 years follow-up (Lustman 1988, Peyrot 1999) with or without treatment. For example, a 5-year follow-up of patients enrolled in an 8-week antidepressant treatment trial found that 92% of patients experienced persistent or recurrent MDD, with 58% experiencing recurrence within 12 months of treatment (Lustman 1997c).

IMPACT OF DEPRESSION ON DIABETES AND PSYCHOSOCIAL OUTCOMES

Depression has been found to be associated with worsened glycemic control and diabetes complications in diagnosed T1D and T2D samples. In a meta-analysis of 25 cross-sectional studies, small-to-medium effect sizes in the relationship between hyperglycemia and depressive symptoms were observed (Lustman 2000a). Recent cross-sectional studies have mirrored this finding among Hispanic adults (Gross 2004), children with T1D (Stewart 2005), and postmenopausal women with a lifetime history of MDD (Wagner 2007b). Prospective studies of changes in depressive symptoms have not shown depression to predict changes in glycemic control among ethnically diverse middle-age and older adults (Gary 2005, Trief 2006). Adherence to self-care behaviors does not appear to be a mediator between depressive symptoms and glycemic control among adults with T1D and T2D (Lustman 2005). A meta-analysis of 27 studies found medium effect sizes in the association between depression and worsened long-term diabetes complications (e.g., macrovascular disease, neuropathy, nephropathy, retinopathy, microvascular disease) in both T1D and T2D samples (de Groot 2001, Clouse 2003). Recent work examining the relationship of depression and diabetic neuropathy is consistent with these findings (Vileikyte 2005).

There is accumulating evidence for negative outcomes associated with comorbid depression including: decreased adherence to diabetes self-care behaviors, such as dietary recommendations, exercise behaviors, and oral hypoglycemic regimens (Ciechanowski 2000, Vickers 2006); decreased quality of life (Jacobson 1997a, Gaynes 2002); decreased social support (Sacco 2006); increased functional disability compared to nondiabetic patients with MDD (Egede 2004, Bruce 2005) as well as significant unemployment and work disability (Von Korff 2005); increased hospitalizations in children with T1D (Stewart 2005); and earlier mortality after adjusting for covariates (e.g., age, diabetes complications) (Katon 2005, Zhang 2005, Ismail 2007). Minor depression may also be associated with lower self-reported health status, cognitive limitations (e.g., confusion, memory loss, difficulty making decisions), and diabetes symptoms (Egede 2002b, Katon 2007, McCollum 2007), although additional evidence is needed to further elucidate this relationship.

Analyses of the economic impact of comorbid depression and diabetes have indicated that individuals with both disorders have higher ambulatory care use, greater prescription expenditures, and higher overall health care expenditures than patients with diabetes alone (Ciechanowski 2000, Egede 2002b, Finkelstein 2003, Jones 2004, Nichols 2007).

DEPRESSION AS A PREDICTOR OF DIABETES

A bidirectional association has been observed for depression and diabetes in which depression has been found to increase the risk of the development of T2D in prospective longitudinal cohorts (Eaton 1996, Knol 2006, Engum 2007) and the presence of diabetes increases the risk of developing depression postdiagnosis (Anderson 2001, Ali 2006, Barnard 2006, Shaban 2006). Some studies have reported as much as a two-fold risk of subsequent T2D in the presence of MDD or moderate depressive symptoms (Eaton 1996, Engum 2007), whereas others report modest or nonsignificant risk estimates over similar periods after adjusting for covariates such as BMI and education (Carnethon 2003, Saydah 2003, Arroyo 2004, Golden 2004, Carnethon 2007). A meta-analysis of nine studies found a 37% increase in risk for T2D with a lifetime history of depressive symptoms (Knol 2006). Evidence from the Third National Health and Nutrition Examination Survey (NHANES III) suggests that a lifetime history of MDD among women under the age of 40 years increased the risk of metabolic syndrome, although additional studies are needed to confirm this finding (Kinder 2004).

TREATMENT METHODS AND PROVIDERS

Depression can be effectively treated in diabetes patients using traditional treatment modalities such as antidepressant medications, individual cognitive behavioral therapy (CBT), and problem-solving therapy (PST). Randomized placebo-controlled trials of tricyclic (e.g., nortriptyline) (Lustman 1997b) and selective serotonin reuptake inhibitor (SSRI) antidepressant medications (e.g., fluoxetine [Lustman 2000b], sertraline [Goodnick 1997], paroxetine [Paile-Hyvarinen 2003]) have been shown to be efficacious in treating depression. An uncontrolled randomized trial comparing fluoxetine and paroxetine showed comparable improvement in depression in a sample of patients with T2D and MDD (Gulseren 2005). Nortriptyline (25–50 mg q.d.) has been found to have a hyperglycemic effect on blood glucose control following treatment. Fluoxetine (40 mg q.d. maximum dose), sertraline (50 mg q.d. maximum dose), paroxetine (20 mg q.d.), and bupropion extended release (150–450 mg q.d.) (Lustman 2007) have been found to be associated with overall improvement in glycemic control and for BMI when bupropion was tested (Lustman 2007). Maintenance treatment using sertraline has been shown to be effective in extending depression remission compared to placebo (Lustman 2006), with sustained hypoglycemic effects observed for one year following depression remission in both placebo and sertraline treatment groups. In this study, younger adults (age <55 years) showed longer periods of symptom remission in the sertraline group compared with placebo and older adults (Williams 2007).

CBT has also been shown to effectively treat depression in patients with T2D in a randomized controlled trial compared to a diabetes education intervention (Lustman 1998). Improvements in A1C in the CBT group were observed at the 6-month follow-up evaluation and exceeded those of the control group.

Recent studies have demonstrated the efficacy of a collaborative care approach utilizing PST (Katon 2004c). In the Pathways study, T1D and T2D participants meeting criteria for MDD or dysthymia (persistent low-grade depressive mood lasting 2 or more years) from nine primary care health settings were randomized to either a case management intervention embedded within a primary care setting or usual care (UC). Patients receiving the case management intervention received a stepped-care approach utilizing education and support for antidepressant medication and/or PST delivered by trained clinical specialist nursing staff (Katon 2004c). Patients receiving the intervention showed greater improvements in adequate dosing of antidepressant medications, less severe depression, higher patient ratings of global improvement, and higher satisfaction with care over a 12-month follow-up period (Katon 2004c). Patients with two or more diabetes complications receiving the intervention showed greater improvements in depression outcomes at follow-up compared with the UC group. Patients with fewer than two diabetes complications showed comparable depression outcomes to the UC group (Kinder 2006). Patient attachment style was shown to be associated with depression treatment success using PST compared to UC (Ciechanowski 2006). Overall, no improvements in glycemic control or adherence to diabetes self-care behaviors were observed from baseline to 6- or 12-month follow-up evaluation (Katon 2004c, Lin 2006). A small decrease in BMI was observed and nonadherence to oral hypoglycemic agents increased over time in the intervention group (Lin 2006).

Participants did not receive diabetes-specific education or adherence support for diabetes self-management that might have contributed to improvement in glycemic outcomes. This treatment approach has been shown to be a cost-effective means of providing treatment for co-occurring depression, with limited additional cost associated with the intervention and significant cost savings associated with non–mental health expenditures over time (Katon 2006, Simon 2007).

A variety of barriers to adequate treatment of depression in patients with diabetes have been identified. These include stigma associated with mental illness and patient perceptions of depressive symptoms as a form of weakness or an inevitable consequence of chronic illness (Egede 2002a); perceived discrimination in medical and mental health care resulting in racial and ethnic disparities in the use of depression treatment (Egede 2002a, de Groot 2006, Wagner 2007a); lack of screening and adequate diagnosis by primary care physicians (Katon 2004a); lack of dose adjustment of antidepressant medications by primary care providers (Katon 2004a); and lack of referrals to psychotherapy services in addition to antidepressant medication treatment (Katon 2004a). Patient satisfaction with the use of antidepressant medications and mental health providers has been shown to be favorable among those who have received depression treatment (Katon 2004c, de Groot 2006).

RECOMMENDATIONS FOR FUTURE RESEARCH

Based on the available literature, a number of areas merit additional research attention to further define the etiology, course, outcomes, and treatment of comorbid depression and diabetes.

1. Little is known about the physiologic factors responsible for apparent increased rates of depression in T1D and T2D. Further research is needed to evaluate the neurochemical, hormonal, immune/inflammatory, and neurological contributors to depression in diabetes.
2. Although there is mounting evidence for increased prevalence of depression in T1D and T2D, the majority of studies have been cross-sectional and uncontrolled in design. Prospective, controlled studies are needed to better characterize the course and impact of clinical depression in diabetes as well as the unique contribution of depression on the development of metabolic syndrome and T2D. Clinical definitions and thresholds should be used to distinguish depression syndromes from short-term emotional states (e.g., adjustment to the diagnosis of diabetes or the development of a complication) and diabetes-related distress.
3. There is currently a paucity of literature addressing rates and correlates of depression among children with T2D and women with gestational diabetes.
4. Although there is strong evidence for the efficacy of one tricyclic antidepressant medication and four SSRI medications, more research is needed to characterize the efficacy of short- and long-term use and relationship to glycemic control of the full spectrum of SSRI and SNRI (serotonin and norepinephrine reuptake inhibitor) antidepressant medications in both adults and children with diabetes.

5. Additional research is needed to evaluate exercise as an efficacious and effective treatment modality for the treatment of depression in patients with T1D and T2D.
6. Additional research is needed to investigate effective means of depression prevention in patients with diabetes.
7. Additional research is needed to establish the cost-effectiveness of all modes of depression treatment in patients with T1D and T2D.

RECOMMENDATIONS FOR SCREENING AND CARE

Depression is a frequent comorbid condition in patients with T1D and T2D. The following recommendations for clinical care are based on the literature and expert opinion (Evans 2005):

1. Depression screening is recommended at every visit for diabetes patients, accompanied by procedures to review patient responses and address clinically significant levels of symptoms. Increased concern is indicated for patients presenting with elevated blood glucose and with worsening diabetes complications and those who report a lifetime history of depression and may therefore be at increased risk for future depressive episodes. Providers may use a variety of brief screening tools to detect depressive symptoms in diabetes patients.
2. Providers are recommended to maintain a low threshold for depression treatment and promote rigorous, ongoing treatment of depression, once identified. Adequate adjustment of dosing for antidepressant medications, well-monitored maintenance therapy, and referrals to mental health services should be routinely provided by health care providers. Coordination of depression and diabetes care across providers is also recommended to ensure adequate depression treatment and follow-up care in light of the persistence and recurrence of depression in diabetes patients and the association with poor medical management.
3. Evidence supports the use of a stepped-care approach (medication and therapy) and monitored maintenance therapy to achieve symptom remission and improvements in glycemic control.
4. Use of a collaborative care approach that integrates therapy and antidepressant medication within primary care settings is suggested. This intervention paradigm has demonstrated the capacity to reduce some barriers, such as social stigma, to the effective treatment of depression in diabetes patients and has been shown to be cost-effective to health care organizations.
5. Incorporation of depression curricula into diabetes education and routine communication with patients about the role of depression in diabetes outcomes is recommended to reduce patient perceptions of stigma associated with mental illness and improve patient awareness of treatment options.
6. Incorporation of depression screening measures into clinical care outcomes within health care organizations is recommended.

BIBLIOGRAPHY

Ali S, Stone MA, Peters JL, Davies MJ, Khunti K: The prevalence of co-morbid depression in adults with type 2 diabetes: a systematic review and meta-analysis. *Diabet Med* 23:1165–1173, 2006

American Psychiatric Association: *Diagnostic and Statistical Manual of Mental Disorders - DSM-IV-TR*. 4th ed. Washington, D.C., American Psychiatric Association, 2000

Anderson RJ, Freedland KE, Clouse RE, Lustman PJ: The prevalence of comorbid depression in adults with diabetes: a meta-analysis. *Diabetes Care* 24:1069–1078, 2001

Arroyo CG, Hu FB, Ryan L, Kawachi I, Colditz G, Speizer F, Manson J: Depressive symptoms and risk of type 2 diabetes in women. *Diabetes Care* 27:129–133, 2004

Asghar S, Hussain A, Alit SMK, Khan AKA, Magnusson A: Prevalence of depression and diabetes: a population-based study from rural Bangladesh. *Diabet Med* 24:872–877, 2007

Barnard KD, Skinner TC, Peveler R: The prevalence of co-morbid depression in adults with type 1 diabetes: systematic literature review. *Diabet Med* 23:445–448, 2006

Beck AT, Steer RA, Brown GK: *BDI-II Beck Depression Inventory Manual*. 2nd ed. San Antonio, TX, The Psychological Corporation, Harcourt, Brace & Company, 1996

Bruce DG, Davis WA, Davis TME: Longitudinal predictors of reduced mobility and physical disability in patients with type 2 diabetes. *Diabetes Care* 28:2441–2447, 2005

Carnethon M, Biggs M, Barzilay JJ, Smith N, Vaccarino V, Bertoni AG, Arnold A, Siscovick D: Longitudinal association between depressive symptoms and incident type 2 diabetes mellitus in older adults: the Cardiovascular Health Study. *Arch Intern Med* 167:802–807, 2007

Carnethon M, Kinder L, Fair J, Stafford R, Fortmann S: Symptoms of depression as a risk factor for incident diabetes: findings from the National Health and Nutrition Examination Epidemiologic Follow-Up Study, 1971–1992. *Am J Epidemiol* 158:416–423, 2003

Ciechanowski PS, Russo JE, Katon WJ, Von Korff M, Simon GE, Lin EHB, Ludman EJ, Young BA: The association of patient relationship style and outcomes in collaborative care treatment for depression in patients with diabetes. *Med Care* 44:283–291, 2006

Ciechanowski PS, Katon WJ, Russo JE: Depression and diabetes: impact of depressive symptoms on adherence, function, and costs. *Arch Intern Med* 160:3278–3285, 2000

Clouse RE, Lustman PJ, Freedland KE, Griffith LS, McGill JB, Carney RM: Depression and coronary heart disease in women with diabetes. *Psychosom Med* 65:376–383, 2003

de Groot M, Doyle T, Hockman E, Wheeler C, Pinkerman B, Shubrook J, Gotfried R, Schwartz F: Depression among type 2 diabetes rural Appalachian clinic attenders. *Diabetes Care* 30: 1602–1604, 2007

de Groot M, Pinkerman B, Wagner J, Hockman E: Depression treatment and satisfaction in a multicultural sample of type 1 and type 2 diabetic patients. *Diabetes Care* 29:549–553, 2006

de Groot M, Anderson RJ, Freedland KE, Clouse RE, Lustman PJ: Association of depression and diabetes complications: a meta-analysis. *Psychosom Med* 63:619–630, 2001

Eaton WW, Armenian H, Gallo J, Pratt L, Ford DE: Depression and risk for onset of type 2 diabetes. *Diabetes Care* 19:1097–1102, 1996

Egede LE: Diabetes, major depression and functional disability among U.S. adults. *Diabetes Care* 27:421–428, 2004

Egede LE, Zheng D: Independent factors associated with major depressive disorder in a national sample of individuals with diabetes. *Diabetes Care* 26:104–111, 2003

Egede LE: Beliefs and attitudes of African Americans with type 2 diabetes toward depression. *Diabetes Educ* 28:258–268, 2002a

Egede LE, Zheng D, Simpson K: Comorbid depression is associated with increased health care use and expenditures in individuals with diabetes. *Diabetes Care* 25:464–470, 2002b

Engum A: The role of depression and anxiety in onset of diabetes in a large population-based study. *J Psychosom Res* 62:31–38, 2007

Erdman HP, Klein MH, Greist JH, Skare SS, Husted JJ, Robins LN, Helzer JE, Goldring E, Hamburger M, Miller JP: A comparison of two computer-administered versions of the NIMH Diagnostic Interview Schedule. *J Psychiatr Res* 26:85–95, 1992

Evans D, Charney DS, Lewis L, Golden RN, Gorman JM, Krishnan KRR, Nemeroff CB, Bremner JD, Carney RM, Coyne JC, Delong MR, et al.: Mood disorders in the medically ill: scientific review and recommendations. *Biol Psychiatry* 58:175–189, 2005

Finkelstein, EA, Bray JW, Chen H, Larson MJ, Miller K, Tompkins C, Keme A, Manderscheid R: Prevalence and costs of major depression among elderly claimants with diabetes. *Diabetes Care* 26:415–420, 2003

Fisher L, Skaff MM, Mullan JT, Arean P, Mohr D, Masharani U, Glasgow R, Laurencin G: Clinical depression versus distress among patients with type 2 diabetes: not just a question of semantics. *Diabetes Care* 30:542–548, 2007

Fisher L, Chesla CA, Mullan JT, Skaff MM, Kanter RA: Contributors to depression in Latino and European-American patients with type 2 diabetes. *Diabetes Care* 24:1751–1757, 2001

Gary TL, Baptiste-Roberts K, Crum RM, Cooper LA, Ford DE, Brancati FL: Changes in depressive symptoms and metabolic control over 3 years among African Americans with type 2 diabetes. *Int J Psychiatry Med* 35:377–382, 2005

Gary TL, Crum RM, Cooper-Patrick L, Ford D, Brancati FL: Depressive symptoms and metabolic control in African-Americans with type 2 diabetes. *Diabetes Care* 23:23–29, 2000

Gaynes BN, Burns B, Tweed D, Erickson P: Depression and health-related quality of life. *J Nerv Ment Dis* 190:799–806, 2002

Golden SH, Williams JE, Ford DE, Yeh H, Sanford CP, Nieto FJ, Brancati FL: Depressive symptoms and the risk of type 2 diabetes. *Diabetes Care* 27:429–435, 2004

Goodnick PJ, Kumar A, Henry JH, Buki VM, Goldberg RB: Sertraline in coexisting major depression and diabetes mellitus. *Psychopharmacol Bull* 33:261–264, 1997

Grandinetti A, Kaholokula J, Crabbe K, Kenui C, Chen R, Chang H: Relationship between depressive symptoms and diabetes among native Hawaiians. *Psychoneuroendocrinology* 25:239–246, 2000

Grey M, Whittemore R, Tamborlane W: Depression in type 1 diabetes children: natural history and correlates. *J Psychosom Res* 53:907–911, 2002

Gross R, Olfson M, Gameroff M, Carasquillo O, Shea S, Feder A, Lantigua R, Fuentes M, Weissman M: Depression and glycemic control in Hispanic primary care patients with diabetes. *J Gen Intern Med* 20:460–466, 2004

Gulseren L, Gulseren S, Hekimsoy Z, Mete L: Comparison of fluoxetine and paroxetine in type II diabetes mellitus patients. *Arch Med Res* 36:159–165, 2005

Helzer JE, Robins LN: The Diagnostic Interview Schedule: its development, evolution and use. *Soc Psychiatry Psychiatr Epidemiol* 23:6–16, 1988

Hermanns N, Kulzer B, Krichbaum M, Kubiak T, Haak T: How to screen for depression and emotional problems in patients with diabetes: comparison of screening characteristics of depression questionnaires, measurement of diabetes-specific emotional problems and standard clinical assessment. *Diabetologia* 49:469–477, 2006

Ismail K, Winkley K, Stahl D, Chalder T, Edmonds M: A cohort study of people with diabetes and their first foot ulcer: the role of depression on mortality. *Diabetes Care* 30:1473–1479, 2007

Jacobson AM, de Groot M, Samson JA: The effects of psychiatric disorders and symptoms on quality of life in patients with type I and type II diabetes mellitus. *Qual Life Res* 6:11–20, 1997a

Jacobson AM, Hauser ST, Willet JB, Wolfsdorf JI, Dvorak R, Herman L, de Groot M: Psychological adjustment to IDDM: 10-year follow-up of an onset cohort of child and adolescent patients. *Diabetes Care* 20:811–818, 1997b

Jones LE, Clarke W, Carney CP: Receipt of diabetes services by insured adults with and without claims for mental disorders. *Medical Care* 42:1167–1175, 2004

Katon W, Lin EHB, Kroenke K: The association of depression and anxiety with medical symptom burden in patients with chronic medical illness. *General Hospital Psychiatry* 29:147–155, 2007

Katon W, Unutzer J, Fan M, Williams JW, Schoenbaum M, Lin EHB, Hunkeller EM: Cost-effectiveness and net benefit of enhanced treatment of depression for older adults with diabetes and depression. *Diabetes Care* 29:265–270, 2006

Katon W, Rutter C, Simon G, Lin EB, Ludman E, Ciechanowski P, Kinder L, Young G, von Korff M: The association of comorbid depression with mortality in patients with type 2 diabetes. *Diabetes Care* 28:2668–2672, 2005

Katon W, Simon G, Russo J, von Korff M, Lin E, Ludman E, Ciechanowski P, Bush T: Quality of depression care in a population-based sample of patients with diabetes and major depression. *Med Care* 42:1222–1229, 2004a

Katon W, Von Korff M, Ciechanowski P, Russo J, Lin E, Simon G, Ludman E, Walker E, Bush T, Young B: Behavioral and clinical factors associated with depression among individuals with diabetes. *Diabetes Care* 27:914–920, 2004b

Katon W, Von Korff M, Lin E, Simon G, Ludman E, Russo J, Ciechanowski P, Walker E, Bush T: The Pathways Study. a randomized trial of collaborative care in patients with diabetes and depression. *Arch Gen Psychiatry* 61:1042–1049, 2004c

Kinder LS, Carnethon MR, Palaniappan LP, King AC, Fortmann SP: Depression and the metabolic syndrome in young adults: findings from the Third National Health and Nutrition Examination Survey. *Psychosom Med* 66:316–322, 2004

Kinder LS, Katon WJ, Ludman E, Russo J, Simon G, Lin EHB, Ciechanowski P, Von Korff M, Young B: Improving depression care in patients with diabetes and multiple complications. *J Gen Intern Med* 21:1036–1041, 2006

Knol MJ, Twisk JW, Beekman AT, Heine RJ, Snoek FJ, Pouwer F: Depression as a risk factor for the onset of type 2 diabetes mellitus: a meta-analysis. *Diabetologia* 49:837–845, 2006

Kokkonen J, Kokkonen ER: Mental health and social adaptation in young adults with juvenile-onset diabetes. *Nord J Psychiatry* 49:175–181, 1995

Kovacs M, Obrosky DS, Goldston D, Drash A: Major depressive disorder in youths with IDDM: a controlled prospective study of course and outcome. *Diabetes Care* 20:45–51, 1997

Kovacs M, Mukerji P, Drash A, Iyengar S: Biomedical and psychiatric risk factors for retinopathy among children with IDDM. *Diabetes Care* 18:1592–1599, 1995

Kroenke K, Spitzer RL, Williams JBW: The PHQ-9: validity of a brief depression severity measure. *J Gen Intern Med* 16:606–613, 2001

Lawrence JM, Standiford DA, Loots B, Klingensmith GJ, Williams DE, Ruggiero A, Liese AD, Bell RA, Waitzfelder BE, McKeown RE: Prevalence and correlates of depressed mood among youth with diabetes: the SEARCH for Diabetes in Youth study. *Pediatrics* 117:1348–1358, 2006

Lin EHB, Katon W, Rutter C, Simon GE, Ludman EJ, Von Korff M, Young B, Oliver M, Ciechanowski PC, Kinder L, Walker E: Effects of enhanced depression treatment on diabetes self-care. *Ann Fam Med* 4:46–53, 2006

Lustman PJ, Williams MM, Sayuk GS, Nix BD, Clouse RE: Factors influencing glycemic control in type 2 diabetes during acute- and maintenance-phase treatment of major depressive disorder with bupropion. *Diabetes Care* 30:459–466, 2007

Lustman PJ, Clouse RE, Nix BD, Freedland KE, Rubin EH, McGill JB, Williams MM, Gelenberg AJ, Ciechanowski PS, Hirsch IB: Sertraline for prevention of depression recurrence in diabetes mellitus: a randomized, double-blind, placebo-controlled trial. *Arch Gen Psychiatry* 63:521–529, 2006

Lustman PJ, Clouse RE, Ciechanowski PS, Hirsch IB, Freedland KE: Depression-related hyperglycemia in type 1 diabetes: a mediational approach. *Psychosom Med* 67:195–199, 2005

Lustman PJ, Anderson RJ, Freedland KE, de Groot M, Carney RM, Clouse RE: Depression and poor glycemic control: a meta-analytic review of the literature. *Diabetes Care* 23:934–942, 2000a

Lustman PJ, Freedland KE, Griffith LS, Clouse RE: Fluoxetine for depression in diabetes: a randomized double-blind placebo-controlled trial. *Diabetes Care* 23:618–623, 2000b

Lustman PJ, Griffith LS, Freedland KE, Kissel SS, Clouse RE: Cognitive behavior therapy for depression in type 2 diabetes mellitus: a randomized, controlled trial. *Ann Intern Med* 129:613–621, 1998

Lustman PJ, Clouse RE, Griffith LS, Carney RM, Freedland KE: Screening for depression in diabetes using the Beck Depression Inventory. *Psychosom Med* 59:24–31, 1997a

Lustman PJ Griffith LS, Clouse RE, Freedland KE, Eisen SA, Rubin EH, Carney RM, McGill JB: Effects of nortriptyline on depression and glycemic control in diabetes: results of a double-blind, placebo-controlled trial. *Psychosom Med* 59:241–250, 1997b

Lustman PJ, Griffith LS, Freedland KE, Clouse RE: The course of major depression in diabetes. *Gen Hosp Psychiatry* 19:138–143, 1997c

Lustman PJ, Griffith LS, Clouse RE: Depression in adults with diabetes. Results of 5-yr follow-up study. *Diabetes Care* 11:605–612, 1988

Lustman PJ, Harper GW, Griffith LS, Clouse RE: Use of the Diagnostic Interview Schedule in patients with diabetes mellitus. *J Nerv Ment Dis* 174:743–746, 1986

McCollum M, Ellis SL, Regensteiner JG, Zhang W, Sullivan PW: Minor depression and health status among US adults with diabetes mellitus. *Am J Manag Care* 13:65–72, 2007

Nichols L, Barton PL, Glazner J, McCollum M: Diabetes, minor depression and health care utilization and expenditures: a retrospective database study. *Cost Effectiveness and Resource Allocation* 5(4), 2007.

Paile-Hyvarinen M, Wahlbeck K, Eriksson JG: Quality of life and metabolic status in mildly depressed women with type 2 diabetes treated with paroxetine: a single-blind randomised placebo controlled trial. *BMC Family Practice* 4(7), 2003

Peyrot M, Rubin RR: Persistence of depressive symptoms in diabetic adults. *Diabetes Care* 22:448–452, 1999

Polonsky WH, Fisher L, Earles J, Dudl RJ, Lees J, Mullan J, Jackson RA: Assessing psychosocial distress in diabetes. *Diabetes Care* 28:626–631, 2005

Pouwer F, Beekman ATF, Nijpels G, Dekker JM, Snoek FJ, Kostense PJ, Heine RJ, Deeg DJH: Rates and risks for co-morbid depression in patients with type 2 diabetes mellitus: results from a community-based study. *Diabetologia* 46:892–898, 2003

Radloff L: The CES-D scale: a self-report depression scale for research in the general population. *Applied Psychological Measurement* 1:385–401, 1977

Robins L, Wing J, Wittchen HU, Helzer JE, Babor TF, Burke J, Farmer A, Jablenski A, Pickens R, Regier DA, et al.: The Composite International Diagnostic Interview: an epidemologic instrument suitable for use in conjunction with different diagnostic systems in different cultures. *Arch Gen Psychiatry* 45:1069–1077, 1988

Roy A, Roy M: Depressive symptoms in African-American type I diabetics. *Depression and Anxiety* 13:28–31, 2001

Sacco WP, Yanover T: Diabetes and depression: the role of social support and medical symptoms. *J Behav Med* 29:523–531, 2007

Saydah SH, Brancati FL, Golden SH, Fradkin J, Harris MI: Depressive symptoms and the risk of type 2 diabetes mellitus in a US sample. *Diabetes/Metabolism Research and Reviews* 19:202–208, 2003

Shaban MC, Fosbury J, Kerr D, Cavan DA: The prevalence of depression and anxiety in adults with type 1 diabetes. *Diabet Med* 23:1381–1384, 2006

Simon GE, Katon WJ, Lin EHB, Rutter C, Manning WG, Von Korff M, Ciechanowski P, Ludman EJ, Young BA: Cost-effectiveness of systematic depression treatment among people with diabetes mellitus. *Arch Gen Psychiatry* 64:65–72, 2007

Spitzer R, Williams JBW, Gibbon M, First MB: The Structured Clinical Interview for DSM-III-R (SCID) - I: history, rationale, and description. *Arch Gen Psychiatry* 49:624–629, 1992

Stewart SM, Rao U, Emslie GJ, Klein D, White PC: Depressive symptoms predict hospitalization for adolescents with type 1 diabetes mellitus. *Pediatrics* 115:1315–1319, 2005

Trief PM, Morin PC, Izquierdo R, Teresi JA, Eimicke JP, Goland R, Starren J, Shea S, Weinstock RS: Depression and glycemic control in elderly ethnically diverse patients with diabetes. *Diabetes Care* 29:830–835, 2006

Vickers KS, Nies MA, Patten CA, Dierkhising R, Smith SA: Patients with diabetes and depression may need additional support for exercise. *Am J Health Behav* 30:353–362, 2006

Vileikyte L, Leventhal H, Gonzale J, Peyrot M, Rubin R, Ulbrecht J, Garrow A, Waterman C, Cavanagh P, Boulton A: Diabetic peripheral neuropathy and depressive symptoms. *Diabetes Care* 28:2378–2383, 2005

Von Korff M, Katon W, Lin EHB, Simon G, Ciechanowski P, Ludman E, Oliver M, Rutter C, Young B: Work disability among individuals with diabetes. *Diabetes Care* 28:1326–1332, 2005

Wagner J, Abbott G: Depression and depression care in diabetes: relationship to perceived discrimination in African Americans. *Diabetes Care* 30:364–366, 2007a

Wagner JA, Tennen H: History of major depressive disorder and diabetes outcomes in diet- and tablet-treated post-menopausal women: a case control study. *Diabet Med* 24:211–216, 2007b

Wagner J, Tsimikas J, Abbott G, de Groot M, Heapy A: Racial and ethnic differences in diabetic patient-reported depression symptoms, diagnosis, and treatment. *Diabetes Research and Clinical Practice* 75:119–122, 2006

Welch GW, Jacobson AM, Polonsky WH: The Problem Areas in Diabetes scale: an evaluation of its clinical utility. *Diabetes Care* 20:760–766, 1997

Williams JBW, Gibbon M, First MB, Spitzer RL, Davies M, Borus J, Howes MJ, Kane J, Pope HG Jr, Rounsaville B, Wittchen H-U: The Structured Clinical Interview for DSM-III-R (SCID) - II: multisite test-retest reliability. *Arch Gen Psychiatry* 49:630–636, 1992

Williams MM, Clouse RE, Nix BD, Rubin EH, Sayuk GS, McGill JB, Gelenberg AJ, Ciechanowski PS, Hirsch IB, Lustman PJ: Efficacy of sertraline in prevention of depression recurrence in older versus younger adults with diabetes. *Diabetes Care* 30:801–806, 2007

Zhang X, Norris SL, Gregg EW, Cheng YJ, Beckles G, Kahn HS: Depressive symptoms and mortality among persons with and without diabetes. *Am J Epidemiol* 161:652–660, 2005

Zhao W, Chen Y, Lin M, Sigal RJ: Association between diabetes and depression: sex and age differences. *Public Health* 120:696–704, 2006

Mary de Groot, PhD, is an Associate Professor of Medicine at the Indiana University School of Medicine in Indianapolis, IN.

Chapter 2
Eating Disorders and Disordered Eating Behavior

Deborah Young-Hyman, PhD, CDE

DEFINITION OF EATING DISORDERS (ED) AND DISORDERED EATING BEHAVIOR (DEB)

The American Psychiatric Association [APA] manual of mental health diagnoses (DSM-IV-TR 2000) (American Psychiatric Association 2000) defines disordered eating behaviors as caloric restriction, excessive exercise, use of laxatives and other forms of pharmacologic purging, binge eating, and, in patients with diabetes, intentional reduction or omission of insulin. DEB cognitions, which also contribute to diagnostic criteria, include preoccupation with weight and size and/or shape. Reflecting the predominant behavior type, major diagnostic categories of ED are anorexia, bulimia, and eating disorders not otherwise specified. Diagnosis of ED vs. DEB is based on the frequency of behavior and cognitions. When threshold frequency is documented, either by self-report or interview, behavior and cognitions reach the level of diagnosis (ED). Less frequent behaviors and cognitions are considered subclinical (DEB). Though behaviors vary, shared characteristics are that the person desires to control weight and change appearance, and the behaviors and cognitions interfere with other activities of daily living and are extreme. Concerns about shape and size drive maladaptive weight management behaviors. Behavioral criteria used in the general population are applied to patients with diabetes with the additional behavior of insulin manipulation (omission or reduction) (Crow 1998).

PATIENTS WITH DIABETES: A VULNERABLE POPULATION

Patients with type 1 and type 2 diabetes have elevated rates of overweight and obesity (Liu 2009). Weight status is strongly associated with DEB in otherwise healthy individuals seeking weight loss and in individuals with type 1 diabetes (T1D), particularly young women (Neumark-Sztainer 2002a, Young-Hyman 2011b, Young-Hyman 2011c). Although there is evidence regarding weight concerns, elevated BMI, and increased rates of binge eating in patients with type 2 diabetes (T2D) (Pinhas-Hamiel 1999, Papelbaum 2005), evidence linking weight, weight concerns, and development of ED and DEB in patients with T2D is scarce.

Behaviors and attitudes such as dietary restraint, food preoccupation (such as carbohydrate monitoring and restriction), portion control, control of blood glucose through selective food intake, and programmed exercise are prescribed components of diabetes treatment and are the cornerstone by which good glycemic control is achieved (American Diabetes Association [ADA] 2007). These treatment behaviors can become DEB when they are used inappropriately for rapid weight loss, carried to excess, interfere with activities of daily living, and/or become a health risk (American Psychiatric Association 2000, Daneman 2002).

Ongoing treatment of diabetes exposes patients to situations known to be triggers for the development of DEB. These include: feeling a loss of autonomy because of the monitoring/reporting of food intake, physical activity, and blood glucose to family members; monitoring by and accountability to health care providers to maintain health and weight (Surgenor 2002); sequelae of the treatment regimen such as changes in attitudes about eating (Steel 1990, Anderson 2002); increased sense of vulnerability and loss of control as a result of altered self and body concept (Steel 1990, Wolman 1994, Erkolahti 2003); and weight gain after the initiation of insulin treatment (Larger 2005). Adhering to treatment may be a predisposing risk factor for the development of DEB in patients with diabetes independent of other psychological, familial, or societal influences (Colton 1999).

Although there remain questions about whether DEB is associated with poorer long-term metabolic control in patients with T1D (Affenito 1997a, Herpertz 1998a, Engstrom 1999, Peveler 2005), the presence of diagnosable ED and behavior categorized as subclinical DEB has been shown to be associated with an increase in complications: retinopathy (Rydall 1997), neuropathy (Steel 1987), transient lipid abnormalities (Affenito 1997b), increased hospitalizations for diabetic ketoacidosis (Rodin 1992), and poorer short-term metabolic control (Rodin 1992, Affenito 1997a, Meltzer 2001). Cross-sectional studies have shown associations between elevated A1C and the presence of diagnosable ED (Wing 1986, Affenito 1997a, Herpertz 1998a), subclinical DEB (Wing 1986), and intentional insulin omission (Jones 2006). Associations between DEB and the complications of T2D have not been extensively examined (Herpertz 1998b, Herpertz 2000, Herpertz 2001, Papelbaum 2005). Refusal to initiate insulin treatment by patients with T2D (psychological insulin resistance) (Davis 2006) may be driven, in part, by concerns about weight gain, but this is anecdotal and has not been systematically tested.

An assessment of DEB should be performed when weight gain, weight loss, and/or worsening glycemic control (including severe hypoglycemia and/or ketoacidosis) cannot be explained by disease processes, changes in care, medication or insulin regimen, a monitored weight-loss program, obvious noncompliance, or psychiatric morbidity, especially in young women (Daneman 2002).

PREVALENCE OF DIAGNOSABLE ED AND SUBCLINICAL DEB

Diagnosable ED has low prevalence in the diabetes population (Ackard 2008). There are varying estimates of the prevalence of diagnosable ED and DEB in individuals with T1D compared with healthy referent populations (Crow 1998, Engstrom 1999). Estimates range from 3.8% (Pollack 1995) to 31% in adolescent and young adult women with T1D (Polonsky 1994). Some studies have found similar rates to the general population and some higher, but assessment methods vary (Rodin 1986–1987, Steel 1989, Fairburn 1991, Peveler 1992, Striegel-Moore 1992, Crow 1998, Herpertz 1998a, Bryden 1999, Engstrom 1999, Meltzer 2001).

Subclinical DEB is increasing in all segments of the U.S. population and Westernized cultures, presumably associated with emphasis on the thinness ideal and concern about overweight/obesity. Prevalence rates of subclinical DEB may be underestimated because dieting behavior is common and there is a stigma attached to self-reporting DEB (Neumark-Sztainer 2002b). The prevailing belief is that the diagnosis of diabetes is associated with elevated rates of DEB when intentional reduction in insulin dose or omission is considered purging behavior to control weight, especially in women with T1D and in adolescent girls (Hudson 1983, Bubb 1991, Rodin 1991, Hockey 1993, Biggs 1994, Pollack 1995, Crow 1998, Affenito 2001). However, a recent study using a population-based healthy comparison sample did not show elevated rates of diagnosable ED in the cohort with diabetes (Ackard 2008).

Bulimic behaviors and insulin omission are the most commonly reported DEB in patients with T1D (Goebel-Fabbri 2008, Alice Hsu 2009), whereas caloric restriction/restraint and binging are more commonly reported by women with T2D (Herpertz 2001, Young-Hyman 2010). Rates of DEB in boys with diabetes have been shown to be considerably lower than those found for women (Meltzer 2001, Neumark-Sztainer 2002a) but may be increasing (Svensson 2003). Higher prevalence of T2D in minority populations could potentially be associated with increased rates of DEB but this relationship has not yet been demonstrated. Studies that compare occurrence of DEB in patients with type 1 versus type 2 diabetes show similar rates; however, types of behaviors reported differ. "Drive for thinness" and "body dissatisfaction" are more common in individuals with T2D. Intentional insulin omission (to cause glycosuria) is more common in patients with T1D (Herpertz 1998b, Herpertz 2001).

Among overweight young women attempting weight loss, both with (type 1) and without diabetes, weight status is a strong predictor of DEB (Striegel-Moore 1992, Vamado 1997, Arriaza 2001, Sherwood 2001, Neumark-Sztainer 2002b, Rodin 2002, Decaluwe 2003, de Man Lapidoth 2006, Shisslak 2006). In studies reporting BMI, type 1 cohorts have been significantly heavier than healthy control subjects, with average BMI above the normal range. Elevation in weight, independent of diagnosis, would in itself predict higher rates of DEB (Engstrom 1999, Jones 2006). However, few studies of diabetes cohorts have compared rates of DEB with healthy control groups matched for age, sex, and weight (Engstrom 1999, Colton 2004, Jones 2006). When subjects matched for BMI were used to compare overweight and obese patients having T2D with obese nondiabetic patients seeking weight loss and an obese nonclinical sample (Battaglia 2006), low levels of binge eating disorder were diagnosed overall (<5% in all groups). However, obese patients with diabetes had the lowest scores on the Eating Disorder Examination, but the highest scores on the Restraint scale (Mannucci 2002). Higher scores on the Restraint scale were attributed to treatment behaviors. Although there is robust documentation that behavior generally considered subclinical DEB using DSM criteria such as binge eating, purging (defined as intentional insulin omission), and caloric restriction are commonly reported by patients with diabetes (Fairburn 1991, Bryden 1999, Jones 2006), it is not known how much these reports reflect cognitions based on attempted adherence to the diabetes care regimen.

Weight gain consequent to good blood glucose control could be a driver of weight concerns (Meltzer 2001, Battaglia 2006) and is known to be a side effect of successful treatment (Steel 1990). Although the presumption is that DEB in this population is associated with elevated BMI levels, only one study stratified the diabetes cohort (both type 1 and 2 diabetes, men and women, age range 18–65 years) by weight status. Three percent of under- and normal weight women had a current ED, whereas 6.8% of the overweight and 10.3% of obese women reported DEB (Herpertz 1998b). These rates are similar to samples with equivalent BMIs seeking weight loss (Vamado 1997). A conflict may exist between the need to control weight and achieve good glycemic control (in patients with both T1D and T2D). In particular, young adult and adolescent women have been shown to use insulin omission specifically for weight control (Biggs 1994, Khan 1996). Fear of improved glycemic control "because I will gain weight" and diabetes-specific distress predict intentional insulin omission (Polonsky 1994). Although one goal of medical nutrition therapy (MNT) is to prevent weight gain (Nathan 2005), supervised weight management programs are not routinely available when weight gain occurs secondary to successful treatment with insulin.

ETIOLOGY OF ED AND DEB IN THE DIABETES POPULATION: PSYCHIATRIC SYMPTOMS, REGIMEN COMPLIANCE (OR NONCOMPLIANCE), OR PHYSIOLOGIC DYSREGULATION

Primary risk factors for ED and DEB (in the nondiabetic population) are weight and size concerns, early eating problems and dieting, the presence of other forms of psychopathology, sexual abuse and other adverse life experiences, and low self-worth (Jacobi 2004). Except for weight concerns and depression, the relationships between these risk factors and occurrence of DEB in the diabetic population have received little attention.

Establishing the occurrence of DEB attributable to having diabetes and managing the disease is complicated by the paucity of studies that concurrently assess psychiatric symptoms, psychological adjustment to illness, and sequelae of the diabetes care regimen. Bryden et al. (1999) tracked BMI along with weight and shape concerns in adolescents and young adults with T1D; as both men and women became overweight, DEB increased. However, baseline and ongoing psychological status, independent of weight concerns, was not assessed. In contrast, Pollock et al. (1995) followed new-onset girls and boys with T1D (ages 8–13 years) from diagnosis for up to 14 years. The presence of DEB, compliance with medical regimen, and psychiatric symptoms were assessed, including weight concerns. Low rates of DSM-III diagnosable ED (3.8%) were found; however "youths with eating problems were nine times more likely to have had a psychiatric disorder than the rest of the patients" (p. 291). A recent study found that onset of insulin restriction in women with T1D was associated with fear of weight gain and problems with the self-management regimen (Goebel-Fabbri 2011). Problematic eating behavior specific to the diabetes care regimen appears to be part of a constellation of pervasive noncompliance associated with higher psychiatric morbidity or poorer adjustment to illness (Pollock 1995, Wilfley 2000, Pollock-BarZiv 2005, Goebel-Fabbri 2011).

Two studies demonstrated an association between psychiatric morbidity and DEB in patients with T2D independent of weight status. In one study, overweight and obese patients had more diagnosable ED, and patients with ED had significantly more anxiety disorders and trended towards being more depressed. In the second, DEB was also strongly associated with psychopathology such as depression, low self-esteem, and general psychopathology but not weight (Herpertz 1998b, Papelbaum 2005). Given the known comorbidity between emotional disorders (depression in particular) (Anderson 2001) and diabetes, and between emotional disorders and DEB in the healthy population (Telch 1998, Stice 1999, Stice 2000, Stice 2001, Stice 2002), DEB could be part of a constellation of poor psychological adjustment and/or poor adjustment to illness, which is comorbid with overweight and T2D (Herpertz 1998a).

Behaviors considered triggers for and pathognomonic of DEB are embedded in the diabetes treatment regimen (Bantle 2006). Lack of success with MNT can leave patients feeling out of control of both eating behavior and glycemia (Surgenor 2002). Feeling out of control of eating behavior, preoccupation with food, and calorie restriction are DSM-IV-TR diagnostic criteria for bulimia, binge eating disorder, and eating disorder not otherwise specified (American Psychiatric Association 2000). Primary criteria for binge eating disorder include subjective self-evaluation of repeatedly eating amounts of food in a short period of time that are "definitely larger than most individuals would eat under similar circumstances." Making this subjective determination (when an amount of food is large or excessive) for an individual with diabetes could be attributable to failure to adhere to MNT prescription, especially in the context of treatment of hypoglycemia. Other possibilities exist for misattribution of adherent behavior as DEB (Polonsky 1999). As caloric restraint is prescribed as part of treatment, inaccuracies in judgment regarding appropriateness of food intake can occur in the context of carbohydrate counting, falling blood glucose level, misjudgment of the causes of symptoms (Johnson 2000, Hay 2003, Davis 2004), or excessive nutrition intake related to exercise.

Hormonal evidence for dysregulation of hunger and satiety in patients with diabetes suggests difficulty controlling food intake and consequent blood glucose levels. Further, nonphysiologic dosing of insulin impacts appetite regulation (Young-Hyman 2010). Hormonal dysregulation (including loss of endogenous insulin and amylin secretion) (Koda 1992, Kruger 1999), dysregulation of incretin production, which contributes to metabolism in the gut (Dupre 2005, Higgins 2007), complications of the disease such as gastroparesis (Parkman 2004), and fluctuations in blood glucose level, particularly hypoglycemia (ADA 2002), may predispose vulnerable patients to adoption of maladaptive weight management strategies (such as insulin manipulation) to control hunger and associated weight gain.

MEASUREMENT OF ED AND DEB

Most studies to date have used measurement tools standardized in the general population to establish the presence of ED and DEB in patients with diabetes. Questionnaires include but are not limited to the Eating Attitudes Test (EAT) 40 (Garner 1979) and EAT-26 (Garner 1982), Eating Disorder Inventory (EDI-3)

(Garner 2004), the Bulimia Test - Revised (BULIT-R) (Thelen 1991), and the Eating Disorder Examination (EDE) (Cooper 1989), which is conducted in interview format. Evaluation tools include items about attitudes and behaviors that are embedded in the diabetes treatment regimen. For example BULIT-R items ("Do you feel you have control over the amount of food you consume?" and "I eat a lot of food when I'm not even hungry.") could refer to the diabetes care regimen (the former by prescription of dietary restraint and the latter by a prescribed meal plan), carbohydrate to insulin ratio, and/or treatment for low blood glucose. Diabetes care providers identified more than twenty questions on the EDI-3 that could be answered in the context of treatment and endorsed independent of weight concerns (Young-Hyman 2010). When questionnaires standardized in healthy populations are used, scores may be elevated in patients with both T1D and T2D, due to the overlap in items which are diagnostic of disordered eating attitudes and DEB and prescribed as part of diabetes treatment (Daneman 1998). When questionnaires or interview techniques standardized in the nondiabetic population are used, it is recommended that questions be modified to address intent of behaviors, including insulin manipulation (Criego 2009). Some studies have expanded the EDE and SCID interview format to include such questions (Peveler 2005).

Two questionnaire exceptions were found: the Diabetes Eating Problems Survey (DEPS), created by Antisdel, Laffel, and Anderson (2001) and refined by Markowitz et al. (2010), and the AHEAD (Assessing Health and Eating among Adolescents with Diabetes) survey (Neumark-Sztainer 2002a). Both include questions regarding the adjustment of insulin specifically for the purposes of weight reduction, and both couch questions in terms of diabetes care and issues related to glycemic control and weight gain due to treatment (Antisdel 2001, Neumark-Sztainer 2002a). However, neither questionnaire has been validated in a clinical population with an independent diagnosis of ED. Findings from a study validating a questionnaire that assesses hunger and satiety in the context of diabetic care, the Diabetes Treatment and Satiety Scale (DTSS-20), suggest that patients with T1D routinely experience contradictory clinical situations (regarding blood glucose levels, usual MNT, and insulin dosing) during which they feel full, hungry, and/or out of control of food intake (Young-Hyman 2011a). It is speculated that the lack of appropriate hunger and satiety cues is related to hormonal dysregulation. (See section regarding physiologic dysregulation of appetite.)

To establish diagnosis of ED or document subclinical DEB, thorough evaluation in the diabetes population should include assessment of adjustment to illness, overall psychological status, weight and shape concerns, specific questions regarding maladaptive use of the insulin or medication regimen to lose weight, and reliability of proprioceptive cues regarding hunger and satiety in the context of blood glucose levels (Young-Hyman 2010).

LIMITATIONS OF CURRENT RESEARCH FINDINGS

Gaps in research regarding the association of DEB and diabetes include: *1*) assessment of DEB in the context of adherence to medical regimen and adjustment to illness; *2*) understanding the contribution of insulin and medication dosing to feelings of hunger and satiety; *3*) dietary prescriptions/medical nutrition therapy as potential sources of information/attitudes leading to feelings of loss of control over food intake; *4)* need for appropriate comparison groups such as healthy-weight matched individuals seeking to prevent weight gain or weight loss, minority comparison groups, and other chronic disease groups with conditions affecting weight/metabolism; *5)* incomplete psychological characterization of samples; *6)* discrimination of preexisting/evolving psychopathology associated with noncompliance; and *7)* the need to use diabetes-specific assessment tools.

Prior studies of the prevalence of DEB in individuals with diabetes have not systematically addressed issues of regimen intensity, responsibility taking for regimen decisions, expectations of health care providers for glycemic and weight outcomes, and eating cognitions associated with medical care. The contributions of diabetes treatment knowledge or regimen adherence to the prevalence or endorsement of DEB are not established. Very few studies were found to have monitored patients from the time of diagnosis to establish the relationships or chronology between psychological symptomatology (depression in particular), DEB, weight gain, or regimen adjustment to prevent weight gain. Studies in adult women have not taken into account use of hormones for birth control or hormone replacement therapy (HRT), which can cause excess weight gain and increase appetite (Abrams 1992, Gallo 2004, Gallo 2006). Last, no studies to date have simultaneously assessed physiologic markers of hormones and incretins contributing to dysregulation of hunger and satiety and symptoms of DEB in the context of diabetes care.

RECOMMENDATIONS FOR SCREENING AND CARE

DEB is accepted as a serious and potentially life-threatening comorbidity of diabetes, despite controversy about diagnosis and prevalence. No published randomized controlled intervention trials of treatment of DEB or ED with diabetes cohorts could be found. Therefore screening recommendations are derived from the extant literature, and treatment recommendations are adapted from DEB interventions with healthy populations (Kelly 2005, Goebel-Fabbri 2009).

If DEB is suspected, *screening* should be implemented as follows:

1. Use diabetes-specific measurement tools to distinguish between behavior that indicates regimen adherence versus DEB to control weight, independent of glycemic control goals (Goebel-Fabbri 2009, Young-Hyman 2011a).
2. Evaluate overall psychological adjustment to establish whether behaviors indicate DEB, psychiatric morbidity, and/or poor adjustment to the diagnosis and requirements of treatment regimen (noncompliance). Patients with known psychiatric morbidity should be screened for DEB when unexplained poor glycemic control, weight gain, and/or weight loss occurs (Kelly 2005).
3. Evaluate insulin and other medication dosing/amount and episodes of hypoglycemia as potential causes for lack of satiety and/or loss of control over food intake. Evaluate accuracy of internal cues indicating need for food or treatment (with medication) in the context of blood glucose level (Goebel-Fabbri 2009).

4. Evaluate potential contributions of dietary prescription and information (MNT) to attitudes and behaviors regarding food intake, including food preoccupation and self-evaluation of actual or subjective dietary restraint and binging (ADA 2007).
5. Assess patients' expectations for achieving good glycemic control: at what cost to psychosocial adjustment, quality of life, eating behaviors, and weight.

If screening indicates DEB, *formal evaluation and care* should be implemented:

1. Refer for psychological/psychiatric evaluation. Once ED/DEB is established by questionnaire/interview, referral for treatment to a mental health professional familiar with the medical management of diabetes and treatment of DEB should be made (ADA 2007).
2. When treatment for DEB is begun, the treating professional as well as key individuals in the patient's social support network in treatment (parents for children and teens, partners or close family/community members for adults) should be incorporated into the diabetes management team (Criego 2009).
3. Depending on severity of symptoms, medications (antidepressant and anti-anxiety) and hospitalization should be considered.
4. Routine monitoring of DEB symptoms at medical management visits is also an integral part of the ongoing treatment process so that appropriate adjustments to the diabetes care regimen can be made (ADA 2007, Criego 2009). Careful evaluation of the contribution of prescribed diabetes care behaviors, knowledge, intent of behavior, and glycemic and weight goals should be conducted. Incorporation of diabetes treatment personnel into the DEB treatment plan helps to ensure that the prescription for regimen behaviors can be adjusted as needed (Goebel-Fabbri 2009).
5. Use of cognitive behavioral therapy, interpersonal therapy, and integrative cognitive therapy with adjunctive pharmacotherapy to address significant psychiatric symptoms are recognized treatment approaches in the nondiabetic population and should be provided to those with diabetes. Based on successful intervention methods, treatment can be individually or group administered by a trained professional (usually a behaviorally trained psychologist, social worker, or dietitian) who is familiar with the treatment of both DEB and diabetes (de Zwaan 2004, Pike 2004, Tantleff-Dunn 2004, Peterson 2004).
6. Interventions should target specific maladaptive behaviors (such as manipulation of insulin or medication omission) to ensure health, and should target cognitions about body image, self-esteem, autonomy, interpersonal relationships, and disease self-efficacy, particularly control of glucose and weight, depending upon symptoms reported, to improve mental health. Recommendations follow procedures used in the general population but with the addition of self-management behavior, which needs to be addressed with the diabetes care team in the context of preserving glycemic control. If metabolic derangements (severe hypoglycemia and ketoacidosis) are found to be associated with DEB, metabolic derangements must first be stabilized via medical management (ADA 2007).

BIBLIOGRAPHY

Abrams J: Lifestyle changes most often suggested for weight complaints: special report: annual pill survey. *Contracept Technol Update* 13:154–156, 1992

Ackard DM, Vik N, Neumark-Sztainer D, Schmitz KH, Hannan P, Jacobs DR Jr: Disordered eating and body dissatisfaction in adolescents with type 1 diabetes and a population-based comparison sample: comparative prevalence and clinical implications. *Pediatr Diabetes* 9:312–319, 2008

Affenito SG, Adams CH: Are eating disorders more prevalent in females with type 1 diabetes mellitus when the impact of insulin omission is considered? *Nutr Rev* 59:179–182, 2001

Affenito SG, Backstrand JR, Welch GW, Lammi-Keefe CJ, Rodriguez NR, Adams CH: Subclinical and clinical eating disorders in IDDM negatively affect metabolic control. *Diabetes Care* 20:182–184, 1997a

Affenito SG, Lammi-Keefe CJ, Vogal S, Backstand JR, Welch GW, Adams CH: Women with insulin-dependent diabetes mellitus (IDDM) complicated by eating disorders are at risk for exacerbated alterations in lipid metabolism. *Eur J Clin Nutr* 51:462–466, 1997b

Alice Hsu YY, Chen BH, Huang MC, Lin SJ, Lin MF: Disturbed eating behaviors in Taiwanese adolescents with type 1 diabetes mellitus: a comparative study. *Pediatr Diabetes* 10:74–81, 2009

American Diabetes Association: Standards of medical care in diabetes: 2007. *Diabetes Care* 30 (Suppl. 1):S4–S41, 2007

American Diabetes Association Task Force for Writing Nutrition Principles and Recommendations for the Management of Diabetes and Related Complications: American Diabetes Association position statement: evidence-based nutrition principles and recommendations for the treatment and prevention of diabetes and related complications. *J Am Diet Assoc* 102:109–118, 2002

American Psychiatric Association: Eating disorders. In *Diagnostic and Statistical Manual of Mental Disorders, DSM-IV-TR*. 4th ed. Washington, DC, American Psychiatric Association, 2000, p. 583-597

Anderson BJ, Vangsness L, Connell A, Butler D, Goebel-Fabbri A, Laffel LM: Family conflict, adherence, and glycaemic control in youth with short duration type 1 diabetes. *Diabet Med* 19:635–642, 2002

Anderson RJ, Freedland KE, Clouse RE, Lustman PJ: The prevalence of comorbid depression in adults with diabetes: a meta-analysis. *Diabetes Care* 24:1069–1078, 2001

Antisdel JE, Laffel LMB, Anderson B: Improved detection of eating problems in women with type 1 diabetes using a newly developed survey (abstract). *Diabetes* 50 (Suppl. 1):A47, 2001

Arriaza CA, Mann T: Ethnic differences in eating disorder symptoms among college students: the confounding role of body mass index. *J Am Coll Health* 49:309–315, 2001

Bantle JP, Wylie-Rosett J, Albright AL, Apovian CM, Clark NG, Franz MJ, Hoogwerf BJ, Lichtenstein AH, Mayer-Davis E, Mooradian AD, Wheeler ML: Nutrition recommendations and interventions for diabetes–2006: a position statement of the American Diabetes Association. *Diabetes Care* 29:2140–2157, 2006

Battaglia MR, Alemzadeh R, Katte H, Hall PL, Perlmuter LC: Brief report: disordered eating and psychosocial factors in adolescent females with type 1 diabetes mellitus. *J Pediatr Psychol* 31:552–556, 2006

Biggs MM, Basco MR, Patterson G, Raskin P: Insulin withholding for weight control in women with diabetes. *Diabetes Care* 17:1186–1189, 1994

Bryden KS, Neil A, Mayou RA, Peveler RC, Fairburn CG, Dunger DB: Eating habits, body weight, and insulin misuse: a longitudinal study of teenagers and young adults with type 1 diabetes. *Diabetes Care* 22:1956–1960, 1999

Bubb JA Pontious SL: Weight loss from inappropriate insulin manipulation: an eating disorder variant in an adolescent with insulin-dependent diabetes mellitus. *Diabetes Educ* 17:29–32, 1991

Colton P, Olmsted M, Daneman D, Rydall A, Rodin G: Disturbed eating behavior and eating disorders in preteen and early teenage girls with type 1 diabetes: a case-controlled study. *Diabetes Care* 27:1654–1659, 2004

Colton P, Rodin GM, Olmsted MP, Daneman D: Eating disturbances in young women with type 1 diabetes mellitus: mechanisms and consequences. *Psychiatric Annals* 29:213–218, 1999

Cooper Z, Cooper PJ, Fairburn CG: The validity of the eating disorder examination and its subscales. *Br J Psychiatry* 154:807–812, 1989

Criego A, Crow S, Goebel-Fabbri AE, Kendall D, Parkin CG: Eating disorders and diabetes screening and detection. *Diabetes Spectrum* 22:143–146, 2009

Crow S, Keel PK, Kendall D: Eating disorders and insulin-dependent diabetes mellitus. *Psychosomatics* 39:233–243, 1998

Daneman D, Rodin G, Jones J, Colton P, Rydall A, Maharaj S, Olmsted M: Eating disorders in adolescent girls and young adult women with type 1 diabetes. *Diabetes Spectrum* 15:83–105, 2002

Daneman D, Olmsted M, Rydall A, Maharaj S, Rodin G: Eating disorders in young women with type 1 diabetes. *Hormone Research* 50 (Suppl. 1):79–86, 1998

Davis S, Alonso MD: Hypoglycemia as a barrier to glycemic control. *J Diabetes Complications* 18:60–68, 2004

Davis SN, Renda SM: Psychological insulin resistance: overcoming barriers to starting insulin therapy. *Diabetes Educ* 32 (Suppl 4):146S–152S, 2006 de Man Lapidoth J, Ghaderi A, Norring C: Eating disorders and disordered eating among patients seeking non-surgical weight-loss treatment in Sweden. *Eat Behav* 7:15–26, 2006

de Zwaan M, Pyle RL, Mitchell JE: Pharmacological treatment of anorexia nervosa, bulimia nervosa, and binge eating disorder. In *Handbook of Eating Disorders and Obesity.* Thompson JK, Ed. Hoboken, NJ, John Wiley & Sons, 2004, p. 186–217

Decaluwe V, Braet C: Prevalence of binge-eating disorder in obese children and adolescents seeking weight-loss treatment. *Int J Obes Relat Metab Disord* 27:404–409, 2003

Dupre J: Glycaemic effects of incretins in type 1 diabetes mellitus: a concise review, with emphasis on studies in humans. *Regul Pept* 128:149–157, 2005

Engstrom I, Kroon M, Arvidsson C-G, Segnestam K, Snellman K, Aman J: Eating disorders in adolescent girls with insulin-dependent diabetes mellitus: a population-based case-control study. *Acta Paediatr* 88:175–180, 1999

Erkolahti RK, Ilonen T, Saarijarvi S: Self-image of adolescents with diabetes mellitus type-I and rheumatoid arthritis. *Nord J Psychiatry* 57:309–312, 2003

Fairburn CG, Peveler RC, Davies B, Mann JI, Mayou RA: Eating disorders in young adults with insulin dependent diabetes mellitus: a controlled study. *BMJ* 303:17–20, 1991

Gallo MF, Lopez LM, Grimes DA, Schulz KF, Helmerhorst FM: Combination contraceptives: effects on weight. *Cochrane Database Syst Rev* CD003987, 2006

Gallo MF, Grimes DA, Schulz KF, Helmerhorst FM: Combination estrogen-progestin contraceptives and body weight: systematic review of randomized controlled trials. *Obstet Gynecol* 103:359–373, 2004

Garner DM: *Eating Disorder Inventory-3 Professional Manual.* Lutz, FL, Psychological Assessment Resources, 2004

Garner DM, Olmsted MP, Bohr Y, Garfinkle PE: The Eating Attitudes Test: psychometric features and clinical correlates. *Psychol Med* 12:871–878, 1982

Garner DM, Garfinkel PE: The Eating Attitudes Test: an index of the symptoms of anorexia nervosa. *Psychol Med* 9:273–279, 1979

Goebel-Fabbri A, Anderson BJ, Fikkan J, Franko DL, Pearson K, Weinger K: Improvement and emergence of insulin restriction in women with type 1 diabetes. *Diabetes Care* 34:545–550, 2011

Goebel-Fabbri A: Disturbed eating behaviors and eating disorders in type 1 diabetes: clinical significance and treatment recommendations. *Curr Diab Rep* 9:133–139, 2009

Goebel-Fabbri A, Fikkan J, Franko DL, Pearson K, Anderson BJ, Weinger K: Insulin restriction and associated morbidity and mortality in women with type 1 diabetes. *Diabetes Care* 31:415–419, 2008

Hay LC, Wilmshurst EG, Fulcher G: Unrecognized hypo- and hyperglycemia in well-controlled patients with type 2 diabetes mellitus: the results of continuous glucose monitoring. *Diabetes Technol Ther* 5:19–26, 2003

Herpertz S, Albus C, Kielmann R, Hagemann-Patt H, Lichtblau K, Köhle K, Mann K, Senf W: Comorbidity of diabetes mellitus and eating disorders: a follow-up study. *J Psychosom Res* 51:673–678, 2001

Herpertz S, Albus C, Lichtblau K, Köhle K, Mann K, Senf W: Relationship of weight and eating disorders in type 2 diabetic patients: a multicenter study. *Int J Eat Disord* 28:68–77, 2000

Herpertz S, Albus C, Wagener R, Kocnar M, Wagner R, Henning A, Best F, Foerster H, Schulze Schleppinghoff B, Thomas W, Köhle K, Mann K, Senf W: Comorbidity of diabetes and eating disorders. Does diabetes control reflect disturbed eating behavior? *Diabetes Care* 21:1110–1116, 1998a

Herpertz S, Wagener R, Albus C, Kocnar M, Wanger R, Best F, Schulze Schleppinghoff B, Filz H, Forster K, Thomas W, Mann K, Kohle K, Senf W: Diabetes mellitus and eating disorders: a multicenter study on the comorbidity of the two diseases. *J Psychosom Res* 44:503–515, 1998b

Higgins SC, Gueorguiev M, Korbonits M: Ghrelin, the peripheral hunger hormone. *Ann Med* 39:116–136, 2007

Hockey S, Brown LJ, Lunt H: Prevalence of insulin self manipulation in young women with insulin dependent diabetes. *N Z Med J* 106:474–476, 1993

Hudson JI, Hudson MS, Wentworth SM: Self-induced glycosuria: a novel method of purging in bulimia. *JAMA* 249:2501, 1983

Jacobi C, Hayward C, de Zwaan M, Kraemer HC, Agras WS: Coming to terms with risk factors for eating disorders: application of risk terminology and suggestions for a general taxonomy. *Psychol Bull* 130:19–65, 2004

Johnson SB, Perwien AR, Silverstein JH: Response to hypo- and hyperglycemia in adolescents with type I diabetes. *J Pediatr Psychol* 25:171–178, 2000

Jones J, Lawson ML, Daneman D, Olmsted MP, Rodin G: Eating disorders in adolescent females with and without type 1 diabetes: cross sectional study. *BMJ* 320:1563–1566, 2006

Kelly SD, Howe CJ, Hendler JP, Lipman TH: Disordered eating behaviors in youth with type 1 diabetes. *Diabetes Educ* 31:572–583, 2005

Khan Y, Montgomery AM: Eating attitudes in young females with diabetes: insulin omission identifies a vulnerable subgroup. *Br J Med Psychol* 69(Pt 4):343–353, 1996

Klingensmith GJ, Ed: *Intensive Diabetes Management*. 3rd ed. Alexandria, VA, American Diabetes Association, 2003, p. 160

Koda JE, Fineman M, Rink TJ, Dailey GE, Muchmore DB, Linarelli LG: Amylin concentrations and glucose control. *Lancet* 339:1179–1180, 1992

Kruger DF, Gatcomb PM, Owen SK: Clinical implications of amylin and amylin deficiency. *Diabetes Educ* 25:389–397, 1999

Larger E: Weight gain and insulin treatment. *Diabetes & Metabolism* 31(4 Pt 2):4S51–4S56, 2005

Liu L, Lawrence JM, Davis C, Liese AD, Pettitt DJ, Pihoker C, Dabelea D, Hamman R, Waitzfelder B, Kahn HS: Prevalence of overweight and obesity in youth with diabetes in USA: the SEARCH for Diabetes in Youth Study. *Pediatric Diabetes* 10:1399–1405, 2009

Mannucci E, Tesi F, Ricca V, Pierazzuoli E, Barciulli E, Moretti S, Di Bernardo M, Travaglini R, Carrara S, Zucchi T, Placidi GF, Rotella CM: Eating behavior in obese patients with and without type 2 diabetes mellitus. *Int J Obes Relat Metab Disord* 26:848–853, 2002

Markowitz J, Butler DA, Volkening LK, Antisdel JE, Anderson BJ, Laffel LM: Brief screening tool for disordered eating in diabetes: internal consistency and external validity in a contemporary sample of pediatric patients with type 1 diabetes. *Diabetes Care* 33:495–500, 2010

Meltzer LJ, Johnson SB, Prine JM, Banks RA, Desrosiers PM, Silverstein JH: Disordered eating, body mass, and glycemic control in adolescents with type 1 diabetes. *Diabetes Care* 24:678–682, 2001

Nathan D, Delahanty L: *Beating Diabetes*. Boston, McGraw-Hill, 2005

Neumark-Sztainer D, Patterson J, Mellin A, Ackard DM, Utter J, Story M, Sockalosky J: Weight control practices and disordered eating behaviors among adolescent females and males with type 1 diabetes: associations with sociodemographics, weight concerns, familial factors, and metabolic outcomes. *Diabetes Care* 25:1289–1296, 2002a

Neumark-Sztainer D, Story M, Hannan PJ, Perry CL, Irving LM: Weight-related concerns and behaviors among overweight and nonoverweight adolescents: implications for preventing weight-related disorders. *Arch Pediatr Adolesc Med* 156:171–178, 2002b

Papelbaum M, Appolinário JC, Moreira Rde O, Ellinger VC, Kupfer R, Coutinho WF: Prevalence of eating disorders and psychiatric comorbidity in a clinical sample of type 2 diabetes mellitus patients. *Rev Bras Psiquiatr* 27:135–138, 2005

Parkman H, Hasler H, Fisher R: American Gastroenterological Association technical review on the diagnosis and treatment of gastroparesis. *Gastroenterology* 127: 1592–1622, 2004

Peterson CB, Wonderlich SA, Mitchell JE, Crow SJ: Integrative cognitive therapy for bulimia nervosa. In *Handbook of Eating Disorders and Obesity*. Thompson JK, Ed. Hoboken, NJ, John Wiley & Sons, 2004, p. 245–262

Peveler RC, Bryden KS, Neil HA, Fairburn CG, Mayou RA, Dunger DB, Turner HM: The relationship of disordered eating habits and attitudes to clinical outcomes in young adult females with type 1 diabetes. *Diabetes Care* 28:84–88, 2005

Peveler RC, Fairburn CG, Boller I, Dunger D: Eating disorders in adolescents with IDDM: a controlled study. *Diabetes Care* 15:1356–1360, 1992

Pike KM, Devlin MJ, Loeb C: Cognitive-behavioral therapy in the treatment of anorexia nervosa, bulimia nervosa, and binge eating disorder. In *Handbook of Eating Disorders and Obesity.* Thompson JK, Ed. Hoboken, NJ, John Wiley & Sons, 2004, p. 130–162

Pinhas-Hamiel O, Standiford D, Hamiel D, Dolan LM, Cohen R, Zeitler PS: The type 2 family: a setting for development and treatment of adolescent type 2 diabetes mellitus. *Arch Pediatr Adolesc Med* 153:1063–1067, 1999

Pollock M, Kovacs M, Charron-Prochownik D: Eating disorders and maladaptive dietary/insulin management among youths with childhood-onset insulin-dependent diabetes mellitus. *J Am Acad Child Adolesc Psychiatry* 34:291–296, 1995

Pollock-BarZiv SM, Davis C: Personality factors and disordered eating in young women with type 1 diabetes mellitus. *Psychosomatics* 46:11–18, 2005

Polonsky WH: *Diabetes Burnout: What to Do When You Can't Take It Anymore.* Alexandria, VA, American Diabetes Association, 1999, p. 348

Polonsky WH, Anderson BJ, Lohrer PA, Aponte JE, Jacobson AM, Cole CF: Insulin omission in women with IDDM. *Diabetes Care* 17:1178–1185, 1994

Rodin G, Olmsted MP, Rydall AC, Maharaj SI, Colton PA, Jones JM, Biancucci LA, Daneman D: Eating disorders in young women with type 1 diabetes mellitus. *J Psychosom Res* 53:943–949, 2002

Rodin GM, Daneman D: Eating disorders and IDDM. A problematic association. *Diabetes Care* 15:1402–1412, 1992

Rodin G, Craven J, Littlefield C, Murray M, Daneman D: Eating disorders and intentional insulin undertreatment in adolescent females with diabetes. *Psychosomatics* 32:171–176, 1991

Rodin GM, Johnson LE, Garfinkel PE, Daneman D, Kenshole AB: Eating disorders in female adolescents with insulin dependent diabetes mellitus. *Int J Psychiatry Med* 16:49–57, 1986–1987

Rydall AC, Rodin GM, Olmsted MP, Devenyi RG, Daneman D: Disordered eating behavior and microvascular complications in young women with insulin-dependent diabetes mellitus.[See comment.] *N Engl J Med* 336:1849–1854, 1997

Sherwood NE, Neumark-Sztainer D: Internalization of the sociocultural ideal: weight–related attitudes and dieting behaviors among young adolescent girls. *Am J Health Promot* 15:228–231, 2001

Shisslak CM, Mays MZ, Crago M, Jirsak JK, Taitano K, Cagno C: Eating and weight control behaviors among middle school girls in relationship to body weight and ethnicity. *J Adolesc Health* 38:631–633, 2006

Steel JM, Lloyd GG, Young RJ, MacIntyre CC: Changes in eating attitudes during the first year of treatment for diabetes. *J Psychosom Res* 34:313–318, 1990

Steel JM, Young RJ, Lloyd GG, MacIntyre CC: Abnormal eating attitudes in young insulin-dependent diabetics. *Br J Psychiatry* 155:515–521, 1989

Steel JM, Young RJ, Lloyd GG, Clarke B: Clinically apparent eating disorders in young diabetic women: associations with painful neuropathy and other complications. *Br Med J (Clin Res Ed)* 294(6576):859–862, 1987

Stice E: Risk and maintenance factors for eating pathology: a meta-analytic review. *Psychol Bull* 128:825–848, 2002

Stice E, Bearman SK: Body-image and eating disturbances prospectively predict increases in depressive symptoms in adolescent girls: a growth curve analysis. *Dev Psychol* 37:597–607, 2001

Stice E, Hayward C, Cameron RP, Killen JD, Taylor CB: Body-image and eating disturbances predict onset of depression among female adolescents: a longitudinal study. *J Abnorm Psychol* 109:438–444, 2000

Stice E, Agras WS, Hammer LD: Risk factors for the emergence of childhood eating disturbances: a five-year prospective study. *Int J Eat Disord* 25:375–387, 1999

Striegel-Moore RH, Nicholson TJ, Tamborlane WV: Prevalence of eating disorder symptoms in preadolescent and adolescent girls with IDDM. *Diabetes Care* 15:1361–1368, 1992

Surgenor L, Horn J, Hudson SM: Links between psychological sense of control and disturbed eating behavior in women with diabetes mellitus: implications for predictors of metabolic control. *J Psychosom Res* 52:121–128, 2002

Svensson M, Engstrom I, Aman J: Higher drive for thinness in adolescent males with insulin-dependent diabetes mellitus compared with healthy controls. *Acta Paediatr* 92:114–117, 2003

Tantleff-Dunn S, Gokee-LaRose J, Peterson RD: Interpersonal psychotherapy for the treatment of anorexia nervosa, bulimia nervosa, and binge eating disorder. In *Handbook of Eating Disorders and Obesity*. Thompson JK, Ed. Hoboken, NJ, John Wiley & Sons, 2004, p. 163–187

Telch CF, Stice E: Psychiatric comorbidity in women with binge eating disorder: prevalence rates from a non-treatment-seeking sample. *J Consult Clin Psychol* 66:768–776, 1998

Thelen MH, Farmer J, Wonderlich S, Smith M: A revision of the bulimia test: the BULIT-R. *Psychological Assessment* 3:119–124, 1991

Vamado PJ, Williamson DA, Bentz BG, Ryan DH, Rhodes SK, O'Neil PM, Sebastian SB, Barker SE: Prevalence of binge eating disorder in obese adults seeking weight loss treatment. *Eat Weight Disord* 2:117–124, 1997

Wilfley D, Friedman MA, Dounchis JZ, Stein RI, Welch RR, Ball SA: Comorbid psychopathology in binge eating disorder: relation to eating disorder severity at baseline and following treatment. *J Consult Clin Psychol* 68:641–649, 2000

Wing R, Nowalk MP, Marcus MD, Keoske R, Finegold D: Subclinical eating disorders and glycemic control in adolescents with type 1 diabetes. *Diabetes Care* 9:162–167, 1986

Wolman C, Resnick MD, Harris LJ, Blum RW: Emotional well-being among adolescents with and without chronic conditions. *J Adolesc Health* 15:199–204, 1994

Young-Hyman D, Davis C, Looney S, Grigsby C, Peterson C: Development of the diabetes treatment and satiety scale (DTSS-20). *Diabetes* 60 (Suppl. 1):A218, 2011a

Young-Hyman D, Laffel L, Markowitz J, Norman J, Muir A, Lindsley K: Evaluating eating disorder risk (EDR) in T1D youth transitioning to insulin pump (CSII) therapy (Rx). *Diabetes* 60 (Suppl. 1):A226, 2011b

Young-Hyman D, Laffel L, Markowitz J, Norman J, Muir A, Lindsley K: Evaluating eating disorder risk at time of teen T1D diagnosis (DX). *Diabetes* 60 (Suppl. 1):A1229, 2011c

Young-Hyman D, Davis C: Disordered eating behavior in individuals with diabetes: importance of context, classification and evaluation. *Diabetes Care* 33:683–689, 2010

Young-Hyman D: Eating Disorders. In *Diagnostic and Statistical Manual of Mental Disorders, DSM-IV-TR*. 4th ed. Washington, DC, American Psychiatric Association, 2000, p. 583–597

Deborah Young-Hyman, PhD, CDE, is Professor of Pediatrics at the Georgia Prevention Center, Institute for Public and Preventive Health, Georgia Health Sciences University, Augusta, GA.

Chapter 3
Hypoglycemia

Linda Gonder-Frederick, PhD, Daniel J. Cox, PhD, ABPP,
Harsimran Singh, PhD, and Jaclyn A. Shepard, PsyD

THE PROBLEM OF HYPOGLYCEMIA: DEFINITIONS AND PREVALENCE

Hypoglycemic episodes, the most common acute complication of diabetes, are almost unavoidable, especially for patients using insulin. Hypoglycemia can be defined both biologically and symptomatically. The biological definition, based on blood glucose (BG) levels, is any reading <3.9 mmol/l (70 mg/dl) (Workgroup on Hypoglycemia, American Diabetes Association [ADA] 2005). This, however, treats all BG levels <70 as symptomatically equal, which is misleading. Symptomatically, hypoglycemia is defined in terms of its impact on the central nervous system. The Diabetes Control and Complications Trial (DCCT) defined three levels of hypoglycemia: mild, moderate, and severe (DCCT Research Group 1997). *Mild* hypoglycemia is characterized by symptoms caused by counterregulatory hormones and mild neuroglycopenia that do not significantly disrupt cognitive-motor functioning and are quickly alleviated by consuming carbohydrates. *Moderate* hypoglycemia can disrupt routine functioning, but the individual maintains the executive capacity to recognize symptoms and initiate treatment.

When mild or moderate episodes are not recognized or treated in a timely manner, *severe* hypoglycemia (SH) can occur. With SH, extreme neuroglycopenia precludes the ability to self-treat due to cognitive impairment, unconsciousness, or seizure. Episodes of SH are inherently dangerous, especially when no one else is present to provide emergency assistance or when the individual is engaging in potentially dangerous activities such as driving a vehicle (Cox 2006b). Mortality due to SH, albeit uncommon, does occur, accounting for an estimated 2 to 4% of deaths in individuals with type 1 diabetes (T1D) (Swade 1997, Allen 2003, Dagogo-Jack 2004, Friedrich 2004, Cox 2006b). Some of these mortalities are associated with nocturnal hypoglycemia, which can lead to what has been called the "dead in bed" phenomenon (Sovik 1999).

There are no definitive statistics on the frequency of hypoglycemia, but it has been estimated that individuals with T1D have an average of two episodes per week, most of these mild or moderate (Allen 2001, Cryer 2003). For SH, estimates of prevalence vary widely across studies. In the DCCT, SH occurred at least once per year in 65% of patients on intensive insulin regimens, with an average of 61.2 episodes per 100 patient years (DCCT Research Group 1997). Other prospective studies have reported frequencies ranging from 4.8 to 19 episodes per 100 patient years (Bognetti 1997, Davis 1997, Allen 2001, Rewers 2002, Leese 2003). However, prevalence rates do not accurately reflect the fact that the majority of episodes are concentrated in a minority subgroup of patients who have frequent and recurrent SH (Cox 1999, Honkasalo 2011). This is true not only for adults, but also for children, where 80 to 100% of episodes occur in 20 to 33% of patients (Bognetti 1997, Rewers 2002). The occurrence of SH is also not evenly distributed across times of day, with 50% or more episodes occurring at night in both children and adults (DCCT Research Group 1991, Bognetti 1997, Davis 1997).

In type 2 diabetes (T2D), some studies have reported a much lower frequency of hypoglycemia, especially when patients on all treatment regimens, including dietary therapy alone and low-dose oral medications, are included in the study (Katakura 2003). Hypoglycemia is less common during the initial years following diagnosis of T2D, presumably due to intact counterregulatory hormone mechanisms (Cryer 2003, Henderson 2003, Zammitt 2005). However, it seems that after insulin use begins, the frequency of hypoglycemia, including SH, is equivalent in T1D and T2D (Holstein 2003, Leese 2003). The use of oral sulfonylureas also greatly increases hypoglycemia in patients with T2D (Chelliah 2004, Steppel 2004, Zammit 2005).

THE IMPACT OF HYPOGLYCEMIA ON PHYSICAL AND EMOTIONAL WELL-BEING

The practical implications of hypoglycemia can range from patients' personal lives to their working and social relationships, with potential negative consequences for their overall quality of life (Cryer 2004, Frier 2008, Singh 2010). Episodes of hypoglycemia are typically associated with negative consequences, including unpleasant symptoms, potential embarrassment, and inconvenience (Gonder-Frederick 1997a, Cox 2002, Jørgensen 2003). Scientific studies of the prevalence of physical injury due to SH are somewhat rare (Graveling 2010, Griffith 2011); however, clinical experience indicates that this is not uncommon. Recent retrospective and prospective surveys have demonstrated that a subgroup of patients is at a higher risk for hypoglycemia-related driving mishaps and automobile accidents (Cox 2003, Sommerfield 2003, Cox 2006b).

In people with T1D, acute hypoglycemia may produce impairment in various cognitive domains, including immediate and visual memory, delayed memory, prospective memory, and visual-motor and spatial skills (Holmes 1984, Wirsén 1992, Draelos 1995, Ewing 1998, Sommerfield 2003, Amiel 2009). There has been concern that frequent episodes of SH may also have long-term negative effects on the brain and cognitive function; however, research in this area has produced mixed results (Wredling 1990, Perros 1997, Deary 2003, Hershey 2003, DCCT Research Group 2007). These equivocal findings may be in part due to sample differences in the age of diabetes onset. Studies examining associations between SH and its impact on cognitive functioning and other development processes have shown that SH may have a more damaging effect on the developing brain in young children with T1D than in older children or adults. Children and adolescents diagnosed with T1D before the age of 5 or 6 years exhibit poorer cognitive function compared with those diagnosed later in life (Ryan 1985, Ryan 1988, Bjørgaas 1996; also see Chapter 5). For older people with T2D, there is increasing evidence to suggest that occurrence of SH is associated with a greater subsequent risk of dementia (Whitmer 2009), but this may be a result of a combination of factors, including chronic hyperglycemia and hypoglycemia (Strachan 2011).

Recurrent hypoglycemia and SH can also have negative impact on psychosocial functioning, health status, and overall quality of life in both individuals with diabetes and their significant others (Gold 1994, Gonder-Frederick 1997a, Davis 2005, Leiter 2005, Nordfeldt 2005a, Laiteerapong 2011, Pettersson 2011, Williams 2011). In adults with diabetes, there is evidence that ongoing problems with SH are associated with chronic mood changes, reduced happiness and energy levels, and feelings of helplessness, anxiety, and depression, and they can be a risk factor for affective disorders (Gold 1997, Strachan 2000, Hermanns 2003, Hermanns 2005). Treatment and management of SH can also pose a significant economic burden for patients and the health care system in terms of health care expenses and indirect costs due to decreased productivity (DCCT Research Group 1995, Lundkvist 2005, Reviriego 2008).

Unpleasant symptoms and experiences related to hypoglycemia can cause considerable anxiety in patients with diabetes and their significant others, which may lead to fear of hypoglycemia (FOH) (Myers 2007, Wild 2007, Gonder-Frederick 2011). High levels of FOH can impair quality of life in families of children with T1D (Nordfeldt 2005b, Jaser 2009, Haugstvedt 2010), and parents can exhibit particularly high levels of fear when their children have experienced seizures or comas (Clarke 1998). High FOH may adversely impact glycemic control in children with T1D, as parents may encourage higher BG levels than clinically desirable to avoid future occurrences (Barnard 2010; also see Chapter 14). In spouses and partners of patients who experience recurrent SH, there are not only higher levels of FOH but also more sleep disturbances (due to anxiety about nocturnal hypoglycemia) and reported marital conflict (Gonder-Frederick 1997a, Stahl 1998, Jørgensen 2003). Although numerous studies have investigated FOH, it has been difficult to empirically document its impact on diabetes management (Wild 2007). However, there is some scientific evidence, and much clinical evidence, that high levels of FOH in individuals with T1D or insulin-treated T2D, as well as in parents of youth with T1D, can contribute to treatment behaviors that maintain higher BG levels (Cox 1987, Cox 1990, Wild 2007, Patton 2008). Survey data have also shown that FOH is the most common reason for not adjusting insulin doses, as hypoglycemia is the most feared complication of intensive insulin therapy (McCrimmon 1994, Reach 2005). FOH is also a primary barrier to exercise in patients with type 1 and type 2 diabetes (Brazeau 2008, Shahar 2008).

RISK FACTORS FOR HYPOGLYCEMIA

All hypoglycemic episodes in diabetes are caused by a surplus of insulin or other BG-lowering medications relative to food intake and physical activity. Physiologically, factors such as greater insulin sensitivity, higher BG variability, and impaired renal function increase the risk for hypoglycemia, as do some medications that delay gastric emptying (Chelliah 2004, Workgroup on Hypoglycemia ADA 2005, Honkasalo 2011). Numerous studies have documented that glycemic control and variables that lower A1C (e.g., more intensive insulin therapy) result in increased risk for hypoglycemia in both youth and adults (Davis 1997, DCCT Research

Group 1997, Allen 2001). Some studies have attempted to go beyond these broad relationships and identify the immediate, discrete precursors of hypoglycemic episodes. This research shows that diabetes management plays a critical role in hypoglycemia risk, with 75% or more episodes being behaviorally induced in people with both T1D and T2D. For youth and adults, the majority of episodes were attributed to reduced food intake, including missed meals, and increased physical activity (Bognetti 1997, Davis 1997, Murata 2005). A recent retrospective study of 84 children and adolescents found that most SH episodes occurred when meals (carbohydrates) were delayed, followed by intense physical activity and excessive insulin administration (Cosmescu 2008). Another retrospective study involving >1,300 adults with T1D and T2D identified daily exercise as a major risk factor for SH (Honkasalo 2011). The occurrence of *unexpected* vigorous activity has also been highlighted as a common precipitant (Clarke 1999).

Clinical experience indicates that many patients have only a rudimentary understanding of the effects of food and exercise on BG levels. Clinicians cannot assume that patients and their caregivers know about more complex behavioral risk factors for hypoglycemia, such as eating foods high in fat content, which can result in a delayed and/or depressed glycemic response, or engaging in elongated sessions of moderate physical activity, which can utilize as much (or more) glucose than shorter bouts of intense exercise. Maladaptive decisions and behaviors leading to hypoglycemia can also occur in patients who are nonadherent or nonconscientious about their diabetes management, including those who may skip meals or snacks, or fail to count carbohydrate content when calculating meal boluses. Psychiatric conditions that result in disordered behavior can also greatly increase patient risk, especially disordered eating behavior characterized by undereating, or binge eating accompanied by purging (Young-Hyman 2010).

For some patients, frequent and recurrent episodes of hypoglycemia may be related to emotional or cognitive problems that contribute to poor decision making and judgments, or risky behaviors in dealing with low BG. Patients may minimize or dismiss the potential seriousness of episodes, experience secondary gain through the care and concern of family members, or perceive delaying treatment as a form of "winning" in a power struggle with diabetes.

Another understudied but important risk factor is patient cognitions: beliefs, attitudes, and judgments about hypoglycemia and its treatment. Clinically, it is not uncommon to encounter patients who believe they can function fine at very low BG levels (e.g., <54 mg/dl) or that hypoglycemia is a necessary part of having good diabetes control. Other beliefs and attitudes can lead patients to have lower personal glycemic thresholds for treating hypoglycemia or a tendency to delay treatment, which greatly increase risk.

Some patients also engage in overtreatment of hyperglycemia, or what is sometimes called diabetes "micro-management," often resulting in insulin over-bolusing or "stacking." These individuals may be highly conscientious in their diabetes management and highly motivated to avoid hyperglycemia and long-term complications. However, high anxiety about hyperglycemia can become maladaptive and lead to extreme behaviors to avoid high BG (e.g., increased insulin dosing), which may increase hypoglycemic episodes (Ritholtz 2008, Singh 2010).

Episodes of SH occur when milder or more moderate levels of hypoglycemia are not recognized and treated quickly enough or adequately. The probability of

SH occurrence has been described in a biopsychobehavioral model that attempts to integrate the complex physiological, psychological, and behavioral processes that determine risk level (Gonder-Frederick 1997b, Cox 1999). The first step of this model is the occurrence of mild or moderate hypoglycemia, which triggers certain physiological reactions, including hormonal counterregulation and neuroglycopenia. These, in turn, cause adrenergic and neuroglycopenic symptoms, followed by patient detection and recognition of these symptoms, which ideally leads to appropriate decision making and self-treatment, thereby avoiding SH.

However, the potential for SH is not avoided when hypoglycemic symptoms are not produced, recognized, or treated in a timely manner, which often occurs when a patient has hypoglycemic-associated autonomic failure (HAAF). With HAAF, frequent low-BG episodes lead to defective counterregulatory (epinephrine) responses to hypoglycemia and reduced hypoglycemic awareness (HA) (Cryer 2002, Cryer 2004, Kubiak 2004). This can cause BG to drop lower during hypoglycemia and fail to produce warning symptoms until levels are very low, which greatly increases the probability for significant neuroglycopenia and mental confusion, possibly preventing timely self-treatment. The relationship between reduced HA and SH risk has been well documented in people with both T1D and T2D, and it has been estimated that up to 60% of SH episodes are not associated with warning symptoms (DCCT Research Group 1991, Cryer 2002, Henderson 2003). Approximately 25% of patients with T1D appear to have some degree of reduced HA (Hepburn 1990, Geddes 2007).

Factors contributing to HAAF, reduced HA, and SH risk include frequent hypoglycemic episodes, intensive insulin regimens, lower A1C levels, longer diabetes duration, physical exercise, suppressed nocturnal counterregulation, and alcohol consumption (Avogaro 1989, Kerr 1990, DCCT Research Group 1991, Davis 1997, DCCT Research Group 1997, Rewers 2002, Cryer 2003, Banarer 2004, Bulsara 2004, Sandoval 2004, Workgroup on Hypoglycemia ADA 2005, Richardson 2005, Schultes 2007). Smoking is another risk factor for SH, although it is unclear at this point whether it is related to HAAF (Hirai 2007). Even in the absence of HAAF and reduced HA, patients may fail to detect early warning signs of hypoglycemia. Field studies have found that both adults and children with T1D may fail to recognize half or more of BG levels lower than 70 mg/dl (3.9 mmol/l) (Clarke 1995, Gonder-Frederick 2008). Another field study prospectively followed adults with T1D with and without a recent history of SH (Cox 1999) over a 6-month period. The study replicated the relationship between HAAF-related factors (e.g., reduced HA, frequent low BG) and SH risk; however, individuals in the high-risk group also showed cognitive and behavioral differences. Specifically, individuals with SH history showed more cognitive impairment during hypoglycemia and a tendency to treat episodes with food rather than faster-acting carbohydrates.

Parents have been shown to demonstrate poor ability to detect low BG in their children (Gonder-Frederick 2008). Factors that can contribute to parents' and their children's failure to detect hypoglycemia include attention and perceptual processes, inaccurate beliefs about low-BG symptoms, and misattribution of symptoms to non-BG-related causes. Emotional distress may also have a negative impact; for example, school-aged children with depressive symptoms show poorer hypoglycemia detection (Gonder-Frederick 2008).

Age is a major factor in SH, with older people and younger children at highest risk (Bognetti 1997, Bulsara 2004, Chelliah 2004). Increased risk in the elderly often occurs due to impaired renal function and/or medications (Chelliah 2004), and the elderly in poor glycemic control have more frequent episodes (Munshi 2011). Adolescents are at higher risk than adults with T1D (DCCT Research Group 1994), and children under 6 years of age are at higher risk than those over 6 years old (Davis 2001). One prospective study has documented the relationship between psychiatric disorders and higher SH risk in older children (Rewers 2002), and another investigated surreptitious intentional insulin overdosing by adolescents with emotional disturbance and family problems (Boileau 2006). A recent study of over 1,000 adults with T1D and T2D found that depression was a risk factor for SH (Honkasalo 2011). In the elderly, cognitive impairment and dementia also significantly increases risk (Brauser 2011). Adults in lower socioeconomic status (SES) groups are at higher risk, including those who are "food-insecure" and vulnerable to experiencing hunger secondary to inability to afford food (Bulsara 2004, Seligman 2010). For children and adolescents, being underinsured significantly increases risk (Ratner 2000, Bulsara 2004).

INTERVENTIONS TO REDUCE SH RISK

Any intervention that reduces the frequency of hypoglycemia and/or improves timely detection and treatment of episodes will be effective in reducing SH risk. Also, interventions that reduce the frequency of hypoglycemia and SH typically reduce FOH. The essential foundation for reducing SH risk is adequate diabetes education to provide patients with an understanding of how imbalances in insulin, food, and physical activity occur, and ways to avoid such imbalances. This type of patient education and training (especially educating patients regarding HA) may not be implemented because of limited personnel resources, despite being part of recommended diabetes self-management education (DSME). Some authors have even suggested that inadequate patient education is a major reason why patients experience increased hypoglycemia when they transition to intensive insulin therapies (Mühlhauser 1993). In addition to hypoglycemia prevention, patients need education on the appropriate treatment of episodes and the importance of responding immediately and appropriately to avoid SH. Such education should include training in hypoglycemic symptomatology, including the physiological basis of symptoms and their impact on the ability to adequately self-treat.

When an individual presents with problems with SH, the first target of intervention is often the insulin regimen. Numerous studies show that long-lasting insulin analogs decrease the occurrence of both diurnal and nocturnal hypoglycemia in people with T1D and T2D (Brunelle 1998, Ratner 2000, Yki-Jarvinen 2000, Davis 2004, Home 2004, Alemzadeh 2005, Rosenstock 2005). Many studies have also demonstrated that continuous subcutaneous insulin infusion (CSII) therapy or insulin pump therapy significantly reduces the frequency of hypoglycemia and SH risk in both adults and children (Boland 1999, Bode 2002, Linkeschova 2002, Litton 2002, Rami 2003, Bulsara 2004, Colquitt 2004). However, two recent meta-analyses of this literature point out that CSII does not always reduce hypoglycemia (Weissberg-Benchell 2003, Hirsch 2005). Other changes in insulin may also be indicated; for example, discontinuing basal insulin doses during exercise may significantly decrease hypoglycemia in children (Tansey 2006). For patients who have tried a variety of different insulin regimens but continue to have serious problems with SH, transplant surgery may be considered. However, there are significant surgical and postoperative complications, and islet cell transplant does not result in long-term insulin independence for the majority of patients (Shapiro 2006, Meloche 2007). And, although glycemic thresholds for counterregulation and symptoms improve after islet cell transplant, the magnitude of the epinephrine response (signaling hypoglycemia) may remain impaired (Rickels 2007).

In addition to reducing episode frequency, interventions can focus on improving the ability to detect hypoglycemia when it occurs. There is research aimed at developing pharmacological agents that increase hypoglycemic awareness (Heller 2008), but these agents are not yet available. Several studies have found that, if patients can rigorously avoid BG levels <70 mg/dl (3.9 mmol/l) for just a few weeks, timely hormonal counterregulation and adrenergic warning symptoms are restored (Cranston 1994, Fanelli 1994). Unfortunately, there have been no large-scale clinical trials evaluating this intervention to determine what proportion of patients might respond to treatment or what types of support programs are needed for patient success. In addition, only one long-term follow-up study has investigated whether a single course of treatment (3-month physician-supervised avoidance of hypoglycemia) produces long-lasting results (Dagogo-Jack 1999).

With recent technological advances in diabetes management, continuous glucose monitoring (CGM) has been increasingly used in the detection and reduction of hypoglycemia. CGM can provide patients with warnings when BG trends indicate that hypoglycemia is imminent (Boland 2001, Chico 2003, Jeha 2004). An early randomized trial (Garg 2006) showed that patients with T1D and insulin-requiring T2D who wore continuous glucose monitors for three consecutive 72-hour periods experienced significant improvements in glycemic excursions compared with patients using traditional BG monitoring. Specifically, those using continuous glucose monitors spent 21% less time in hypoglycemia and 26% more time within BG target range. More recent clinical trials have focused on the impact of longer-duration use of continuous glucose monitors on hypoglycemic risk. In a recent study of both adults and youth with T1D who did CGM for 26 weeks, time spent in hypoglycemia was significantly shorter and time spent in euglycemia (normal glucose content) was significantly longer compared with control subjects using self-monitoring of blood glucose (SMBG) (Battelino 2011). Though these results are promising, other findings suggest that CGM may not effectively reduce hypoglycemia for all patients. Results from the Juvenile Diabetes Research Foundation (JDRF) trial did not find a statistically significant difference in time spent in hypoglycemia or in the frequency of SH over 6 months of CGM as compared with SMBG for any age-group (JDRF Continuous Glucose Monitoring Study Group 2008). However, adults in this study were able to achieve better glycemic control without increasing hypoglycemic risk.

Sensor-augmented pump (SAP) therapy, which integrates CGM use and insulin pump therapy, is a first step toward the development of a closed-loop control system (or "artificial pancreas") and one of the newest diabetes technologies aimed at reducing hyperglycemia while preventing hypoglycemia. A number of studies, including two large clinical trials (Sensor-Augmented Pump Therapy for A1C

Reduction [STAR 3]; Sensing With Insulin Pump Therapy to Control HbA1c [SWITCH]), are underway to evaluate the feasibility and efficacy of SAP therapy with adults and, most recently, youth with T1D (Fisher 2006, Kordonouri 2010, Conget 2011, Scaramuzza 2011). Early findings have indicated beneficial effects on metabolic control in both adults and children, including improved A1C (Hermanides 2011, Scaramuzza 2011), without increasing hypoglycemia (Buse 2011, Slover 2011). A possible negative effect on diabetes management is overtreating hypoglycemia due to delays in glucose feedback (Wolpert 2007, Block 2008). When this technology is introduced, however, this time lag should be addressed in the context of its use (see Chapter 11).

Because diabetes management behaviors play a critical role in hypoglycemia and SH, it is not surprising that *behavioral* interventions are effective in reducing risk. The behavioral intervention receiving the most scientific study is Blood Glucose Awareness Training (BGAT), designed to improve patients' ability to recognize symptoms and other cues that signal low BG and to anticipate the effect of treatment factors such as insulin, food, and physical activity on glucose levels (Cox 1989, Gonder-Frederick 2000, Cox 2006a, Cox 2008). BGAT is a structured, manualized training program that integrates diabetes didactics, self-monitoring and self-assessment strategies, and evaluation of personal diabetes management behaviors. A recent article reviewed 15 studies of BGAT in the U.S. and Europe showing that the intervention can have numerous treatment benefits, such as improved hypoglycemia detection, decreased frequency of low BG and SH, and reduced FOH (Cox 2006a). Patients who complete BGAT after initiating intensive insulin therapy have been shown to maintain integrity of counterregulation and avoid the typical increase in frequency of hypoglycemia with improved diabetes control (Kinsley 1999).

Despite evidence for its effectiveness, BGAT is not widely disseminated. It is an intensive and demanding training program, there are reimbursement issues, and there are not enough trained and experienced health care professionals to offer BGAT. To make it more widely available, BGAT has been translated for Internet delivery as BGATHome, and the initial tests are encouraging (Cox 2008). A similar psychobehavioral intervention, also using strategies such as BG symptom diaries and BG estimation with accuracy evaluation, has been developed and tested in controlled trials in Germany (Kubiak 2006, Hermanns 2010). Long-term follow-up after this intervention found significantly lower rates of SH in the experimental group with no increase in A1C.

There is also compelling evidence that less-intensive behavioral interventions may be effective, suggesting that more effort should be directed at developing, testing, and disseminating these types of programs. For example, structured outpatient education specifically designed to teach patients about the causes, effects, and treatment of hypoglycemia may prevent the increased risk associated with intensive insulin regimens (Plank 2004, Samann 2005). Another intervention combined a case-management approach with psychoeducation, and it decreased episodes of SH by 60% (Svoren 2003). Also encouraging are studies from Norway showing that mass distribution of patient education materials (videotapes and brochures) reduced episodes of SH without compromising metabolic control in children with T1D. This randomized, controlled trial followed more than 200 pediatric patients over a 24-month period and found that episodes of SH were reduced from 45 to 24% in the experimental intervention group (Nordfeldt 2003, Norfeldt 2005a).

The successful results of these relatively simple interventions focusing on didactics suggest that inadequate patient education is an underrecognized but major risk factor for SH. The positive findings for several educational and behavioral interventions, combined with the difficulty of finding these for many patients, suggest that programs with demonstrated effectiveness at reducing SH risk are underimplemented in diabetes health care. Such programs are likely to be cost-effective because of the significant financial burden of hypoglycemia on the individual and the health care system (Brito-Sanfiel 2010). Given its impact on the quality of life, emotional well-being, and physical safety and health of people with diabetes, the problem of hypoglycemia has not received the attention it deserves, and the availability of interventions to reduce episodes is inadequate. Clearly, much more effort on several fronts, including research, clinical care, e-health efforts, and diabetes advocacy, needs to be directed at finding ways to implement effective interventions to address the problem of hypoglycemia in diabetes.

RECOMMENDATIONS FOR CARE

1. Hypoglycemia is common in patients with both T1D and T2D, and patients should be assessed at each clinical encounter to determine whether this is a problem area for them. If there are problems, more detailed assessment should be conducted to determine whether or not referral is needed for patient education or other interventions, following the example of a comprehensive hypoglycemia interview provided by Cradock and Frier (2010). Often patients are reluctant to discuss SH episodes with health care professionals due to fears that their ability to engage in certain activities and/or occupations (e.g., driving, piloting airplanes) will be restricted (Davis 1997, DCCT Research Group 1997, Leese 2003, Workgroup on Hypoglycemia ADA 2005, Zammitt 2005).
2. FOH is common and should be periodically assessed in both patients and family members, including parents of children with diabetes, especially following distressing or traumatic episodes of SH. When patients present with chronically high BG levels, the possibility of very high FOH should be considered (Gonder-Frederick 1997b, Nordfeldt 2005b, Wild 2007, Barnard 2010).
3. During hypoglycemia assessments at clinic visits, potential problems in diabetes management behaviors related to episodes (e.g., missed meal, increased physical activity, variable work schedule that changes insulin dosing schedule) should be identified to guide patient counseling/education (Bognetti 1997, Workgroup on Hypoglycemia ADA 2005, Honkasalo 2011).
4. Individuals who exhibit risky behavior associated with increased episodes of hypoglycemia that are found to be associated with clinically significant emotional or cognitive problems will benefit from referral to a psychotherapist or counselor with expertise in diabetes management and behavioral intervention.

5. Beliefs about hypoglycemia and its treatment need to be assessed to identify attitudes and behaviors that increase risk. Some questions that may be helpful include: "How low does your BG need to be before you believe you need to raise it?" and "How low does your BG need to be before it affects your ability to think and function?"

6. When concerns regarding hyperglycemia appear to be contributing to increased hypoglycemic events, the practitioner might consider additional education sessions with a diabetes educator and modification of the care regimen that encourages more monitoring as well as compensatory strategies such as modification of the patient's MNT.

7. Hypoglycemic awareness/detection should be assessed at each clinic visit given that hormonal counterregulation and symptom thresholds can change over time. Assess ability to recognize hypoglycemia in patients who do not report traditional hypoglycemic unawareness, because even these patients may fail to detect up to 50% of episodes. Ability to recognize hypoglycemia should also be assessed in pediatric patients as well as their parents, since research indicates that poor ability to identify low BG may be a risk factor for SH (Cox 1999, Cryer 2002, Workgroup on Hypoglycemia ADA 2005, Gonder-Frederick 2008).

8. Patients with comorbid psychiatric or cognitive problems, as well as those in lower-SES groups, may warrant closer monitoring for problems with SH given their higher risk level (Rewers 2002, Seligman 2010, Honkasalo 2011).

9. Ideally, all patients should receive comprehensive education on hypoglycemia, including its causes, its impact on cognitive functioning, and the need for immediate treatment. For the subset of patients who have recurrent problems with hypoglycemia, this education should be a continuing part of clinical care. Education regarding HAAF and the impact of frequent episodes of mild hypoglycemia on the ability to counterregulate and recognize warning symptoms should be provided, with care taken to present information in a manner that translates to behavior change strategies. Further, routine screening regarding incidence and identification may need to be accompanied by suggestions regarding accessible treatment resources (such as print or web-based information) when the practitioner is not able to provide these ongoing services.

10. Patients should be assessed for frequency of mild hypoglycemic events during clinic visits given that these can be a risk factor for HAAF and SH. Education regarding the impact of frequent mild hypoglycemia on symptoms and hormonal response should be provided to patients who have one or more weekly episodes, and the possibility of following a regimen aimed at avoiding these events to improve counterregulation should be discussed with the patient (Cranston 1994, Heller 2008).

11. CGM or SAP therapy should be considered for patients who have recurrent SH due to hypoglycemic unawareness, problems with nocturnal hypoglycemia, very high levels of FOH, or hypoglycemia that interferes with quality of life, and for those who live alone. Given the complexity of these technologies, patients considering using CGM or SAP therapy

should receive comprehensive and systematic training from diabetes educators (Hermanides 2011, JDRF Research Group 2011).

12. Some of the strategies used in BGAT and BGATHome (e.g., BG Awareness Diaries) have been published previously for use by health care providers including psychologists, diabetes educators, nurses, and physicians (Cox 2006a) and can be suggested as intervention resources, especially when trained providers are not geographically available.

ACKNOWLEDGMENTS

This manuscript was supported in part by NIH/NIDDK Grants R01DK60039 and R21DK080896. The authors thank Karen Vajda and Kelli McFarling for their editorial assistance.

BIBLIOGRAPHY

Alemzadeh R, Berhe T, Wyatt DT: Flexible insulin therapy with glargine insulin improved glycemic control and reduced severe hypoglycemia among preschool-aged children with type 1 diabetes mellitus. *Pediatrics* 115:1320–1324, 2005

Allen C, LeCaire T, Palta M, Daniels K, Meredith M, D'Alession DJ: Risk factors for frequent and severe hypoglycemia in type 1 diabetes. *Diabetes Care* 24:1878–1881, 2001

Allen KV, Frier BM: Nocturnal hypoglycemia: clinical manifestations and therapeutic strategies toward prevention. *Endocr Prac* 9:530–543, 2003

Amiel SA: Hypoglycemia: from the laboratory to the clinic. *Diabetes Care* 32:1364–1371, 2009

Avogaro AJ, Bristow D, Bier DM, Cobelli C, Toffolo G: Stable-label intravenous glucose tolerance test minimal model. *Diabetes* 38:1048–1055, 1989

Banarer S, Cryer PE: Hypoglycemia in type 2 diabetes. *Med Clin North Am* 88:1107–1116, 2004

Barnard K, Thomas S, Royle P, Noyes K, Waugh N: Fear of hypoglycaemia in parents of young children with type 1 diabetes: a systematic review. *BMC Pediatr* 10:50, 2010

Battelino T, Phillip M, Bratina N, Nimri R, Oskarsson P, Bolinder J: Effect of continuous glucose monitoring on hypoglycemia in type 1 diabetes. *Diabetes Care* 34:795–800, 2011

Bjørgaas M, Sand T, Gimse R: Quantitative EEG in type 1 diabetic children with and without episodes of severe hypoglycemia: a controlled, blind study. *Acta Neurol Scand* 93:398–402, 1996

Block JM, Buckingham B: Use of real-time continuous glucose monitoring technology in children and adolescents. *Diabetes Spectr* 21:84–90, 2008

Bode BW, Tamborlane WV, Davidson PC: Insulin pump therapy in the 21st century: strategies for successful use in adults, adolescents, and children with diabetes. *Postgrad Med* 111:69–77, 2002

Bognetti E, Brunelli A, Meschi F, Viscardi M, Bonfanti R, Chiumello G: Frequency and correlates of severe hypoglycaemia in children and adolescents with diabetes mellitus. *Eur J Pediatr* 156:589–591, 1997

Boileau P, Aboumrad B, Bougnères P: Recurrent comas due to secret self-administration of insulin in adolescents with type 1 diabetes. *Diabetes Care* 29:430–431, 2006

Boland E, Monsod T, Delucia M, Brandt CA, Fernando S, Tamborlane WV: Limitations of conventional methods of self-monitoring of blood glucose: lessons learned from 3 days of continuous glucose sensing in pediatric patients with type 1 diabetes. *Diabetes Care* 24:1858–1862, 2001

Boland EA, Grey M, Oesterle A, Fredrickson L, Tamborlane WV: Continuous subcutaneous insulin infusion: a new way to lower risk of severe hypoglycemia, improve metabolic control, and enhance coping in adolescents with type 1 diabetes. *Diabetes Care* 22:1779–1784, 1999

Brauser D: Elderly dementia patients at serious risk for hypoglycemia. Paper presented at the annual meeting of the American Association for Geriatric Psychiatry (AAGP), San Antonio, TX, Abstract NR-20, March 2011

Brazeau A-S, Rabasa-Lhoret R, Strychar I, Mircescu H: Barriers to physical activity among patients with type 1 diabetes. *Diabetes Care* 31:2108–2109, 2008

Brito-Sanfiel M, Diago-Cabezudo JI, Calderon A: Economic impact of hypoglycemia on healthcare in Spain. *Expert Rev Pharmacoecon Outcomes Res* 10:649–660, 2010

Brunelle RL, Llewelyn J, Anderson JH Jr, Gale EAM, Koivisto VA: Meta-analysis of the effect of insulin lispro on severe hypoglycemia in patients with type 1 diabetes. *Diabetes Care* 21:1726–1731, 1998

Bulsara MK, Holman CD, Davis EA, Jones TW: The impact of a decade of changing treatment on rates of severe hypoglycemia in a population-based cohort of children with type 1 diabetes. *Diabetes Care* 27:2293–2298, 2004

Buse JB, Dailey G, Ahmann AA, Bergenstal RM, Green JB, Peoples T, Tanenberg RJ, Yang Q: Baseline predictors of A1C reduction in adults using sensor-augmented pump therapy or multiple daily injection therapy: the STAR 3 experience. *Diabetes Technol Ther* 13:601–606, 2011

Chelliah A, Burge MR: Hypoglycaemia in elderly patients with diabetes mellitus: causes and strategies for prevention. *Drugs Aging* 21:511–530, 2004

Chico A, Vidal-Rios P, Subira M, Novials A: The continuous glucose monitoring system is useful for detecting unrecognized hypoglycemias in patients with type 1 and type 2 diabetes but is not better than frequent capillary glucose measurements for improving metabolic control. *Diabetes Care* 26:1153–1157, 2003

Clarke WL, Cox DJ, Gonder-Frederick LA, Julian D, Kovatchev B, Young-Hyman D: The biopsychobehavioral model of risk of severe hypoglycemia II: self-management behaviors. *Diabetes Care* 22:580–584, 1999

Clarke WL, Gonder-Frederick LA, Snyder AL, Cox DJ: Maternal fear of hypoglycemia in their children with insulin dependent diabetes mellitus. *J Pediatr Endocrinol Metab* 11:189–194, 1998

Clarke WL, Cox DJ, Gonder-Frederick LA, Julian D, Schlundt D, Polonsky W: Reduced awareness of hypoglycemia in adults with IDDM: a prospective study of hypoglycemic frequency and associated symptoms. *Diabetes Care* 18:517–522, 1995

Colquitt JL, Green C, Sidhu MK, Hartwell D, Waugh N: Clinical and cost-effectiveness of continuous subcutaneous insulin infusion for diabetes. *Health Technol Assess* 8:1–171, 2004

Conget I, Battelino T, Giménez M, Gough H, Castañeda J, Bolinder J; SWITCH Study Group: The SWITCH study (sensing with insulin pump therapy to control HbA(1c)): design and methods of a randomized controlled crossover trial on sensor-augmented insulin pump efficacy in type 1 diabetes suboptimally controlled with pump therapy. *Diabetes Technol Ther* 13:49–54, 2011

Cosmescu A, Felea D, Mătăsaru S: [Severe hypoglycemia in children and adolescents suffering from type 1 diabetes mellitus]. *Rev Med Chir Soc Med Nat Iasi* 112:955–958, 2008

Cox DJ, Ritterband L, Magee J, Clarke W, Gonder-Frederick L: Blood glucose awareness training delivered over the internet. *Diabetes Care* 31:1527–1528, 2008

Cox DJ, Gonder-Frederick L, Ritterband L, Patel K, Schachinger H, Fehm-Wolfsdorf G, Hermanns N, Snoek F, Zrebiec J, Polonksy W, Schlundt D, Kovatchev B, Clarke WL: Blood glucose awareness training: what is it, where is it, and where is it going? *Diabetes Spectr* 19:43–49, 2006a

Cox DJ, Kovatchev B, Vandecar K, Gonder-Frederick L, Ritterband L, Clarke W: Hypoglycemia preceding fatal car collisions. *Diabetes Care* 29:467–468, 2006b

Cox DJ, Penberthy JK, Zrebiec J, Weinger K, Aikens JE, Frier BM, Stetson B, DeGroot M, Trief P, Schaechinger H, Hermanns N, Gonder-Frederick L, Clarke WL: Incidence of driving mishaps and their correlates among drivers with diabetes. *Diabetes Care* 26:2329–2334, 2003

Cox DJ, Gonder-Frederick L, McCall A, Kovatchev B, Clarke WL: The effects of glucose fluctuation on cognitive function and QOL: the functional costs of hypoglycaemia and hyperglycaemia among adults with type 1 or type 2 diabetes. *Int J Clin Pract Suppl* 129:20–26, 2002

Cox DJ, Gonder-Frederick L, Kovatchev B, Young-Hyman D, Donner TW, Julian DM, Clarke W: Biopsychobehavioral model of severe hypoglycemia II: understanding the risk of severe hypoglycemia. *Diabetes Care* 22:2018–2025, 1999

Cox DJ, Gonder-Frederick L, Antoun B, Clarke WL, Cryer P: Psychobehavioral metabolic parameters of severe hypoglycemic episodes. *Diabetes Care* 13:458–459, 1990

Cox DJ, Gonder-Frederick L, Lee JH, Julian DM, Carter WR, Clarke WL: Effects and correlates of blood glucose awareness training among patients with IDDM. *Diabetes Care* 12:313–318, 1989

Cox DJ, Irvine A, Gonder-Frederick L, Nowacek G, Butterfield J: Fear of hypoglycemia: quantification, validation, and utilization. *Diabetes Care* 10:617–621, 1987

Cradock S, Frier B: Determining the risk of hypoglycaemia people with type 2 diabetes: an approach for clinical practice. *Br J Diabetes Vasc Dis* 10:44–46, 2010

Cranston I, Lomas J, Maran A, Macdonald I, Amiel SA: Restoration of hypoglycaemia awareness in patients with long-duration insulin-dependent diabetes. *Lancet* 344:283–287, 1994

Cryer PE: Diverse causes of hypoglycemia-associated autonomic failure in diabetes. *N Engl J Med* 350:2272–2279, 2004

Cryer PE, Davis SN, Shamoon H: Hypoglycemia in diabetes. *Diabetes Care* 26:1902–1912, 2003

Cryer PE: Hypoglycaemia: the limiting factor in the glycaemic management of type I and type II diabetes. *Diabetologia* 45:937–948, 2002

Dagogo-Jack S: Hypoglycemia in type 1 diabetes mellitus: pathophysiology and prevention. *Treat Endocrinol* 3:91–103, 2004

Dagogo-Jack S, Fanelli CG, Cryer PE: Durable reversal of hypoglycemia unawareness in type 1 diabetes. *Diabetes Care* 22:866–867, 1999

Davis CL, Delamater AM, Shaw KH, La Greca AM, Edison MS, Perez-Rodriguez JE, Nemery R: Parenting styles, regimen adherence, and glycemic control in 4- to 10-year-old children with diabetes. *J Pediatr Psychol* 26:123–129, 2001

Davis EA, Keating B, Byrne G, Russell M, Jones TW: Hypoglycemia: incidence and clinical predictors in a large population-based sample of children and adolescents with IDDM. *Diabetes Care* 20:22–25, 1997

Davis RE, Morrissey M, Peters JR, Wittrup-Jensen K, Kennedy-Martin T, Currie CJ: Impact of hypoglycaemia on quality of life and productivity in type 1 and type 2 diabetes. *Curr Med Res Opin* 21:1477–1483, 2005

Davis S, Alonso MD: Hypoglycemia as a barrier to glycemic control. *J Diabetes Complications* 18:60–68, 2004

Deary IJ, Sommerfield AJ, McAulay V, Frier B: Moderate hypoglycaemia obliterates working memory in humans with and without insulin treated diabetes. *J Neurol Neurosurg Psychiatry* 74:278–279, 2003

Diabetes Control and Complications Trial Research Group: Long-term effect of diabetes and its treatment on cognitive function. *N Engl J Med* 356:1842–1852, 2007

Diabetes Control and Complications Trial Research Group: Hypoglycemia in the Diabetes Control and Complications Trial. *Diabetes* 46:271–286, 1997

Diabetes Control and Complications Trial Research Group: Resource utilization and costs of care in the Diabetes Control and Complications Trial. *Diabetes Care* 18:1468–1478, 1995

Diabetes Control and Complications Trial Research Group: Effect of intensive diabetes treatment on the development and progression of long-term complications in adolescents with insulin-dependent diabetes mellitus: Diabetes Control and Complications Trial. *J Pediatr* 125:177–188, 1994

Diabetes Control and Complications Trial Research Group: Epidemiology of severe hypoglycemia in the Diabetes Control and Complications Trial. *Am J Med* 90:450–459, 1991

Draelos MT, Jacobson AM, Weinger K, Widom B, Ryan CM, Finkelstein DM, Simonson DC: Cognitive function in patients with insulin-dependent diabetes mellitus during hyperglycemia and hypoglycemia. *Am J Med* 98:135–144, 1995

Ewing FM, Deary IJ, McCrimmon RJ, Strachan MWJ, Frier BM: Effect of acute hypoglycemia on visual information processing in adults with type 1 diabetes mellitus. *Physiol Behav* 64:653–660, 1998

Fanelli C, Pampanelli S, Epifano L, Rambotti AM, Ciofetta M, Modarelli F, Di Vincenzo A, Annibale B, Lepore M, Lalli C: Relative roles of insulin and hypoglycaemia on induction of neuroendocrine responses to, symptoms of, and deterioration of cognitive function in hypoglycaemia in male and female humans. *Diabetologia* 37:797–807, 1994

Fisher LK, Halvorson M: Future developments in insulin pump therapy: progression from continuous subcutaneous insulin infusion to a sensor-pump system. *Diabetes Educ* 32 (Suppl. 1):47S–52S, 2006

Friedrich LV, Dougherty R: Fatal hypoglycemia associated with levofloxacin. *Pharmacother* 24:1807–1812, 2004

Frier BM: How hypoglycaemia can affect the life of a person with diabetes. *Diabetes Metab Res Rev* 24:87–92, 2008

Garg S, Zisser H, Schwartz S, Bailey T, Kaplan R, Ellis S, Jovanovic L: Improvement in glycemic excursions with a transcutaneous, real-time continuous glucose sensor: a randomized controlled trial. *Diabetes Care* 29:44–50, 2006

Geddes J, Wright RJ, Zammitt NN, Deary IJ, Frier B: An evaluation of methods of assessing impaired awareness of hypoglycemia in type 1 diabetes. *Diabetes Care* 30:1868–1870, 2007

Gold AE, Frier BM, MacLeod KM, Deary IJ: A structural equation model for predictors of severe hypoglycaemia in patients with insulin-dependent diabetes mellitus. *Diabet Med* 14:309–315, 1997

Gold AE, Deary IJ, Jones RW, O'Hare JP, Reckless JPD, Frier BM: Severe deterioration in cognitive function and personality in five patients with long-standing diabetes: a complication of diabetes or a consequence of treatment? *Diabet Med* 11:499–505, 1994

Gonder-Frederick L, Schmidt K, Vajda K, Greear M, Singh H, Shepard J, Cox D: Psychometric properties of the Hypoglycemia Fear Survey-II for adults with type 1 diabetes mellitus. *Diabetes Care* 34:801–806, 2011

Gonder-Frederick L, Zrebiec J, Bauchowitz A, Lee J, Cox D, Kovatchev B, Ritterband L, Clarke W: Detection of hypoglycemia by children with type 1 diabetes 6 to 11 years of age and their parents: a field study. *Pediatrics* 121:e489–e495, 2008

Gonder-Frederick L, Cox DJ, Clarke W: Helping patients understand, recognize, and avoid hypoglycemia. In *Practical Psychology for Diabetes Clinicians.* Anderson BJ, Rubin RR, Eds. Alexandria, VA, American Diabetes Association, 2002, p. 113–124

Gonder-Frederick L, Cox DJ, Clarke W, Julian D: Blood glucose awareness training. In *Psychology in Diabetes Care.* Snoek F, Skinner TC, Eds. London, John Wiley and Sons, 2000, p. 169–206

Gonder-Frederick L, Cox DJ, Kovatchev B, Julian D, Clarke W: The psychosocial impact of severe hypoglycemic episodes on spouses of patients with IDDM. *Diabetes Care* 20:1543–1546, 1997a

Gonder-Frederick L, Cox DJ, Kovatchev B, Schlundt D, Clarke W: A biopsychobehavioral model of risk of severe hypoglycemia. *Diabetes Care* 20:661–669, 1997b

Graveling AJ, Frier B: Risks of marathon running and hypoglycaemia in type 1 diabetes. *Diabet Med* 27:585–588, 2010

Griffith R, Tengnah C: Legal basis for standards of driving with diabetes. *Br J Community Nurs* 16:19–22, 2011

Haugstvedt A, Wentzel-Larsen T, Graue M, Søvik O, Rokne B: Fear of hypoglycaemia in mothers and fathers of children with type 1 diabetes is associated with poor glycaemic control and parental emotional distress: a population-based study. *Diabet Med* 27:72–78, 2010

Heller SR: Minimizing hypoglycemia while maintaining glycemic control in diabetes. *Diabetes* 57:3177–3183, 2008

Henderson JN, Allen KV, Deary IJ, Frier BM: Hypoglycaemia in insulin-treated type 2 diabetes: frequency, symptoms and impaired awareness. *Diabet Med* 20:1016–1021, 2003

Hepburn DA, Patrick AW, Eadington DW, Ewing DJ, Frier B: Unawareness of hypoglycaemia in insulin-treated diabetic patients: prevalence and relationship to autonomic neuropathy. *Diabet Med* 7:711–717, 1990

Hermanides J, Nørgaard K, Bruttomesso D, Mathieu C, Frid A, Dayan CM, Diem P, Fermon C, Wentholt IM, Hoekstra JB, Devries JH: Sensor-augmented pump therapy lowers HbA(1c) in suboptimally controlled type 1 diabetes: a randomized controlled trial. *Diabet Med.* doi: 10.1111/j.1464-5491.2011.03256.x

Hermanns N, Kulzer B, Krichbaum M, Kubiak T, Haak T: Long-term effect of an education program (HyPOS) on the incidence of severe hypoglycemia in patients with type 1 diabetes. *Diabetes Care* 33:e36, 2010

Hermanns N, Kulzer B, Krichbaum M, Kubiak T, Haak T: Affective and anxiety disorders in a German sample of diabetic patients: prevalence, comorbidity and risk factors. *Diabet Med* 22:293–300, 2005

Hermanns N, Kubiak T, Kulzer B, Haak T: Emotional changes during experimentally induced hypoglycaemia in type 1 diabetes. *Biol Psychol* 63:15–44, 2003

Hershey T, Lillie R, Sadler M, White NH: Severe hypoglycemia and long-term spatial memory in children with type 1 diabetes mellitus: a retrospective study. *J Int Neuropsychol Soc* 9:740–750, 2003

Hirai FE, Moss SE, Klein BEK, Klein R: Severe hypoglycemia and smoking in a long-term type 1 diabetic population: Wisconsin Epidemiologic Study of Diabetic Retinopathy. *Diabetes Care* 30:1437–1441, 2007

Hirsch IB: Insulin analogues. *N Engl J Med* 352:174–183, 2005

Holmes CS, Koepke KM, Thompson RG, Gyves PW, Weydert JA: Verbal fluency and naming performance in type 1 diabetes at different blood glucose concentrations. *Diabetes Care* 7:454–459, 1984

Holstein A, Egberts E-H: Risk of hypoglycaemia with oral antidiabetic agents in patients with type 2 diabetes. *Exp Clin Endocrinol Diabetes* 111:405–414, 2003

Home P, Bartley P, Russell-Jones D, Hanaire-Brouton H, Heeg J-E, Abrams P, Landin-Olsson M, Hylleberg B, Lang H, Draeger E; Study to Evaluate the Administration of Detemir Insulin Efficacy, Safety and Suitability (STEADINESS) Study Group: Insulin detemir offers improved glycemic control compared with NPH insulin in people with type 1 diabetes: a randomized clinical trial. *Diabetes Care* 27:1081–1087, 2004

Honkasalo MT, Elonheimo OM, Sane T: Severe hypoglycaemia in drug-treated diabetic patients needs attention: a population-based study. *Scand J Prim Health Care.* doi: 10.3109/02813432.2011.580090

Jaser SS, Whittemore R, Ambrosino JM, Lindemann E, Grey M: Coping and psychosocial adjustment in mothers of young children with type 1 diabetes. *Child Health Care* 38:91–106, 2009

Jeha GS, Karaviti LP, Anderson B, Smith EO, Donaldson S, McGirk T, Haymond MW: Continuous glucose monitoring and the reality of metabolic control in preschool children with type 1 diabetes. *Diabetes Care* 27:2881–2886, 2004

Jørgensen HV, Pedersen-Bjergaard U, Rasmussen AK, Borch-Johnsen K: The impact of severe hypoglycemia and impaired awareness of hypoglycemia on relatives of patients with type 1 diabetes. *Diabetes Care* 26:1106–1109, 2003

Juvenile Diabetes Research Foundation Continuous Glucose Monitoring Study Group, Tamborlane WV, Beck RW, Bode BW, Buckingham B, Chase HP, Clemons R, Fiallo-Scharer R, et al.: Continuous glucose monitoring and intensive treatment of type 1 diabetes. *N Engl J Med* 359:1464–1476, 2008

Katakura M, Naka M, Kondo T, Nishii N, Komatsu M, Sato Y, Yamauchi K, Hiramatsu K, Ikeda M, Aizawa T, Hashizume K: Prospective analysis of mortality, morbidity, and risk factors in elderly diabetic subjects: Nagano study. *Diabetes Care* 26:638–644, 2003

Kerr D, Macdonald IA, Heller SR, Tattersall RB: Alcohol causes hypoglycaemic unawareness in healthy volunteers and patients with type 1 (insulin-dependent) diabetes. *Diabetologia* 33:216–221, 1990

Kinsley BT, Weinger K, Bajaj M, Levy CJ, Simonson DC, Quigley M, Cox DJ, Jacobson AM: Blood glucose awareness training and epinephrine responses to hypoglycemia during intensive treatment in type 1 diabetes. *Diabetes Care* 22:1022–1028, 1999

Kordonouri O, Pankowska E, Rami B, Kapellen T, Coutant R, Hartmann R, Lange K, Knip M, Danne T: Sensor-augmented pump therapy from the diagnosis of childhood type 1 diabetes: results of the Paediatric Onset Study (ONSET) after 12 months of treatment. *Diabetologia* 53:2487–2495, 2010

Kubiak T, Hermanns N, Schreckling H-J, Kulzer B, Haak T: Evaluation of a self-management-based patient education program for the treatment and prevention of hypoglycemia-related problems in type 1 diabetes. *Patient Educ Couns* 60:228–234, 2006

Kubiak T, Hermanns N, Schreckling H-J, Kulzer B, Haak T: Assessment of hypoglycaemia awareness using continuous glucose monitoring. *Diabet Med* 21:487–490, 2004

Laiteerapong N, Karter AJ, Liu JY, Moffet HH, Sudore R, Schillinger D, John PM, Huang ES: Correlates of quality-of-life in older adults with diabetes: the Diabetes and Aging Study. *Diabetes Care.* doi: 10.2337/dc10-2424

Leese GP, Wang J, Broomhall J, Kelly P, Marsden A, Morrison W, Frier BM, Morris A: Frequency of severe hypoglycemia requiring emergency treatment in type 1 and type 2 diabetes: a population-based study of health service resource use. *Diabetes Care* 26:1176–1180, 2003

Leiter LA, Yale J-F, Chiasson J-L, Harris SB, Kleinstiver P, Sauriol L: Assessment of the impact of fear of hypoglycemic episodes on glycemic and hypoglycemic management. *Can J Diabetes* 29:186–192, 2005

Linkeschova R, Raoul M, Bott U, Berger M, Spraul M: Less severe hypoglycaemia, better metabolic control, and improved quality of life in type 1 diabetes mellitus with continuous subcutaneous insulin infusion (CSII) therapy: an observational study of 100 consecutive patients followed for a mean of 2 years. *Diabet Med* 19:746–751, 2002

Litton J, Rice A, Friedman N, Oden J, Lee MM, Freemark M: Insulin pump therapy in toddlers and preschool children with type 1 diabetes mellitus. *J Pediatr* 141:490–495, 2002

Lundkvist J, Berne C, Bolinder B, Jönsson L: The economic and quality of life impact of hypoglycemia. *Eur J Health Econ* 6:197–202, 2005

McCrimmon RJ, Frier BM: Hypoglycaemia, the most feared complication of insulin therapy. *Diabetes Metab* 20:503–512, 1994

Meloche RM: Transplantation for the treatment of type 1 diabetes. *World J Gastroenterol* 13:6347–6355, 2007

Mühlhauser I, Berger M: Diabetes education and insulin therapy: when will they ever learn? *J Intern Med* 233:321–326, 1993

Munshi MN, Segal AR, Suhl E, Staum E, Desrochers L, Sternthal A, Giusti J, McCarthy R, Lee Y, Bonsignore P, Weinger K: Frequent hypoglycemia among elderly patients with poor glycemic control. *Arch Intern Med* 171:362–364, 2011

Murata GH, Duckworth WC, Shah JH, Wendel CS, Mohler MJ, Hoffman RM: Hypoglycemia in stable, insulin-treated veterans with type 2 diabetes: a retrospective study of 1662 episodes. *J Diabetes Complications* 19:10–17, 2005

Murata GH, Hoffman RM, Shah JH, Wendel CS, Duckworth WC: A probabilistic model for predicting hypoglycemia in type 2 diabetes mellitus. *Arch Intern Med* 164:1445–1450, 2004

Myers VH, Boyer BA, Herbert JD, Barakat LP, Scheiner G: Fear of hypoglycemia and self-reported posttraumatic stress in adults with type I diabetes treated by intensive regimens. *J Clin Psychol Med Settings* 14:11–21, 2007

Nordfeldt S, Johansson C, Carlsson E, Hammersjo J-A: Persistent effects of a pedagogical device targeted at prevention of severe hypoglycaemia: a randomized, controlled study. *Acta Paediatr* 94:1395–1401, 2005a

Nordfeldt S, Ludvigsson J: Fear and other disturbances of severe hypoglycaemia in children and adolescents with type 1 diabetes mellitus. *J Pediatr Endocrinol Metab* 18:83–91, 2005b

Nordfeldt S, Johansson C, Carlsson E, Hammersjo J-A: Prevention of severe hypoglycaemia in type I diabetes: a randomised controlled population study. *Arch Dis Child* 88:240–245, 2003

Patton SR, Dolan LM, Henry R, Powers SW: Fear of hypoglycemia in parents of young children with type 1 diabetes mellitus. *J Clin Psychol Med Settings* 15:252–259, 2008

Perros P, Frier BM: The long-term sequelae of severe hypoglycemia on the brain in insulin-dependent diabetes mellitus. *Horm Metab Res* 29:197–202, 1997

Pettersson B, Rosenqvist U, Deleskog A, Journath G, Wändell P: Self-reported experience of hypoglycemia among adults with type 2 diabetes mellitus (Exhype). *Diabetes Res Clin Pract* 92:19–25, 2011

Plank J, Kohler G, Rakovac I, Semlitsch BM, Horvath K, Bock G, Kraly B, Pieber TR: Long-term evaluation of a structured outpatient education programme for intensified insulin therapy in patients with type 1 diabetes: a 12-year follow-up. *Diabetologia* 47:1370–1375, 2004

Rami B, Nachbaur E, Waldhoer T, Schober E: Continuous subcutaneous insulin infusion in toddlers. *Eur J Pediatr* 162:721–722, 2003

Ratner RE, Hirsch IB, Neifing JL, Garg SK, Mecca TE, Wilson C, on behalf of the U.S. Study Group of Insulin Glargine in Type 1 Diabetes: Less hypoglycemia with insulin glargine in intensive insulin therapy for type 1 diabetes. *Diabetes Care* 23:639–643, 2000

Reach G, Zerrouki A, Leclercq D, d'Ivernois J-F: Adjusting insulin doses: from knowledge to decision. *Patient Educ Couns* 56:98–103, 2005

Reviriego J, Gomis R, Marañés JP, Ricart W, Hudson P, Sacristán JA: Cost of severe hypoglycaemia in patients with type 1 diabetes in Spain and the cost-effectiveness of insulin lispro compared with regular human insulin in preventing severe hypoglycaemia. *Int J Clin Pract* 62:1026–1032, 2008

Rewers A, Chase HP, Mackenzie T, Walravens P, Roback M, Rewers M, Hamman RF, Klingensmith G: Predictors of acute complications in children with type 1 diabetes. *JAMA* 287:2511–2518, 2002

Richardson T, Weiss M, Thomas P, Kerr D: Day after the night before: influence of evening alcohol on risk of hypoglycemia in patients with type 1 diabetes. *Diabetes Care* 28:1801–1802, 2005

Rickels MR, Schutta MH, Mueller R, Kapoor S, Markmann JF, Naji A, Teff KL: Glycemic thresholds for activation of counterregulatory hormone and symptom responses in islet transplant recipients. *J Clin Endocrinol Metab* 92:873–879, 2007

Ritholz M: Is continuous glucose monitoring for everyone? Consideration of psychosocial factors. *Diabetes Spectr* 21:287–289, 2008

Rosenstock J, Dailey G, Massi-Benedetti M, Fritsche A, Lin Z, Salzman A: Reduced hypoglycemia risk with insulin glargine: a meta-analysis comparing insulin glargine with human NPH insulin in type 2 diabetes. *Diabetes Care* 28:950–955, 2005

Ryan C: Does moderately severe hypoglycemia cause cognitive dysfunction in children? *Pediatric Diabetes* 5:59–62, 2004

Ryan C: Neurobehavioral complications of type 1 diabetes: examination of possible risk factors. *Diabetes Care* 11:86–93, 1988

Ryan C, Vega A, Drash A: Cognitive deficits in adolescents who developed diabetes early in life. *Pediatrics* 75:921–927, 1985

Samann A, Mühlhauser I, Bender R, Kloos C, Muller UA: Glycaemic control and severe hypoglycaemia following training in flexible, intensive insulin therapy to enable dietary freedom in people with type 1 diabetes: a prospective implementation study. *Diabetologia* 48:1965–1970, 2005

Sandoval DA, Guy DL, Richardson MA, Ertl AC, Davis SN: Effects of low and moderate antecedent exercise on counterregulatory responses to subsequent hypoglycemia in type 1 diabetes. *Diabetes* 53:1798–1806, 2004

Scaramuzza AE, Iafusco D, Rabbone I, Bonfanti R, Lombardo F, Schiaffini R, Buono P, Toni S, Cherubini V, Zuccotti GV; Diabetes Study Group of the Italian Society of Paediatric Endocrinology and Diabetology: Use of integrated real-time continuous glucose monitoring/insulin pump system in children and adolescents with type 1 diabetes: a 3-year follow-up study. *Diabetes Technol Ther* 13:99–103, 2011

Schultes B, Jauch-Chara K, Gais S, Hallschmid M, Reiprich E, Kern W, Oltmanns KM, Peters A, Fehm HL, Born J: Defective awakening response to nocturnal hypoglycemia in patients with type 1 diabetes mellitus. *PLoS Med* 4:e69, 2007

Seligman HK, Davis TC, Schillinger D, Wolf MS: Food insecurity is associated with hypoglycemia and poor diabetes self-management in a low-income sample with diabetes. *J Health Care Poor Underserved* 21:1227–1233, 2010

Shahar J: Helping your patients become active. *Diabetes Spectr* 21:59–62, 2008

Shapiro AM, Ricordi C, Hering BJ, Auchincloss H, Lindblad R, Roberston RP, Secchi A, et al.: International trial of the Edmonton protocol for islet transplantation. *N Engl J Med* 355:1318–1330, 2006

Singh H, Gonder-Frederick L, Shepard J, Cox DJ: Hypoglycemia-related cognitive dysfunction and its consequences in diabetes. *Int Diabetes Monit* 22:238–242, 2010

Slover RH, Welsh JB, Criego A, Weinzimer SA, Willi SM, Wood MA, Tamborlane WV: Effectiveness of sensor-augmented pump therapy in children and adolescents with type 1 diabetes in the STAR 3 study. *Pediatr Diabetes*. doi: 10.1111/j.1399-5448.2011.00793.x

Sommerfield AJ, Deary IKJ, McAulay V, Frier BM: Moderate hypoglycemia impairs multiple memory functions in healthy adults. *Neuropsychology* 17:125–132, 2003

Sovik O, Thordarsen H: Dead in bed syndrome in young diabetic patients. *Diabetes Care* 22 (Suppl. 2):B40–B42, 1999

Stahl M, Berger W, Schachinger H, Cox D: Spouse's worries concerning diabetic partner's possible hypoglycemia. *Diabet Med* 15:619–620, 1998

Steppel JH, Horton ES: Beta-cell failure in the pathogenesis of type 2 diabetes mellitus. *Curr Diab Rep* 4:169–175, 2004

Strachan MWJ, Reynolds RM, Marioni RE, Rice JF: Cognitive function, dementia and type 2 diabetes mellitus in the elderly. *Nat Rev Endocrinol* 7:108–114, 2011

Strachan MWJ, Deary IJ, Ewing FM, Frier BM: Recovery of cognitive function and mood after severe hypoglycemia in adults with insulin-treated diabetes. *Diabetes Care* 23:305–312, 2000

Svoren BM, Butler D, Levine B-S, Anderson BJ, Laffel LM: Reducing acute adverse outcomes in youths with type 1 diabetes: a randomized, controlled trial. *Pediatrics* 112:914–922, 2003

Swade TF, Emanuele NV: Alcohol and diabetes. *Compr Ther* 23:135–140, 1997

Tansey MJ, Tsalikian E, Beck RW, Mauras N, Buckingham BA, Weinzimer SA, Janz KF, et al., on behalf of The Diabetes Research in Children Network (DirecNet) Study Group: The effects of aerobic exercise on glucose and counterregulatory hormone concentrations in children with type 1 diabetes. *Diabetes Care* 29:20–25, 2006

Weissberg-Benchell J, Antisdel-Lomaglio J, Seshadri R: Insulin pump therapy: a meta-analysis. *Diabetes Care* 26:1079–1087, 2003

Whitmer RA, Karter AJ, Yaffe K, Quesenberry CP, Selby JV: Hypoglycemic episodes and risk of dementia in older patients with type 2 diabetes mellitus. *JAMA* 301:1565–1572, 2009

Wild D, von Maltzahn R, Brohan E, Christensen T, Clauson P, Gonder-Frederick L: A critical review of the literature on fear of hypoglycemia in diabetes: implications for diabetes management and patient education. *Patient Educ Couns* 68:10–15, 2007

Williams SA, Pollack MF, Dibonaventura M: Effects of hypoglycemia on health-related quality of life, treatment satisfaction and healthcare resource utilization in patients with type 2 diabetes mellitus. *Diabetes Res Clin Pract* 91:363–370, 2011

Wirsén A, Tallroth G, Lindgren M, Agardh C-D: Neuropsychological performance differs between type 1 diabetic and normal men during insulin-induced hypoglycaemia. *Diabet Med* 9:156–165, 1992

Wolpert HA: Use of continuous glucose monitoring in the detection and prevention of hypoglycemia. *J Diabetes Sci Technol* 1:146–150, 2007

Workgroup on Hypoglycemia, American Diabetes Association: Defining and reporting hypoglycemia in diabetes: a report from the American Diabetes Association Workgroup on Hypoglycemia. *Diabetes Care* 28:1245–1249, 2005

Wredling R, Levander S, Adamson U, Lins P-E: Permanent neuropsychological impairment after recurrent episodes of severe hypoglycaemia in man. *Diabetologia* 33:152–157, 1990

Yki-Jarvinen H, Dressler A, Ziemen M, on behalf of the HOE 901/3002 Study Group: Less nocturnal hypoglycemia and better post-dinner glucose control with bedtime insulin glargine compared with bedtime NPH insulin during insulin combination therapy in type 2 diabetes. *Diabetes Care* 23:1130–1136, 2000

Young-Hyman DL, Davis CL: Disordered eating behavior in individuals with diabetes: importance of context, evaluation, and classification. *Diabetes Care* 33:683–689, 2010

Zammitt N, Frier BM: Hypoglycemia in type 2 diabetes: pathophysiology, frequency, and effects of different treatment modalities. *Diabetes Care* 28:2948–2961, 2005

Linda Gonder-Frederick, PhD, is an Associate Professor in the Department of Psychiatry and Neurobehavioral Sciences at the University of Virginia School of Medicine in Charlottesville, VA.

Daniel J. Cox, PhD, ABPP, is a clinical psychologist and professor in the Department of Psychiatry and Neurobehavioral Sciences and the Department of Internal Medicine at the University of Virginia in Charlottesville, VA.

Harsimran Singh, PhD, is a Research Scientist in the Department of Psychiatry and Neurobehavioral Sciences at the University of Virginia School of Medicine in Charlottesville, VA.

Jaclyn A. Shepard, PsyD, is an Assistant Professor in the Department of Psychiatry and Neurobehavioral Sciences at the University of Virginia School of Medicine in Charlottesville, VA.

Chapter 4

Cognitive Difficulties in Children with Type 1 Diabetes

CLARISSA S. HOLMES, PhD

Research into the cognitive status of youth with diabetes has grown over the last quarter of a century and increased in sophistication. Incorporation of neuroimaging techniques allows better understanding of physiological correlates and substrates of emerging cognitive patterns. Discussion of neuroimaging results is beyond the scope of this chapter but the reader is referred to several recent reviews (Musen 2008a, Holmes 2010). Despite these scholarly gains in understanding the relation between diabetes and cognitive status in youth, familial differences and demographic factors, such as social class status, still remain primary factors that account for significant individual differences in cognition, consistent with results from the general population (Overstreet 1997a, Sattler 2001).

INTELLECTUAL PERFORMANCE

Children with type 1 diabetes (T1D) generally have average or above average intellectual functioning (intelligence quotient [IQ] >85). With an average score of 100 and a standard deviation of 15, individual and family differences in IQ exist, similar to those in the general population (Overstreet 1997a, Northam 2001, Gaudieri 2008). Although overall IQ scores of children with T1D are in the average range, they are slightly lower, by ~3 points, than scores of children without diabetes. A group difference of this magnitude has little clinical significance, although it is of scientific interest.

The Wechsler scales are the most commonly used ability tests in school systems. Different versions are available: for young children <7 years old, the *Wechsler Intelligence Scale for Preschoolers* (WPPSI-III) (Wechsler 2002); for school-age youth 6–16 years old, the *Wechsler Intelligence Scale for Children*–IV (WISC-IV) (Wechsler 2003); and for older adolescents over age 16 years, the *Wechsler Adult Intelligence Scale* (WAIS-IV) (Wechsler 2008). Other scales are available but are less commonly in use, such as the *Kaufman Assessment Battery for Children*–Second Edition (K-ABC–II) (Kaufman 2004) and the *Differential Ability Scales*–Second Edition (DAS-II) (Elliot 2007).

LEARNING DISORDERS

For most children with diabetes, academic achievement is at grade level (McCarthy 2002) or consistent with IQ (Overstreet 1997b). However, ~5% of children in the general population experience learning disorders in reading, mathematics, or written language with achievement that is substantially below expectation for age, schooling, and level of intelligence (American Psychiatric Association [APA] 2000). Some children with diabetes, especially those with disease risk factors, may show a higher incidence of learning problems (Holmes 1992, Lin 2010).

ASSESSMENT OF ACHIEVEMENT AND LEARNING DISORDERS

Diagnostic criteria for learning disorders vary by local educational/school districts. However, the national *Diagnostic and Statistical Manual of Mental Disorders IV* (DSM IV) criteria of the APA (2000) include the following: average intelligence with academic achievement *substantially* below IQ, age, or schooling. Often evidence of cognitive "processing" or neuropsychological difficulties (i.e., attention, memory, learning processing problems) is present. A broad survey of skills in language, executive function/planning and attention, visual spatial functioning, memory and learning, and sensorimotor skills is commonly assessed with *A Developmental Neuropsychological Assessment*–Second Edition (NEPSY-II) (Korkman 2007). Specialized measures of processing skills such as memory can be assessed with the *Wechsler Memory Scale*–Third Edition (WMS-III) (Wechsler 1997), the *Wide Range Assessment of Memory and Learning*–Second Edition (WRAML-II) (Sheslow 2003), and the *Children's Memory Scale* (CMS) (Cohen 1997). Often these more specialized neuropsychological tests are administered by referral only to a specially trained neuropsychologist outside of the school system. Criteria for special classroom assistance typically require a "clinical threshold" to be reached, usually performance on individually administered achievement tests that is 15 or more points (1–2 standard deviations) *below* expectation for IQ (APA 2000). Widely used achievement tests available in most school systems include the *Woodcock Johnson Tests of Achievement* (WJ-III-ACH) (Woodcock 2001), the *Wide Range Achievement Test*–Fourth Edition (WRAT-4) (Wilkinson 2006), and the *Wechsler Individual Achievement Test*–Third Edition (WIAT-III) (Wechsler 2009). Like IQ tests, these measures typically provide standardized scores with an average score of 100 and a standard deviation of 15. For most children with diabetes, learning disorders are likely to be "subclinical" and below the level of severity required for formal diagnosis (APA 2000). Medical insurance often covers the cost of psycho-educational assessment administered by qualified personnel. Local school psychologists provide another cost-free option, although this latter option may entail a long wait for services. Finally, parents may be referred to a licensed private psychologist or a clinic-based psychologist such as in a mental health agency. Reevaluation of learning status is required every three years for children formally diagnosed with learning disorders.

REMEDIAL SERVICES

Studies from the early 1990s document a higher incidence of academic classroom assistance for children with diabetes (Hagan 1990, Holmes 1992). Medical management recommendations were modified for younger children, particularly those under the age of 5 years (Ryan 1985, Rovet 1988) to avoid episodes of severe hypoglycemia that lead to seizures or unconsciousness (Silverstein 2005). In the last 10 years there have been few or conflicting studies of the incidence of specialized classroom assistance in diabetic youth (Crawford 1995). Thus, earlier studies may no longer accurately reflect the current incidence of special classroom placement.

The Education of All Handicapped Children Act of 1974 (PL 94-142), now called the Individuals with Disabilities Education Act (IDEA), mandates that all states provide a free appropriate public education (FAPE) in the least restrictive environment for children with a handicapping condition, such as special educational or learning needs, to receive federal funds. Services may be mandated based on borderline or lower intellectual abilities or a significant discrepancy between an individually administered IQ score and an achievement test score along with cognitive processing difficulties, such as clinically significant memory problems. If an individual meets these criteria, services may be provided and an Individual Education Plan (IEP) formulated. An IEP documents the special services or accommodations to be provided for a child in the classroom. Only children with diabetes who have a clinically diagnosable learning disability will qualify for these intensive school services. More information about IDEA is available at www. ed.gov/offices/OSERS/OSEP or through the American Diabetes Association (ADA) at http://www.diabetes.org/living-with-diabetes/parents-and-kids/diabetes-care-at-school/written-care-plans.

Most children with diabetes qualify for a broader, less intensive range of educational services or accommodations through the Education Rehabilitation Act of 1973. This Act forbids discrimination against individuals on the basis of a "disability," which can include temporary disabilities such as a broken leg. Under Section 504 of the Act, students with medical conditions can receive accommodations to participate in academic and extracurricular activities the same as other students. Diagnosis with a formal learning disability is not required to receive educational accommodations with a 504 Plan. Often the foundation of a 504 Plan is a Diabetes Medical Management Plan (DMMP) or physician's order that prescribes recommended school-based medical care plans. The DMMP is the medical basis for an Individualized Health Plan (IHP), written by the school nurse, which specifies what, where, when, and by whom diabetes care tasks will be provided in school. The IHP provides medical care at school but not educational accommodations. A diabetes 504 Plan provides written guidelines for diabetes-related educational accommodations that are protected under federal law. Common services and exceptions may include storing and administering insulin and blood glucose monitoring equipment or supplies at school as well as allowing students to carry and eat snacks in the classroom. More frequent school absences are permitted to accommodate routine medical visits, and extra bathroom breaks or trips to the water fountain are usually allowed. Private schools that receive federal funds must also be responsive to these student-related requests. A teacher, psychologist, school nurse, or principal can organize a 504 meeting. Before a meeting, parents can write a letter that explains their child's diabetes-related needs and how they can be accommodated in school. If necessary, a physician can write a letter to explain unusual medical needs. More information is available about 504 Plans at http://www.isbe.net/spec-ed/pdfs/parent_guide/ch15-section_504.pdf or via the American Diabetes Association at http://www.diabetes.org/living-with-diabetes/parents-and-kids/diabetes-care-at-school/written-care-plans.

NEUROPSYCHOLOGICAL SKILLS ASSOCIATED WITH LEARNING PROBLEMS

Despite generally average IQ scores, subgroups of children may have a higher risk for specific cognitive processing problems or neuropsychological difficulties, in areas such as visual spatial or memory skills. Clinically significant difficulties are defined as more than 15 points below intellectual level (1–2 standard deviations). The following difficulties have been described in subgroups of children with diabetes; individuals may or may not be affected.

CHRONIC DISEASE–RELATED FINDINGS

Earlier disease onset, defined by some authors as <5 years and by others as <7 years, is related to greatest skill disruption, compared with other groups of diabetic children, with lowest scores (4 to 6 points) in mental processing speed, verbal memory, and learning. Differences of this magnitude could be clinically detectable in school performance and may be perceived by children as frustrating and as relative weaknesses compared with their other stronger skills. Slightly lower (2 to 3 points) nonverbal/visual spatial skills, visual memory and learning, and academic achievement are found in children with later disease onset (Ryan 1985, Rovet 1990, Northam 2001, Gaudieri 2008). However, these differences may become greater, up to 7 points, with longer disease duration in adults who had early disease onset (Ferguson 2005).

Longer disease duration, defined as greater than 5 years but usually less than 8 or 9 years in pediatric populations, is related to mildly lower spatial and visual/perceptual skills (2 to 3 points), compared with shorter disease duration under 5 years. Cross-sectional and longitudinal studies indicate that lower verbal memory and failure to make expected developmental gains in vocabulary and other areas of verbal school achievement may be detectable as soon as 2 years after diagnosis with diabetes (Ryan 1985, Rovet 1990, Northam 2001).

RECURRENT SEVERE HYPOGLYCEMIA AND CHRONIC HYPERGLYCEMIA

Severe hypoglycemia that results in seizures or unconsciousness may have differential age-related effects on the brain, with greater visual spatial and diffuse brain and skill impact on children below the age of 5 or 6 years (Hannonen 2003, Hershey 2003). For older children, controversy exists regarding whether severe hypoglycemia affects verbal memory and, if so, at what glycemic threshold. Clinically, detrimental lasting effects may be seen only with multiple severe hypoglycemic episodes (i.e., over five) or episodes that may interact with a sensitive period of child brain development (i.e., under age 5). At the other end of the glucose continuum, recurrent/protracted hyperglycemia or poorer metabolic control (defined by elevated glycosylated hemoglobin levels >9.0%) is associated with significantly lower general and verbal intellectual ability (7 points) compared with those in better metabolic control (Kaufman 1999, Lynch 2006, Perantie 2008). Significantly poorer visual and verbal learning is found compared with children in better metabolic control (Greer 1996, Lynch 2006), along with significant academic under-achievement. In preschool children, protracted hyperglycemia, reflected in higher A1C levels, relates to lower general cognitive ability, poorer receptive language scores, and slower fine motor speed (Patino-Fernandez 2010). In older elementary school–age children, chronic poorer metabolic control has been found to relate to lower academic achievement and poorer attention/memory (Kaufman 1999). Poorer metabolic control may interact with each of the previous disease risk factors and amplify effects.

ACUTE DISEASE–RELATED FINDINGS

Beyond these generally chronic cognitive effects (Gaudieri 2008, Bade-White 2009), evidence of acute, transient cognitive disruption is associated with some diabetes conditions. Acute mild hypoglycemia, defined as >50 mg/dl and <90 mg/dl, is related to transient slowing/disruption in higher-ordered executive functioning (attention, planning, complex decision making) as well as slowed verbal fluency, memory, and motor speed. Accuracy is usually intact (Reich 1990, Ryan 1990, Gonder-Frederick 2009). In the classroom, a hypoglycemic child will have trouble attending to and encoding new information to be recalled. The child may appear sleepy or lethargic. Speed of responding and other cognitive function may not return to normal (prehypoglycemic) levels for up to 45 min once euglycemia is achieved. Despite disrupted blood glucose levels, no evidence of increased rates of attention deficit hyperactivity disorder is reported in association with diabetes. Clinically, attention problems that occur with mild transient hypoglycemia are consistent with the inattentive subtype of attention deficit disorder (Bade-White 2009), although *the condition should not be diagnosed if it is secondary to hypoglycemia, i.e., an underlying medical problem.* The diagnosis of inattention subtype due to attention deficit disorder would be accurate in the absence of fluctuations in blood glucose, particularly hypoglycemia. Acute transient hypoglycemia that involves seizures or unconsciousness is "severe" and falls under the guidelines for severe recurrent hypoglycemia.

In contrast to hypoglycemia, acute hyperglycemia, defined as a blood glucose level of >300 mg/dl, is relatively unstudied in children, but initial evidence shows an association with slightly lower verbal memory and vocabulary scores as well as reduced speed of cognitive functioning, similar to the effects of acute hypoglycemia (Gonder-Frederick 2009).

ASSESSMENT OF NEUROPSYCHOLOGICAL STATUS

Evaluation of neuropsychological status and associated academic performance should follow generally accepted guidelines for identifying children in need of academic assistance. Specialty tests in memory and other neuropsychological skills are available (Lezak 2001). Although tests can be administered by any licensed psychological practitioner, interpretation of results will be more accurate when provided by a trained neuropsychologist or specialist who works with children who have diabetes. Neuropsychological difficulties often co-occur with learning disorders in specific academic areas such as reading or mathematics. State and federal guidelines mandate formal recertification or reassessment of youth diagnosed with learning disorders every three years (Education Rehabilitation Act of

1973). Adoption of testing guidelines also is appropriate with subclinical learning problems. Generally, if a child has learning difficulties of a magnitude that impedes daily or classroom functioning, the youth should be referred to a pediatric or child psychologist. This recommendation includes children who consistently under-achieve in a school subject or who have difficulty with memory or other cognitive processing skills. A teacher or parent referral for a psychoeducational screening can help determine the cause of the problem. A screening test of reading, math, and written skills can be administered by an educational specialist. If a problem is found, follow-up comprehensive testing is necessary to qualify for assistive school services. Medical insurance often covers the cost of psychoeducational assessment administered by qualified personnel. Local school psychologists provide another cost-free option, although this latter choice may entail a longer wait for services.

ASSESSMENT CONSIDERATIONS

For children with diabetes it is important to first rule out or otherwise address more common medically related issues of school absences, poorer glycemic con-trol, and glucose fluctuations in the classroom, all of which may relate to lower academic achievement as well as memory and attention problems.

During psychological assessment, psychologists should first make sure a child is able to perform blood glucose tests and treat episodes of hypoglycemia. A child should bring a glucose meter to the assessment session, ideally along with a small snack of juice and crackers, in case they should be needed. Glucose testing should occur immediately before psychological testing is begun to maximize optimal per-formance. Even mild hypoglycemia (blood glucose level >60 and <90 mg/dl) can adversely impact psychological test performance and scores. If moderate or severe hypoglycemia (blood glucose level ≤50 mg/dl) is detected, psychological testing should be rescheduled for another day to allow time for recovery of optimal cog-nitive status. However, steps should be taken if mild hypoglycemia is suspected during psychological assessment. The assessment should be paused, a blood check should be performed by the child with the child's own equipment, and a snack should be consumed by the child. Packets of peanut butter crackers and juice boxes provide a good supplement to a test kit. After ingestion of 15 grams of car-bohydrate and a 15-min wait, a child should retest his or her blood glucose level to confirm euglycemia, and psychological testing can proceed.

TREATMENT OF LEARNING DISORDERS

Treatment recommendations for learning disorders should be selected with con-sideration of a child's underlying cognitive strengths and weaknesses as well as the affected academic area. Traditionally, learning problems, if present, may be han-dled either with remediation strategies that promote acquisition of delayed skills (deficit-focused) or with compensation strategies that focus on residual abilities and environmental strategies to facilitate optimal skill use (strength-focused) (Kanne 2010). Often a combination of techniques is utilized, but most of the treat-ment literature has studied individuals with frank neurologic difficulty (Raskin 2010) typically not seen in youth with diabetes. Although these strategies reflect current thinking (Kanne 2010, Raskin 2010), they lack empirical validation of treatment efficacy. Currently no studies exist with youth who have diabetes. Thus recommendations for remediation are based on general recommendations for children with learning disorders.

RECOMMENDATIONS FOR INTERVENTION

1. **Circumvention of the problem**. Clinical experience suggests that it is better to teach to "strengths" rather than to drill to remediate "weaknesses." For example, spatial weaknesses can be minimized by giving oral directions rather than a written or drawn map or by adoption of a phonetic versus sight word reading approach.
2. **Assistive learning devices**. Dependent upon the problem, use of assistive learning devices can be helpful. For example, for isolated memory problems, use of a calculator can help compensate for memory difficulty with math facts and provide an opportunity for practice and recognition learning.
3. **Reduced psychomotor efficiency** could necessitate untimed or supplemental time allowances on tests.
4. **Avoid stigmatization** of children. All individuals have cognitive strengths and weaknesses; the peaks and valleys simply may be a little farther apart for a small percentage of children with diabetes who have diagnosable or subclinical learning disorders.
5. **Help the child, family, and academic providers** to understand differences between transient cognitive deficits associated with fluctuations in glucose and diagnosed learning differences.
6. **Self-esteem difficulties** may be present. If they are persistent or severe, psychological treatment should be sought with a school counselor or trained therapist to reassure a child of his or her strengths and to place relative weaknesses in perspective. Children with diabetes are already coping with an altered sense of self because of their illness, which could increase vulnerability to low sense of self-worth (see Chapter 14).

PREVENTION OR MINIMIZATION OF COGNITIVE DIFFICULTIES

The majority of youth with diabetes do not have learning problems that rise to the level of clinical or subclinical learning disorders. However, transient disruption of memory/attention or slowed psychomotor efficiency could occur relatively routinely in the classroom in conjunction with temporary changes in blood glucose concentrations. Subsequent frustration could impede academic performance. Long-term longitudinal study suggests youth with diabetes have higher dropout rates in secondary school compared with nondiabetic counterparts (Lin 2010), a finding that merits replication.

Disease care has been related to youth memory status. Better isolated memory, even in the average range, relates to more daily blood glucose checks independent of the powerful effects of IQ and social class status (Soutor 2004). Strategies that minimize transient glucose fluctuations and secondary variations in memory and attention plausibly could avoid diminished daily disease care and academic difficulties. Similarly, chronically poorer glycemic control, as indexed by A1C, is consistently related to lower academic achievement (Overstreet 1997b, Kaufman 1999, McCarthy 2002). In some cases, this association occurs independently of social class considerations, such that normalization of the brain's chronic metabolic milieu may help avoid cognitive difficulties and lowered school achievement.

Adolescents at study entry in the Diabetes Control and Complications Trial (DCCT) and the Epidemiology of Diabetes Interventions and Complications (EDIC) research who maintained better glycemic control over the 18.5-year study course experienced only mild psychomotor slowing at middle-aged follow-up (Musen 2008b). Efforts to normalize blood glucose levels (Silverstein 2005) with more frequent blood glucose monitoring and meals/snacks (Holmes 2006) and intensive insulin regimens are associated with beneficial glycemic effects regardless of youth "self-management competence" or diabetes knowledge.

Importantly, "forgetting" to perform a specific treatment behavior, such as blood glucose monitoring, is a common self-care compliance issue across a variety of pediatric regimens (Meyers 2006) and youth (Donnelly 1987, Modi 2006). Instances of forgetting self-care behaviors should be handled matter-of-factly because they are a common issue in pediatric and adult medical populations across a broad spectrum of illnesses. Rather than assuming either noncompliance and/or cognitive processing deficits, health care providers can identify patterns of behavior or circumstances surrounding repeated instances of "forgotten behaviors" to facilitate modification of environmental and behavioral cues to maximize the occurrence of the self-care behaviors. Alternatively, explanations may exist, suggesting that the behavior is not literally forgotten, but may be, for example, embarrassing or inconvenient (see Chapter 14). In contrast, memory problems that affect school achievement (e.g., difficulty remembering math facts) should be monitored carefully and considered for possible psychoeducational evaluation.

Early disease onset and hyperglycemia have been implicated in poorer cognitive outcomes in children and adolescents. However, main drivers of academic functioning in this population are identified as socioeconomic environment and IQ. Cognitive deficits in children with diabetes reach the level of diagnosis at about the same rate as the general population. There is a paucity of research that discriminates among metabolically induced problems versus behavioral noncompliance to the medical regimen versus cognitive deficits. There have been no tests of systematic interventions for learning or memory problems in the population of children with diabetes. Therefore generally accepted approaches, including thorough evaluation of deficits, compensatory learning strategies, and assistive devices, are suggested. Once learning difficulties are identified, systematic re-evaluation of them is recommended. The following strategies are provided as expert clinical recommendations to facilitate memory of disease care behaviors that may lead to better metabolic control.

1. **Assessment.** When forgotten behaviors become a barrier to disease management, care should be taken to establish cause, when possible discriminating between disease-specific neurocognitive sequelae (such as memory "lapse" during hypoglycemic episodes), nonadherence versus cognitive deficits or learning disorders, or poor psychological adjustment to illness

(such as depression) that is reflected in noncompliance with self-care behaviors. If behavioral deficits are disease related, such as to poor glycemic control, the medical management team should be informed and included in remediation efforts.

2. **Assistive aides**. Knowledgeable family members who remain involved in youth disease care can help minimize memory and other cognitive demands on youth and help maintain better disease care. This usually takes the form of increased parental or caretaker monitoring of self-management behaviors. If parent-youth interactions become strained, assistance of a health care provider could be beneficial.

3. **Assistive memory devices**. Depending upon the problem, use of assistive memory devices can be helpful. For example, for isolated instances of forgetting to check blood glucose levels, use of a wrist watch with an alarm, a phone with an alarm, or an established routine, such as always checking blood glucose levels before eating, can facilitate daily incorporation of regular disease care tasks.

BIBLIOGRAPHY

American Psychiatric Association: *Diagnostic and Statistical Manual of Mental Disorders*. 4th Ed. (DSM-IV). Washington, DC, American Psychiatric Association, 2000

Bade-White PA, Obrzut JE: The neurocognitive effects of type 1 diabetes mellitus in children and young adults with and without hypoglycemia. *Journal of Developmental and Physical Disabilities* 21:425–440, 2009

Cohen MJ: *Children's Memory Scale*. San Antonio, TX, The Psychological Corporation, 1997

Crawford SG, Kaplan BJ, Field, LL: Absence of an association between insulin-dependent diabetes mellitus and developmental learning difficulties. *Hereditas* 122:73–78, 1995

Donnelly JE, Donnelly WJ, Thong YH: Parental perceptions and attitudes toward asthma and its treatment: a controlled study. *Social Science and Medicine* 24:431–437, 1987

Elliott CD: *Differential Ability Scales*. 2nd Ed. San Antonio, TX, Harcourt Assessment, 2007

Ferguson SC, Blane A, Wardlaw J, Frier BM, Perros P, McCrimmon RJ, Deary IJ: Influence of an early-onset age of type 1 diabetes on cerebral structure and cognitive function. *Diabetes Care* 28:1431–1437, 2005

Gaudieri PA, Greer TF, Chen R, Holmes CS: Cognitive function in children with type 1 diabetes. *Diabetes Care* 31:1892–1897, 2008

Gonder-Frederick LA, Zrebeic JF, Bauchowitz AU, Ritterband LM, Magee JC, Cox DJ, Clarke WL: Cognitive function is disrupted by both hypo- and hyperglycemia in school-aged children with type 1 diabetes: a field study. *Diabetes Care* 32:1001–1006, 2009.

Hagan JW, Barclay CR, Anderson BJ, Freeman DJ, Segal SS, Bacon G, Goldstein GW: Intellective functioning and strategy use in children with insulin-dependent diabetes mellitus. *Child Development* 61:1714–1727, 1990

Hannonen R, Tupola S, Ahonen T, Riikonen R: Neurocognitive functioning in children with type-1 diabetes with and without episodes of severe hypoglycemia. *Developmental Medicine & Child Neurology* 45:262–268, 2003

Hershey T, Lillie R, Sadler M, White NH: Severe hypoglycemia and long-term spatial memory in children with type 1 diabetes mellitus: a retrospective study. *Journal of the International Neuropsychological Society,* 9:740–750, 2003

Hershey T, Bhargava N, Sadler M, White NH, Craft S: Conventional versus intensive diabetes therapy in children with type 1 diabetes. *Diabetes Care* 22:1318–1324, 1999

Holmes CS, Morgan KL, Powell PW: Neuropsychological sequelae of type 1 and type 2 diabetes. In *Handbook of Medical Neuropsychology: Applications of Cognitive Neuroscience*. Armstrong CL, Morrow L, Eds. New York, Springer, 2010, p. 415–430

Holmes CS, Chen RS, Streisand R, Marschall D, Soutor SA, Swift E, Cant C: Predictors of youth diabetes care behaviors and metabolic control: a structural equation modeling approach. *Journal of Pediatric Psychology* 31:770–784, 2006

Holmes CS, Dunlap WS, Chen RS, Cornwell JM: Gender differences in the learning status of diabetic children. *Journal of Consulting and Clinical Psychology* 60:698–704, 1992

Kanne SM, Grissom MO, Farmer JE: Interventions for children with neuropsychological disorders. In *Pediatric Neuropsychology: Research, Theory, and Practice*. Yeates KW, Ris MD, Taylor HG, Pennington BR, Eds. New York, Guilford Press, 2010

Kaufman FR, Epport K, Engilman R, Halvorson M: Neurocognitive functioning in children diagnosed with diabetes before age 10 years. *Journal of Diabetes and Its Complications* 13:31–38, 1999

Kaufman AS, Kaufman NL: *Kaufman Assessment Battery for Children*. 2nd ed. Circle Pines, MN, American Guidance Service, 2004

Korkman M, Kirk U, Kemp S: *A Developmental Neuropsychological Assessment*. 2nd ed. San Antonio, TX, The Psychological Corporation, 2007

Kovacs M, Ryan C, Obrosky DS: Verbal intellectual and visual memory performance of youths with childhood-onset insulin-dependent diabetes mellitus. *Journal of Pediatric Psychology* 19:475–483, 1994

Lezak MD, Howieson DB, Loring DW: *Neuropsychological Assessment*. 4th ed. New York, Oxford University Press, 2001

Lin A, Northam EA, Rankins D, Werther GA, Cameron FJ: Neuropsychological profiles of young people with type 1 diabetes 12 yr after disease onset. *Pediatric Diabetes* 11:235–243, 2010

McCarthy AM, Lindgren S, Mengeling MA, Tsalikian E, Engvall JC: Effects of diabetes on learning in children. *Pediatrics* 109:1–10, 2002

Meyers KEC, Thomson PD, Weiland H: Noncompliance in children and adolescents after renal transplantation. *Transplantation* 62:186–189, 1996

Modi AC, Quittner AL: Barriers to treatment adherence for children with cystic fibrosis and asthma: what gets in the way? *Journal of Pediatric Psychology* 31:846–858, 2006

Musen G: Cognition and brain imagining in type 1 diabetes. *Current Diabetes Rep* 8:132–137, 2008a

Musen G, Jacobson AM, Ryan CM, Cleary PA, Waberski BH, et al.: Impact of diabetes and its treatment on cognitive function among adolescents who participated in the Diabetes Control and Complications Trial. *Diabetes Care* 31:1933–1938, 2008b

Northam EA, Lin A: Hypoglycaemia in childhood onset type 1 diabetes: part villain, but not the only one. *Pediatric Diabetes* 11:134–141, 2010

Northam EA, Anderson PJ, Jacobs R, Hughes M, Warner GL, Werther GA: Neuropsychological profiles of children with type 1 diabetes 6 years after disease onset. *Diabetes Care* 24:1541–1546, 2001

Overstreet S, Holmes CS, Dunlap WP, Frentz J: Sociodemographic risk factors to disease control in children with diabetes. *Diabetic Medicine* 14:153–157, 1997a

Overstreet S, Holmes CS, Dunlap WP, Frentz J: Sociodemographic risk factors to intellectual and academic functioning in children with diabetes. *Intelligence* 24:367–380, 1997b

Patino-Fernandez AM, Dellamater AM, Applegate EB, Brady E, Eidson M, Nemery R, Gonzalez-Mendoza L, Richton S: Neurocognitive functioning in preschool-age children with type 1 diabetes mellitus. *Pediatric Diabetes* 11:424–430, 2010

Perantie DC, Lim A, Wu A, Weaver P, et al.: Effects of prior hypoglycemia and hyperglycemia on cognition in children with type 1 diabetes mellitus. *Pediatric Diabetes* 9:87–95, 2008

Raskin SA: Current approaches to cognitive rehabilitation. In *Handbook of Medical Neuropsychology*. Armstrong CL, Morrow L, Eds. New York, Springer, 2010

Reich JN, Kaspar C, Puczynski MS, Puczynski S, Cleland J, Dellángela K, Emanuele MA: Effect of hypoglycemic episode on neuropsychological functioning in diabetic children. *Journal of Clinical and Experimental Neuropsychology* 12:613–626, 1990

Rovet JF, Ehrlich RM, Czuchta D: Intellectual characteristics of diabetic children at diagnosis and one year later. *Journal of Pediatric Psychology* 15:775–788, 1990

Rovet JF, Ehrlich RM, Hoppe M: Specific intellectual deficits in children with early onset diabetes mellitus. *Child Development* 59:226–234, 1988

Ryan CM, Atchison J, Puczynski S, Puczynski M, Arslanian S, Becker D: Mild hypoglycemia associated with deterioration of mental efficiency in children with insulin-dependent diabetes mellitus. *Journal of Pediatrics* 117:32–38, 1990

Ryan CM, Vega A, Drash A: Cognitive deficits in adolescents who developed diabetes early in life. *Pediatrics* 75:921–927, 1985

Sattler JM: *Assessment of Children: Cognitive Applications.* 4th ed. New York, Sattler, 2001

Sheslow D, Adams W: *Wide Range Assessment of Memory and Learning.* 2nd ed. Wilmington, DE, Wide Range, 2003

Silverstein J, Klingensmith G, Copeland K, Plotnick L, Kaufman F, Laffel L, Deeb L, Grey M, Anderson B, Holzmeister LA, Clark N: Care of children and adolescents with type 1 diabetes: a statement of the American Diabetes Association. *Diabetes Care* 28:186–212, 2005

Soutor S, Chen RS, Streisand R, Kaplowitz P, Holmes CS: Memory matters: developmental differences in predictors of chronic disease care behaviors. *Journal of Pediatric Psychology* 29:493–505, 2004

Wechsler D: *Wechsler Individual Achievement Test.* 3rd ed. San Antonio, TX, NCS Pearson, 2009

Wechsler D: *Wechsler Adult Intelligence Scale.* 4th ed. San Antonio, TX, Harcourt Assessment, 2008

Wechsler D: *Wechsler Intelligence Scale for Children.* 4th ed. San Antonio, TX, Harcourt Assessment, 2003

Wechsler D: *Wechsler Primary and Preschool Scale of Intelligence.* 4th ed. San Antonio, TX, Harcourt Assessment, 2002

Wechsler D: *Wechsler Memory Scale.* 3rd ed. San Antonio, TX, Harcourt Assessment, 1997

Wilkinson GS, Robertson GJ: *Wide Range Achievement Test.* 4th ed. Lutz, FL, Psychological Assessment Resources, 2006

Woodcock RW, McGrew KS, Mather N: *Woodcock-Johnson III Tests of Achievement.* Itasca, IL, Riverside Publishing, 2001

Clarissa S. Holmes, PhD, is a Professor of Psychology, Pediatrics, and Psychiatry at Virginia Commonwealth University in Richmond, VA. She also has an appointment as an Adjunct Professor of Psychiatry at Georgetown University in Washington, DC.

Chapter 5
Neurocognitive Dysfunction in Adults with Diabetes

Christopher M. Ryan, PhD

Compelling evidence that diabetes has neurocognitive consequences that are characterized by functional and structural damage to the central nervous system (CNS) was first presented nearly 50 years ago when brain autopsies were conducted on 16 young and middle-aged adults with very poorly controlled childhood-onset diabetes (Reske-Nielsen 1963, Reske-Nielsen 1965). During life, these individuals showed evidence of mental impairment and/or neurological abnormalities and all had severe micro- and macrovascular biomedical complications, including blindness, renal insufficiency, and coronary disease. At autopsy, the neuropathological studies showed diffusely distributed demyelination—particularly in the cranial nerves, optic chiasm, and multiple white matter tracts—excessive gliosis in gray matter and basal ganglia, and marked vascular changes throughout the brain. This was considered to be evidence of "diabetic encephalopathy" because the degree of brain pathology appeared to be associated with the clinical severity of diabetes-related retinal and renal complications and was quite different from that associated with other medical or neurological disorders.

Since 1965, hundreds of studies have systematically evaluated brain function and structure in children and adults with diabetes, yet not one has described the extensive neuropathological abnormalities that were noted in the cases studied by Reske-Nielsen and colleagues. Because most of their patients had developed diabetes in the 1930s and 1940s, when the quality of care was particularly poor, it is tempting to regard those cases as a historical aberration that may not accurately reflect the types of CNS changes that are most commonly seen in patients today. Nevertheless, those early observations provide a "proof of principle" that under certain circumstances, the integrity of the brain *can be* dramatically affected by diabetes.

Recent studies have demonstrated that although brain dysfunction is indeed associated with diabetes, its magnitude is modest in most instances, and its manifestations vary somewhat, depending on whether the individual has type 1 or type 2 diabetes. This chapter draws on results from neuropsychological, electrophysiological, cerebrovascular, neuroimaging, and neurometabolic assessments to identify diabetes-associated "neurocognitive phenotypes" in adults. Included in this selective review of that literature is a discussion of plausible biomedical risk factors, likely pathophysiological mechanisms, and implications for clinical practice.

Given the importance of level of evidence, it is somewhat disheartening that randomized clinical trials with cognitive outcomes are so infrequent (e.g., Ryan 2006b, Diabetes Control and Complications Trial / Epidemiology of Diabetes Interventions and Complications (DCCT/EDIC) Study Research Group 2007) and that meta-analyses of the cognitive literature focused on diabetic adults are limited to a single, albeit excellent, paper (Brands 2005). Most of the studies referenced in this chapter do, however, meet the evidence level B criteria: they are well-designed descriptive cohort studies that use multiple measures of cognitive function (or other appropriate measures of brain function or structure), incorporate adequate assessments of subjects' metabolic and biomedical status, include reasonable numbers of demographically similar nondiabetic comparison subjects, and have adequate statistical power to detect "moderate" effect sizes—e.g., Cohen's $d \geq 0.4$). The fact that a consistent pattern of results emerges across studies—despite differences in subject populations, outcome measures, and statistical approaches—provides a moderately high level of confidence in the robustness of these findings.

ADULTS WITH TYPE 1 DIABETES

Cognitive Manifestations

Studies of adults with type 1 diabetes (T1D) provide us with an opportunity to examine the extent to which a very long duration of diabetes—usually 20 to 30 years—as well as the development of clinically significant complications affects cognition and brain structure. If one examines large groups of diabetic adults—regardless of complications or other disease-related characteristics—one typically finds the magnitude of cognitive dysfunction to be similar to that seen in diabetic adolescents. When compared with their nondiabetic counterparts, diabetic adults perform more poorly on measures of intelligence, attention, psychomotor speed, cognitive flexibility, and visual perception. Table 5.1 summarizes results from a meta-analysis of 33 case/control studies that were restricted to adults 18 to 50 years of age (Brands 2005) and illustrates the circumscribed nature of diabetes-associated cognitive dysfunction. It is clear that not all cognitive domains are equally affected, insofar as performance is normal on measures of language skills, learning, and memory.

This work, and results from other more recent studies, makes four important points: First, the degree of diabetes-associated cognitive dysfunction is modest, at best, with effect sizes ranging from 0.3 to 0.8 standard deviation units. Second, learning and memory skills—often considered the cognitive domains most sensitive to early brain dysfunction (Winblad 2004)—are entirely unaffected in this patient population, despite 20 or more years of diabetes. Third, this pattern of deficits is analogous to that reported in children with T1D (Gaudieri 2008). Because virtually all adults with T1D were diagnosed during childhood or adolescence, it is challenging to establish the age at which these cognitive changes first appear in the absence of prospective studies across the lifespan. Fourth, the tasks on which diabetic adults typically perform worse—including most tests of fluid intelligence, attention, cognitive flexibility, psychomotor speed, and visuoperception—almost invariably require rapid responding. That latter observation has led to the conclusion that mental slowing may be the fundamental deficit associated with T1D (Ryan 2005), and this is evident not only in adults, but in toddlers (Patiño-Fernández 2010) and children (Northam 2001) with T1D.

Table 5.1. Cognitive characteristics of adults with type 1 diabetes, based on a meta-analysis of published papers. Standardized effect sizes (Cohen's *d*) for each cognitive domain reflect differences between diabetic and nondiabetic patients.

Domain	Effect Size	Significance (P)	Total N	Studies
Overall Cognition	0.40	<0.001	660	16
Intelligence				
■ Crystalized	0.80	<0.01	276	5
■ Fluid	0.50	<0.01	168	4
Language	0.05	NS	144	4
Attention				
■ Visual	0.40	<0.001	195	5
■ Sustained	0.30	<0.01	217	3
Learning and Memory				
■ Working Memory	0.10	NS	244	8
■ Verbal Learning	0.20	NS	204	5
■ Verbal Delayed Memory	0.30	NS	157	3
■ Visual Learning	0.10	NS	187	5
■ Visual Delayed Memory	0.10	NS	157	4
Psychomotor Speed	0.60	<0.05	368	8
Cognitive Flexibility	0.50	<0.001	364	9
Visual Perception	0.40	<0.001	202	5

Adapted from Brands et al. 2005 (Figure 1)

Older adults with T1D show an even more circumscribed pattern of cognitive dysfunction, with even more modest effects. In the single study that addresses this issue, diabetic patients performed significantly more poorly than similarly aged (mean = 61 years) nondiabetic peers on only a single cognitive domain (speed of information processing; $d = 0.34$) (Brands 2006). Whether this reflects the fact that the diabetic subjects tended to be diagnosed in early adulthood rather than childhood, or whether the nondiabetic comparison subjects are also beginning to develop medical conditions that may also interfere with cognitive function—like hypertension (Reitz 2007, Obisesan 2008) and atherosclerosis (Romero 2009)—are plausible interpretations but remain unproven.

Electrophysiological Characteristics

Consistent with evidence of slowed cognition are results demonstrating that diabetes is also associated with slowed brain wave activity, as measured by electroencephalogram (EEG) (Hyllienmark 2005) and by sensory and event-related evoked-potential (Seidl 1996) techniques in children and adults (Virtaniemi 1993, Brismar 2002). When studied at rest during the euglycemic state, well-controlled diabetic young adults showed a reduction in fast wave brain (alpha, beta, and gamma) activity that is most apparent in the temporal regions of the brain, as well as an increase in slow wave (delta and theta) activity in several frontal regions (Brismar 2002). This was unrelated to either degree of metabolic control or past history of severe hypoglycemia, but within individual subjects, a greater degree of slow wave brain activity was associated with slower peripheral nerve conduction velocity. This latter relationship is consistent with the view that diabetes induces both a peripheral neuropathy and a "central neuropathy" (Dejgaard 1991). If neural slowing (peripherally and centrally) is a key manifestation of diabetes, one would also expect to find correlations between the degree of EEG slowing and cognitive slowing. Unfortunately, neither this nor any other study has measured both variables systematically in the same subjects.

Cerebrovascular Outcomes

Cerebral blood flow (CBF) is altered in adults with T1D, with both decreases and increases in degree of perfusion appearing most frequently in frontal and frontotemporal brain regions (Keymeulen 1995, Vázquez 1999, Jiménez-Bonilla 2001). In one large study, 82% of the middle-aged sample of diabetic subjects showed evidence of hypoperfusion in one or more regions of interest, as compared with only 10% of control subjects; similarly, 58% of the diabetic subjects manifested hyperperfusion, compared with 20% of control subjects (Quirce 1997). These results, obtained with single photon emission computerized tomography (SPECT), found changes in cerebral perfusion that appeared in essentially all brain regions, with the greatest effects occurring in the cerebellum, frontal, and frontotemporal regions. None of those subjects had significant cardiovascular disease but many had evidence of retinopathy, leading to the conclusion that changes in cerebral perfusion occur in association with the microvascular complications of diabetes.

Additional support for that view comes from a smaller study that measured cerebral glucose utilization with positron emission tomography (PET) in diabetic patients with and without peripheral neuropathy (Ziegler 1994). Significant reductions in regional cerebral metabolism rate were limited to those patients with complications. These findings, as well as data from cerebrovascular reactivity studies (Fülesdi 1997), support the view that diabetes induces pathological changes in the cerebral microvasculature—particularly in the brain resistance arterioles. Although unproven, it is likely that the underlying pathophysiological mechanisms are similar or identical to those underlying the development of diabetic microvascular complications. The extent to which these cerebrovascular changes are associated with alterations in cognition has not, unfortunately, been studied in diabetic subjects. Research with other patient populations (e.g., stroke) has, however, demonstrated that cerebrovascular changes—particularly hypoperfusion—can have a marked impact on cognitive functioning (Sabri 1999).

Brain Structure Anomalies

Sophisticated neuroimaging research has rarely included large numbers of adults with T1D, but the extant studies have repeatedly demonstrated the presence of modest structural changes, particularly in cortical gray matter (for review, see Jongen 2008). In what remains the largest study to date, 82 young adults with T1D and 36 healthy comparison subjects were assessed with magnetic resonance imaging (MRI) techniques that measured brain density with voxel-based morphometry (VBM)—a well-established, semi-automated quantitative methodology. Diabetic subjects showed reductions in gray matter density in multiple brain regions that included the left posterior cingulate, the left superior temporal gyrus, and the right parahippocampal gyrus (Musen 2006). These values were ~4 to 5% lower than those from healthy control subjects and were correlated with lifetime A1C values but were unrelated to cognitive test scores or recurrent hypoglycemia. Because subjects with clinically significant proliferative diabetic retinopathy were excluded, it is difficult to draw strong conclusions about possible relationships between structural changes and microangiopathy in this study, although secondary analyses showed statistically significant correlations between brain density measures and severity of subclinical retinopathy. Stronger support for a relationship between vascular complications and brain structure comes from a smaller case-control study that explicitly recruited diabetic patients with advanced proliferative diabetic retinopathy and compared them to diabetic adults without microvascular disease (Wessels 2006). Patients with retinopathy had marked reductions in gray matter density in frontal gyri, occipital lobe, and cerebellum, and these were unrelated to A1C values, diabetes duration, age at diagnosis, or blood pressure.

White matter changes appear to be more elusive—at least when traditional neuroimaging techniques are used along with clinical rating systems (Jongen 2008). However, the development and refinement of diffusion tensor imaging (DTI) procedures has led to the recognition that white matter microstructural abnormalities are present in middle-aged adults with long-standing T1D. Diffusion tensor imaging is a neuroimaging technique that measures the directionality of water diffusion in tissues. When the water molecules are constrained by barriers (e.g., cell membranes, fibres, myelin), the diffusion rate is greater in one direction; analysis of the degree of "anisotropic diffusion" yields a measure of the integrity of highly organized and constrained tissues like white matter. In their seminal study, Kodl et al. (2008) compared 25 diabetic adults in good metabolic control with demographically similar nondiabetic subjects and found abnormalities in the integrity of several white matter tracts, particularly the posterior corona radiata and the optic radiations, which were correlated with several disease-related parameters, including longer duration of diabetes and higher A1C values. Moreover, as might be expected from our current understanding of brain-behavior relationships, there was a robust relationship between the magnitude of these structural abnormalities and performance on several cognitive tasks that required visuospatial analysis and eye-hand coordination (Kodl 2008). Although secondary analyses noted that these effects tended to be greater in those diabetic subjects with microvascular complications, the sample size was quite small, and the severity of the complications was limited. Given the possibility that white matter abnormalities may underlie the mental slowing that is characteristically found in many diabetic patients, it makes much sense for a broader use of DTI techniques in future research studies.

Neurochemical Abnormalities

Perturbations in brain chemistry have been noted in both adolescents (Northam 2009) and adults (Mäkimattila 2004, Lyoo 2009) with T1D. Proton magnetic resonance spectroscopy (1H-MRS) has demonstrated, in a large sample of young adults with diabetes, marked differences between diabetic and nondiabetic subjects in brain glucose levels, as well as in levels of key neurotransmitters (Lyoo 2009). As a group, the 123 diabetic subjects had prefrontal glucose concentrations that were 89% higher than values from 38 healthy nondiabetic comparison subjects. Moreover, a linear relationship was noted between lifetime glycemic control and these prefrontal glucose values. Levels of brain neurotransmitters (operationalized as a composite measure of glutamate, glutamine, and γ-aminobutyric acid [Glx]) were higher by 9%, as compared with control subjects, and again a dose-response relationship was found between lifetime A1C and Glx values. Cognitive performance was also significantly compromised in this group of diabetic subjects, with three domains—memory, executive function, and psychomotor speed—most affected.

Glutamate is ordinarily an excitatory neurotransmitter, but, when present in excess, tends to accumulate in extracellular space, exerting an excitotoxic effect on neurons. If this subsequently were to lead to neuronal necrosis, one might expect to find a relationship between degree of cognitive dysfunction and levels of Glx. This study showed exactly that: higher levels of Glx were most strongly correlated with poorer performance on measures of memory and executive function. Although there was no statistically reliable relationship between brain glucose levels and cognitive performance when all diabetic subjects were studied, results from a secondary analysis that compared those in better vs. worse (A1C ≥8%) control revealed that within the more poorly controlled subgroup, higher levels of brain glucose were associated with slower performance on measures of psychomotor speed. Taken together, this series of findings demonstrates the value of magnetic resonance spectroscopy and illustrates the extent to which diabetes can affect brain glucose, neurometabolites, and cognition.

Magnetic resonance spectroscopy has also been successful in revealing the presence of neuronal necrosis and demyelination in a group of middle-aged adults with microvascular complications. Compared with healthy control subjects, diabetic adults with retinopathy had higher levels of choline-containing compounds (Cho—a marker of myelin metabolism and other phospholipid cell membranes) that were most evident in white matter and thalamus. Myo-inositol (mI—a marker of glial proliferation or activation) was also increased in white matter, whereas levels of glucose were increased in all brain regions (Mäkimattila 2004). Longer duration of poorer metabolic control (A1C months) was inversely correlated with two markers of neuronal integrity—*N*-acetylaspartate and glutamate—as well as with Cho in white matter. These findings have been interpreted as evidence of axonal injury, demyelination, and other neuronal pathology, as well as increased membrane proliferation secondary to gliosis that may be mediated by the microvascular changes that occur secondary to chronic hyperglycemia. Consistent with that possibility are the negative data from an earlier study (Perros 1997) that found no evidence of cerebral metabolic abnormalities but had explicitly excluded patients with significant microvascular complications.

Biomedical Risk Factors

Adults with T1D show a distinctive neurocognitive phenotype. They perform somewhat more poorly than their nondiabetic peers on measures of verbal intelligence, attention, psychomotor speed, and cognitive flexibility but show normal levels of performance on measures of learning and memory. Other changes in brain function include a significant slowing in neural transmission, as measured by EEG and other techniques across multiple brain regions, as well as unusual alterations in cerebral blood flow, with some brain regions showing marked hypoperfusion whereas others show hyperperfusion. Brain structure is also affected, with small (~5%) reductions in the density of gray matter in multiple brain regions, as well as alterations in the integrity of white matter—particularly the long tracts of axons that connect one cortical region with another cortical or subcortical region. Neurochemical alterations are also present: brain glucose levels are elevated, as are levels of certain metabolites that are indicative of damage to neurons, axons, and supporting glial cells.

Earlier authors (Deary 1993, Gold 1993) had attributed these manifestations primarily to the consequences of repeated episodes of moderately severe hypoglycemia. That interpretation was quite consistent with data from animal studies (Auer 1984, Auer 2004) and clinical case reports (Auer 1989, Chalmers 1991, Fujioka 1997) demonstrating that *profound* hypoglycemia (blood glucose values <1.5 mmol/l for an extended period of time) can induce cortical changes in multiple brain regions, including involvement of the frontal and temporal cortex as well as the basal ganglia, hippocampus, and brainstem. More recent studies, focusing on episodes of *moderate* recurrent hypoglycemia, have typically failed to find robust relationships between cognition (or other measures of brain integrity) and the occurrence of one or more hypoglycemic events (Brands 2005). For example, data from the 1,144 subjects participating in the DCCT/EDIC Cognitive Follow-Up Study (2007) showed that experiencing one or more episodes of severe hypoglycemia during the 18.5 years of follow-up was not associated with changes in performance over time in any of eight cognitive domains. On the other hand, subjects who had a history of poorer metabolic control (A1C values >8.8%) did show a significant decline over time, but only on tasks requiring psychomotor speed. Similarly, data from a systematic meta-analysis of published papers failed to find any relationship between recurrent hypoglycemia and performance on cognitive tests (Brands 2005). Unfortunately, one of the difficulties in examining relationships between hypoglycemia and neurocognitive outcomes is the challenge of quantitating number and severity of the hypoglycemic episodes. Virtually all studies—with the exception of the DCCT—have been forced to rely on either medical record data (notoriously incomplete) or on the individual's recall of events that may have occurred years earlier (notoriously unreliable). Thus, it is impossible to completely dismiss the possibility that moderately severe hypoglycemia has contributed to some extent to these neurocognitive manifestations, although the larger, more recent studies that have examined this carefully have failed to find compelling evidence for that view (Kramer 1998, DCCT/EDIC Study Research Group 2007). On the other hand, a very large number of studies—using various measures of brain integrity—have found that microvascular complications and other indicators of chronic hyperglycemia are associated with a greatly increased risk of neurocognitive dysfunction (Wessels 2008).

In one early longitudinal study, young and middle-aged adults with T1D were followed over a 7-year period (Ryan 2003) and compared with a group of healthy nondiabetic peers. Cognitive changes occurred during the follow-up period, but they were limited to a single domain—psychomotor speed—and were restricted to those subjects who either had evidence of a clinically significant microvascular complication (e.g., proliferative diabetic retinopathy) at baseline, or who were diagnosed with a clinically significant complication during the follow-up period. Those with no complications at either time point showed no deterioration over time. Taking a multivariate approach to identify possible biomedical variables of decline in psychomotor speed, those researchers found that the presence of microvascular complications at baseline accounted for 12% of the variance, the development of new microvascular and new macrovascular complications accounted for an additional 17% and 7% of the variance, respectively, and systolic blood pressure as well as diabetes duration each independently accounted for between 8% and 9% of the variance.

Those longitudinal findings are consistent with cross-sectional data from younger adults with T1D (Ferguson 2003). Not only was the presence of background diabetic retinopathy in that study predictive of cognitive dysfunction (particularly on measures of fluid intelligence, attention, concentration, and speed of information processing), but these early microvascular changes were also associated with small focal white matter abnormalities that were most evident in the basal ganglia—a region that has been identified as critical for the transfer and organization of information across multiple cortical and subcortical brain regions (Stocco 2010).

Very recent analyses from the DCCT/EDIC Cognitive Study also provide compelling evidence for a link between microvascular disease and cognition (Jacobson 2011). Sophisticated statistical modeling identified five variables that independently predicted decline in psychomotor speed over the 18.5-year follow-up period: older age, lower education, higher lifetime A1C, and two clinically significant microvascular complications: proliferative diabetic retinopathy and presence of renal complications. In addition, a marker of early macrovascular disease (increased carotid intima media thickening) was marginally associated with slower performance, but factors like hypertension, hypercholesterolemia, or waist circumference were unrelated to cognitive outcomes in the final statistical model. Taken together, this work demonstrates that microvascular disease is an especially salient risk factor for cognitive dysfunction in otherwise healthy middle-aged adults with T1D. The fact that the magnitude of those relationships is modest, at best, may reflect the relatively good metabolic control of DCCT/EDIC participants and/or the careful monitoring and excellent access to health care that they received.

Virtually all larger studies linking cognition with microvascular complications in diabetic patients have implicated retinopathy as the strongest biomedical predictor. Interestingly, studies of *nondiabetic* adults have also found evidence that the presence of retinal microaneurysms may double the risk of cognitive impairment in middle-aged adults. This is most evident on measures of memory, psychomotor speed, and so-called frontal lobe tests (Wong 2002, Lesage 2009). Multiple studies have repeatedly demonstrated that retinal microvascular abnormalities are also associated with an increased risk of cerebral atrophy (Wong 2003) and subclinical cerebral infarction (Cooper 2006)—especially when blood pressure is also elevated. Those findings, along with the well-established structural homology between the retinal and cerebral blood supply, indicate that retinal microvascular abnormalities may serve as a surrogate marker of cerebral microangiopathy. Thus, the use of digitized fundus photography may not only provide information about the integrity of the retinal vasculature but may also provide a noninvasive assessment of the cerebral microcirculation (Wong 2001, Longstreth 2006). One could imagine the following chain of events occurring in diabetic adults in poor metabolic control. Chronic hyperglycemia leads to microvascular disease, which, if it affects the cerebral microvasculature to the same extent as it affects the retina and kidney, reduces cerebral blood flow and induces a cerebral hypoperfusion that contributes to the development of brain abnormalities by reducing the efficient delivery of glucose and other nutrients to brain tissue (de la Torre 2004, Ryan 2006a).

Unfortunately, this model does not explain why diabetic subjects—especially those diagnosed in childhood—begin to show evidence of neurocognitive dysfunction within 2 years of diagnosis, long before the onset of even subclinical microvascular complications (Northam 1998). An additional series of metabolic processes, not yet fully identified, may be initiated at around the time of diagnosis (Northam 2006, Ryan 2008) and may influence brain development in such a way that increases the susceptibility of some diabetic subjects to subsequent brain insults or challenges like those associated with diabetic microangiopathy (Biessels 2008).

ADULTS WITH TYPE 2 DIABETES

Cognitive Manifestations

Early studies on patients with type 2 diabetes (T2D) were conducted to test the hypothesis that diabetes caused an acceleration of the aging process (Kent 1976). Because memory changes are one of the earliest manifestations of normal aging (Verhaeghen 1997), those early studies focused on learning and memory skills and found that, indeed, the ability to learn new information and retain it over an extended period of time (30 min or more) was significantly compromised in older adults with T2D (Perlmuter 1984). These basic observations have been replicated and extended since that time (Strachan 1997, Asimakopoulou 2002, Allen 2004, Awad 2004, Kumari 2005, Arvanitakis 2006, Biessels 2006, Gold 2007, Saczynski 2008, Ruis 2009, Reijmer 2010), and it is now clear that relative to age-matched nondiabetic adults, people with T2D tend to perform more poorly on measures requiring mental and motor speed, executive functioning and problem-solving, and learning and memory. Effect sizes are modest at best—Cohen's *d* typically ranges between 0.25 and 0.5 standard deviation units—and are similar to those reported in adults with T1D. The presence of learning and memory deficits is the cognitive characteristic that most clearly differentiates adults with T2D from those with T1D.

In reviewing the very large literature on this topic, there is a high degree of variability across studies in terms of the cognitive domains that are most affected and also in terms of the magnitude of between-group effects. To some extent, this may reflect the heterogeneity of the aging population: older people recruited into these studies may vary appreciably in their educational experiences and may also have a variety of other comorbid medical conditions (e.g., hypertension, vascular disease, overweight/obese), mood (e.g., depression) and metabolic disturbances (e.g., insulin resistance or hyperinsulinemia), and genetic characteristics (e.g., apolipoprotein E4 [APOE4]) that are known to influence performance on cognitive tests (Flory 2000, Waldstein 2003, Hassing 2004, Elias 2005, Watari 2006, Dik 2007, Reitz 2007, Cukierman-Yaffe 2009, Qiu 2009, Tiehuis 2009, Abbatecola 2010, Bruehl 2010, Cavalieri 2010). As a consequence, more recent studies have tended to take these types of confounding variables into account and have consistently found only modest differences on measures of cognitive functioning between older adults with and without diabetes. This phenomenon is nicely illustrated with data from three studies that recruited very different types of subjects (Table 5.2).

Table 5.2. Effect size (Cohen's *d*) for diabetic–nondiabetic comparisons for three cognitive domains reported in three studies. Study 1 included a total of 100 subjects (Ryan 2000); Study 2 included a total of 106 subjects (van den Berg 2010); Study 3 included a total of 136 subjects (van Harten 2007).

	Study 1: Mean Age = 50	Study 2: Mean Age = 66	Study 3: Mean Age = 73	Mean Value Across 3 Studies
Processing Speed	0.50	0.37	0.43	0.43
Executive Function	0.45	0.25	0.37	0.36
Learning / Memory	0.23	0.16	0.37	0.25

Study 1 (Ryan 2000) focused on middle-aged adults (age range: 34 to 65 years; mean = 50 years) and recruited 50 of them from a diabetes research registry along with 50 of their nondiabetic friends or family members. Study 2 (van den Berg 2010) reported data from 68 older diabetic adults (age range: 56 to 80 years; mean = 66 years) recruited from general practitioners' offices and from 38 nondiabetic subjects who were friends, family members, or acquaintances; subjects were evaluated at two points, 4 years apart. Study 3 (van Harten 2007) recruited 92 elderly (age range: 60+ years; mean = 73 years) patients with type 2 diabetes from a department of internal medicine and compared them with 44 age-matched healthy spouses or outpatients treated for back pain or peripheral nerve problems. All subjects in all three studies completed a basic medical evaluation and were assessed with similar neurocognitive test measures that were assigned to three broad cognitive domains: speed of information processing, executive function, and learning and memory. Table 5.2 shows that within the same cognitive domain, the performance of diabetic and nondiabetic subjects varies appreciably, depending on the demographic and biomedical characteristics of the subjects studied. Nevertheless, across these different cohorts, certain domains are consistently more sensitive to the effects of diabetes than others, with processing speed being most strongly affected (mean *d* = 0.43) followed by

executive function (mean d = 0.36). Learning and memory skills appear to be least affected (mean d = 0.25), but this may reflect the fact that these skills are very strongly influenced by other biomedical complications—particularly hypertension (van den Berg 2009)—that are commonly associated with T2D. Indeed, in the study that showed the largest statistically significant effect in the learning/memory domain (van Harten 2007), subsequent statistical adjustment for hypertension led to nonsignificant differences.

Because longer duration of diabetes and poorer metabolic control are the two variables that are most consistently associated with poorer performance in these cross-sectional studies (Ryan 2000, van Harten 2007), one might expect to see an accelerated rate of cognitive decline in diabetic patients, relative to control subjects, in longitudinal follow-up studies. Somewhat surprisingly, data from two recent studies of older adults have found no evidence for that possibility. For example, Study 2 followed the diabetic and nondiabetic subjects over a 4-year period, and although performance on measures of executive function (but not processing speed or memory) continued to decline over time, the two groups of subjects declined in parallel: there was no group-by-time interaction (van den Berg 2010). A similar pattern was noted in another study that followed a group of the "oldest old" (85-year-old adults with and without diabetes) over a 5-year period" (van den Berg 2006). Although the diabetic subjects earned scores lower than nondiabetic comparison subjects on tests requiring rapid responding, there was no evidence of a differential decline in performance on the part of the diabetic subjects. These findings suggest that the as-yet unknown pathophysiological processes that underlie the development of diabetes-related cognitive dysfunction may not be continuous in the same way that degenerative processes, like those underlying Alzheimer's disease, inexorably lead to dementia. Rather, it is possible that the development of cognitive dysfunction occurs in a time-limited fashion, perhaps during a specific window of opportunity or critical period (Biessels 2008).

The data just reviewed are at variance with results from several large-scale longitudinal studies suggesting that diabetes greatly increases the risk of developing dementia (for reviews, see Cukierman 2005, Biessels 2006, Haan 2006, Whitmer 2007, Kloppenborg 2008), although this remains controversial (Strachan 2008, Messier 2009). A comprehensive discussion of this topic is beyond the scope of this chapter, but findings from an excellent systematic review (Biessels 2006) of 14 very-high-quality epidemiologic studies indicate that the risk of dementia is increased in patients with diabetes. For Alzheimer's disease, diabetes is associated with an increase in risk that ranges from 50 to 100%, whereas the diabetes-associated increase in risk for vascular dementia ranges from 100 to 150%. Multiple endocrine, metabolic, and vascular abnormalities have been linked to both diabetes and dementia—including ischemic cerebrovascular disease, hyperglycemia-associated neurotoxicity (glucose toxicity), changes in insulin and amyloid metabolism, increased oxidative stress, and increased release of inflammatory factors like C-reactive protein, interleukin-6, and tumor-necrosis factor-α (Haan 2006, Whitmer 2007). At the present time, however, the causal pathway that underlies the statistical associations between T2D and dementia remains unknown.

Our focus on older adults with T2D has ignored the growing recognition that children and adolescents are also at an elevated risk for T2D, largely because of the Western epidemic of obesity (Shaw 2007). To date, a single study has systematically evaluated a small group of morbidly obese adolescents with T2D and compared them with demographically similar obese adolescents without either diabetes or insulin resistance (Yau 2010). Despite having been diagnosed with diabetes for a relatively brief period of time (mean = 23.4 months), the diabetic subjects performed more poorly than their nondiabetic peers in multiple neurocognitive domains. Effect sizes were nearly twice as large as what has been previously reported for either type 1 or type 2 diabetic adult patients, and ranged from $d = 1.3$ (IQ score) to $d = 0.7$ (verbal memory, psychomotor speed, executive function). Structural brain abnormalities were also present, with reductions in whole brain and frontal white matter volumes as well as significant gray and white matter microstructural alterations in multiple brain regions. Although diabetic subjects did not have clinical evidence of vascular abnormalities, the authors speculate that these structural and functional brain changes may be a consequence of subclinical vascular alterations, changes in glucose and lipid metabolism, and insulin abnormalities. What is clear from this work is that these diabetes-associated neurocognitive abnormalities may develop over a relatively short period of time in adolescents whose brains are still undergoing normal development.

Electrophysiological Characteristics

Older adults with T2D show evidence of neural slowing on recordings of sensory-evoked potentials (Pozzessere 1998), event-related potentials (Kurita 1996, Hissa 2002), and resting EEGs (Mooradian 1988), similar to what has been reported in those with T1D. Longer evoked potential latencies appear relatively soon after diagnosis (Pozzessere 1988) and are especially prominent in patients with peripheral neuropathy (Várkoni 2002). This phenomenon is also quite stable over time. Despite marked increases in A1C values over a 4-year period (from 6.7 to 7.5%), visual evoked potential latencies did not show a corresponding worsening over time (Moreo 1995). Event-related potential latencies—measured while subjects are paying attention to incoming stimuli and identifying infrequently occurring targets—are consistently delayed by 4 to 11% in both older (Hissa 2002) and younger (Dey 1995, Kurita 1996) adults with T2D. Having diabetes appears to be sufficient to induce these changes, since neither degree of metabolic control nor duration of diabetes was correlated with the latency measures.

Electroencephalogram (EEG) recordings from patients with T2D show evidence of neural slowing at rest that is similar to what has been reported previously for children and adults with T1D. In one of the few reports using this methodology, alpha activity was reduced and theta power—indicative of more slow-wave activity—was increased, particularly at central and parietal electrodes (Mooradian 1988). Delta power was also increased somewhat but the very small sample size (13 diabetic and 8 control subjects) limits the sensitivity and generalizability of these findings.

Cerebrovascular Outcomes

Reduced cerebral blood flow is a well-established phenomenon in older adults with T2D. One early study, using SPECT techniques, demonstrated a 15% reduction in CBF in both hemispheres in all brain regions studied (Nagamachi 1994). The magnitude of this effect was associated with disease severity, defined in terms of type of treatment. For example, those with the most severe form of diabetes, treated with insulin, showed significantly lower CBF values in the frontal lobe as compared with those with a less severe form of diabetes that was treated with dietary changes.

More recent research, using continuous arterial spin labeling MRI techniques, has also noted marked reductions in CBF in diabetic patients (mean age = 60 years), as compared with healthy control subjects (Last 2007). Although for all subjects, CBF in the parietal-occipital region was higher than in either the frontal or temporal regions, the diabetic group had significantly lower CBF values than control subjects. Evidence of cortical and subcortical atrophy was present in diabetic subjects, who showed smaller gray and white matter volumes and larger cerebrospinal fluid (CSF) volumes. Reductions in CBF were correlated with brain volume, and both were associated with markers of chronic hyperglycemia (retinopathy, hypertension, and elevated A1C values). These results, which are similar to those previously reported on patients with T1D (Vázquez 1999, Sabri 2000, Jiménez-Bonilla 2001), provide the best evidence to date that there are robust interrelationships among cortical and subcortical atrophy, cerebral perfusion, and biological markers of chronic hyperglycemia.

Unfortunately, the relationship between cerebral blood flow and cognitive test performance remains poorly understood. In one of the few studies to measure both CBF and cognition in diabetic and nondiabetic adults (Tiehuis 2008), total CBF was associated with better performance on tasks requiring rapid information processing, attention, and executive function in both groups of subjects. Diabetic subjects performed worse than control subjects on measures of cognitive function, had smaller brain volumes, and had lower absolute CBF values. However, when absolute CBF values were corrected for brain volume, the corrected CBF values were similar for the two groups. These unexpected findings suggest that diabetic subjects' relatively poorer cognitive performance is not obviously related to corrected total CBF—at least under resting conditions. It remains to be determined whether other vascular mechanisms (e.g., abnormalities in cerebrovascular reactivity in response to a vascular challenge [Last 2007]) are responsible for diabetes-related neurocognitive dysfunction.

Brain Structure Anomalies

Cerebral atrophy and white matter lesions have been reported frequently in studies of older adults with T2D (Araki 1994, den Heijer 2003, Manschot 2006, Kumar A 2008, Kumar R 2008, de Bresser 2010), but the details vary considerably, depending on the nature of the patient population and the neuroimaging techniques employed (van Harten 2006, Jongen 2008).

Results from a large sample of diabetic and nondiabetic adults recruited from the community showed that T2D was associated with smaller gray matter volumes (~22 ml reduction), greater subcortical atrophy (~7 ml increase in lateral ventricle volume), and larger white matter lesion volume (~57% increase) (Jongen 2007). Structural changes were ascertained by means of an automated evaluation of the magnetic resonance (MR) images and were found to be significantly (and unexpectedly) more prominent in women than in men, associated with higher A1C values and older age but unrelated to hypertension, diabetes duration, or hypercholesterolemia. An earlier qualitative analysis of MRI data from essentially this same subject sample also showed that poorer cognitive function, particularly on measures of information processing speed and abstract reasoning, was correlated with degree of cortical atrophy and white matter lesions (Manschot 2006). Furthermore, degree of cortical atrophy was positively associated with the presence of micro- and macrovascular complications and negatively associated with the use of lipid-lowering medications (Manschot 2007).

When identical neuroimaging and neurocognitive assessment parameters (Brands 2006, Manschot 2006) were used to compare type 2 diabetic subjects with type 1 subjects matched on the basis of age (mean = 61 years), sex, and estimated IQ, significantly greater cortical atrophy and more deep white matter lesions were found in those with T2D, with effect sizes ranging from 0.5 to 0.66 (Brands 2007). What makes this especially noteworthy is that as a group, the type 2 subjects were in better metabolic control, had diabetes for a significantly shorter period of time (7 vs. 34 years), and had lower rates of clinically significant microvascular disease (laser-treated retinopathy: 8 vs. 38%). Because they had higher rates of macrovascular disease and more atherosclerotic risk factors (e.g., hypercholesterolemia, triglycerides, hypertension, higher BMI), it is likely that the pathophysiological processes underlying the development of brain anomalies in patients with T2D may be qualitatively different from those associated with T1D. This work strongly implicates atherosclerotic risk factors, but other studies of somewhat older subjects with prediabetes suggests that impaired glucose and/or insulin regulation may also contribute to the development of the brain anomalies associated with T2D (Convit 2003, Convit 2005).

Hippocampal atrophy is also evident in patients with T2D, and these changes may appear relatively early in the course of the disease. Diabetic adults 45 to 70 years of age with no clinical evidence of microvascular complications had significantly smaller hippocampal volumes than age-matched healthy control subjects (5.4 vs. 6.2 cm^3; d = 1.4) but had similar frontal/temporal brain volumes (Gold 2007). Immediate memory performance was also impaired, and these scores were correlated with hippocampal volume (r = 0.25). The best predictor of hippocampal atrophy was A1C, which explained 33% of the variance in multivariate modeling; neither hypertension nor dyslipidemia had an impact on outcomes.

Because only the hippocampus showed any volumetric reductions in this study, the authors suggest that that structure—which has not been evaluated specifically in many other recent neuroimaging studies (Akisaki 2006, Manschot 2006, Musen 2006, Jongen 2007, Last 2007)—may be particularly vulnerable to diabetes-related metabolic and vascular changes. This possibility is consistent with other data demonstrating the sensitivity of the hippocampus to metabolic events like hypoglycemia (Gold 2007) and is reinforced by the very strong relationship between hippocampal volume and metabolic control that was noted in relatively young older adults with no evidence of white matter hyperintensities or other brain anomalies (Gold 2007). Since an earlier study of elderly nondiabetic adults with impaired glucose tolerance noted a similar pattern of results (Convit 2003), it is plausible that the CNS changes found in adults with T2D may be largely a consequence of the metabolic and microvascular changes associated with insulin resistance, glucose dysregulation, and the efficient transport of glucose into brain structures (Kumari 2000, Convit 2005).

Significant hippocampal atrophy has also been found in older adults with diabetes in both the Rotterdam Study (den Heijer 2003) and the Honolulu-Asia Aging Study (Korf 2006). Not only did the diabetic subjects in that latter study have a two-fold increased risk of hippocampal atrophy compared with those without diabetes, but an ancillary autopsy study demonstrated a synergism between diabetes and the presence of the APOE ε4 allele (Peila 2002), a well-known genetic risk factor for Alzheimer's disease (Kim 2009). Participants with both conditions had higher numbers of neuritic plaques in the hippocampus, more neurofibrillary tangles in the hippocampus and cortex, and a greatly elevated risk of cerebral amyloid angiopathy as compared with either condition alone. Cognitive evaluations also indicated that the diagnosis of T2D greatly increased the risk of manifesting Alzheimer's disease or vascular dementia, particularly in those carrying the APOE ε4 allele.

Progression of cortical atrophy over time in people with T2D has only recently been studied (de Bresser 2010), and it is now clear that although detectable increases in cerebral atrophy are evident over a 4-year period, the magnitude of this effect is extremely small. At baseline, diabetic patients had smaller total brain volumes (1.36%) and larger CSF volume (0.98%) than demographically similar nondiabetic comparison subjects but were comparable on two other measures: lateral ventricle volume and white matter hyperintensities. Four years later, the 55 diabetic subjects showed a relatively greater increase (0.11%) on only a single measure of cerebral atrophy: volume of lateral ventricles. The strongest predictor of change over time within the diabetic subjects was age and a history of hypertension; neither A1C nor any other metabolic variable was associated with brain volume changes. These neuroimaging findings are similar to the cognitive data that were also collected on these subjects (van den Berg 2010) and were discussed earlier. Together, they provide no support for the hypothesis that diabetes accelerates the rate of brain degeneration similar to that seen in patients with Alzheimer's disease (Schott 2005). It remains to be determined as to whether larger changes would appear had subjects been followed for a longer period of time, been older at the time of assessment (mean age = 65 years), been in poorer metabolic control (mean A1C = 7.0%), or had more vascular complications.

Neurochemical Abnormalities

Adults with T2D who are evaluated with proton magnetic resonance spectroscopy show alterations in certain brain metabolites that differ somewhat from what has been reported in older adolescents and adults with T1D (Kreis 1992, Mäkimattila 2004, Lyoo 2009, Northam 2009). Changes in myo-inositol (mI) concentrations are most prominent, particularly in frontal white matter, with increases ranging from 16% (left hemisphere) to 26% (right hemisphere) in relatively healthy patients in good metabolic control (A1C = 7.1%) (Ajilore 2007). Although not associated with glycosylated hemoglobin values, the mI values were correlated with scores on the Cerebrovascular Risk Factor Scale, suggesting that this frontal gliosis is secondary to cerebrovascular changes. Several other neurometabolites were measured, including N-acetyl-aspartate (NAA), glutamate, glutamine, and choline, but those values did not differ between diabetic and nondiabetic subjects—contrary to what has been reported in studies of type 1 diabetic adults (Lyoo 2009).

Other investigators studying insulin-treated type 2 diabetic patients who were in poorer metabolic control (A1C = 8.0) have also found mI concentrations elevated in both white and gray matter, as well as increases in gray matter choline (Cho) values (Geissler 2003). Again, there was no correlation between those brain metabolites and A1C values, but there was a strong association with complications. Subjects with peripheral neuropathy had higher Cho as well as higher white matter mI concentrations, as compared with those without neuropathy. In addition, there were strong correlations between neuropathy, white matter abnormalities, and duration of diabetes, consistent with the view that changes in brain metabolites reflect gliosis that may, in turn, be secondary to osmolarity changes and/or cerebral deposition of amylin. Glutamate/glutamine levels were not measured in this study; NAA was measured but found to be similar to values in nondiabetic comparison subjects. Taken together, the differences between these studies and those performed on patients with T1D suggest that the neurometabolic changes occurring in the brain may vary appreciably across these two disorders, with the greatest changes appearing in adults with T1D. Needed is more research using MRS techniques to directly compare people with the two types of diabetes and carefully ascertain the nature and extent of biomedical complications.

Biomedical Risk Factors

Phenomenologically, the neurocognitive characteristics of older adults (and adolescents) with T2D are similar to those of adults (and children) with T1D. Both groups show evidence of mental and motor slowing—this is a nearly ubiquitous finding—and both show performance decrements on measures of attention and executive function that are similar in magnitude (d = ~0.3 to 0.4). A primary distinguishing feature is that people with T2D often (but not invariably) perform more poorly on measures of learning and memory, whereas deficits related to memory are rarely reported in those with T1D. Like their type 1 counterparts, adults with T2D also show evidence of neural slowing, cerebral hypoperfusion, more cortical atrophy and microstructural abnormalities in white matter tracts, and similar—but not identical—alterations in brain neurometabolites.

The biomedical risk factors underlying the development of neurocognitive complications in people with T2D remain poorly understood, although many candidates have been proffered. We know that chronic hyperglycemia and longer duration of diabetes are both strongly associated with the appearance of cognitive dysfunction, as is the presence of vascular risk factors (e.g., hypertension, hypercholesterolemia, and obesity) and micro- and macrovascular complications (Wessels 2008, Reijmer 2010). Insulin dysregulation, commonly seen in patients with T2D, may also have an impact on neurocognitive processes via multiple mechanisms (for reviews see Craft 2004, Cole 2007, McNay 2007, Cardoso 2009, Hallschmid 2009). Several recent papers have also suggested that hypoglycemia may adversely affect cognition in people with T2D (Zammitt 2005), and this may be a key risk factor for the subsequent development of dementia (Whitmer 2009). Table 5.3 summarizes some of the most plausible potential routes to the brain dysfunction associated with T2D (MacLullich 2008). Unfortunately, until researchers conduct studies with large numbers of diabetic and nondiabetic adults who receive both thorough neurocognitive and biomedical/metabolic assessments, the relative contribution of each of these candidate predictor variables will remain unknown.

Table 5.3. Potential Routes of CNS Damage in Type 2 Diabetes

Altered Glucose Levels

- Hypoglycemic episodes
- Protein glycation
- Altered neuronal calcium homeostasis
- Increased vasopressin

Vascular Disease

- Microvascular disease
- Macrovascular disease
- Endothelial dysfunction
- Inflammation
- Oxidative stress
- Altered blood-brain barrier permeability

Insulin Resistance

- Altered CNS glucose utilization
- Deficits in CNS insulin signaling
- β-amyloid accumulation
- Tau phosphorylation

Modified from MacLullich (2008).

If poor metabolic control—broadly defined—is a major risk factor for the development of neurocognitive complications, one would expect that efforts to improve control would lead to a corresponding improvement in cognition. Support for that view has come from the single large-scale randomized clinical trial designed to test that hypothesis (Ryan 2006b). Older adults with T2D treated with metformin were randomized to receive one of two add-on regimens. They received either a thiazolidinedione insulin sensitizer—rosiglitazone—or a sulfonylurea—glyburide—and were followed for 6 months. Cognitive testing was performed prior to randomization and at the end of the study, and fasting plasma glucose (FPG) values were measured over time. Marked improvement in performance on a challenging working memory test was associated with improvements in FPG, regardless of which drug was used; moreover, there was a linear relationship between the magnitude of improvement in FPG and the number of errors made on the working memory test. This study provides the first strong evidence that diabetes-associated cognitive dysfunction may be reversible.

RECOMMENDATIONS FOR CLINICAL PRACTICE

Diabetes-associated cognitive dysfunction is mild in most instances and rarely meets criteria for clinically significant impairment. Nevertheless, the reduction in mental efficiency that is commonly seen in adults (and children) regardless of type of diabetes may be sufficient to "take the edge off" and disrupt optimal performance in the classroom, workplace, and home. Although no prospective studies have documented the exact onset of changes in mental efficiency, preliminary evidence suggests that these changes begin early in the disease course and can worsen over time (Biessels 2008). That is, patients with diabetes may experience subtle changes in performance relatively soon after diagnosis, but those who are in chronically poorer metabolic control and who develop complications may experience continuing neurocognitive decline. If a patient reports that he or she is experiencing declining performance in school, at work, or in the ability to perform activities of daily living including diabetes self-management behaviors, or if the patient asks about the impact of diabetes on functioning, the following approach to screening and evaluation is suggested:

1. **Initiate an open-ended discussion with the patient to document the patient's cognitive complaints and current level of functioning, particularly focusing on perception of deficits relative to prior performance**. Clinicians should ask patients to describe their experiences in a phenomenological fashion and provide concrete examples of the types of errors they have made or the sorts of changes in mental efficiency that they have observed. Whenever possible, obtain confirmation of cognitive decline from individuals in the patient's environment. Patients should also describe the frequency of these events and how they impact daily activities. It is also important to gather information on the patient's concurrent affective state (depressed; anxious; stressed), metabolic status at the time of an occurrence (e.g., hypoglycemic or recently hypoglycemic), and overall level of metabolic control.

2. **Identify other potential biomedical etiologic sources for declining cognitive performance**. Common conditions include hypertension, hypercholesterolemia, obesity, and poor sleep quality (Waldstein 2003, Gunstad 2010, Waters 2011).

3. **Counsel the patient about possible causes of cognitive dysfunction.** Acute hypoglycemia is a well-known cause of transient cognitive dysfunction, and patients should be made aware of how this can cause temporary reductions in mental efficiency (Warren 2005, Frier 2008). Mood can also interfere with cognitive function (Elderkin-Thompson 2003). Patients should be made aware of the relationship between cognitive dysfunction and chronically poor control—especially when it is associated with clinically significantly microvascular complications (Jacobson 2011). Making the connection between improved control and improved cognitive function may motivate patients to work more actively to improve glycemia. Patients can be counseled that they may be able to reduce the severity of their cognitive problems or prevent these problems from becoming more debilitating (Ryan 2006b).

4. **If the patient reports having marked difficulties with daily activities and/or carrying out the tasks necessary for disease management, refer for evaluation/services from a clinical neuropsychologist.** The neuropsychologist can systematically document cognitive strengths and weaknesses, establish degree of impairment, and work with the health care team to identify factors other than diabetes that may disrupt cognitive functioning. Because of the costs of such an assessment, one should have some evidence, corroborated by other individuals familiar with the patient, that the person is showing changes in cognition.

5. **Be cautious in recommending cognitive remediation services.** No study has examined whether cognitive rehabilitation is effective in reversing diabetes-associated cognitive dysfunction, but studies of other conditions have suggested that these approaches may have modest value when applied to patients with well-documented cognitive dysfunction (Cicerone 2005, Rohling 2009). Referrals should be made only after a comprehensive neuropsychological evaluation has been completed. On the other hand, do recommend focusing clinical efforts on improving glycemic control.

6. **Once cognitive decline has been identified, ongoing monitoring by qualified personnel is suggested.** In addition to monitoring neurocognitive function, if decline continues, other biomedical explanations should be ruled out.

7. **Patients may need assistance accommodating to their new "normal" level of functioning.** If dysphoria or anxiety accompanies cognitive impairment, psychotropic medication may be indicated (Petrak 2009).

BIBLIOGRAPHY

Abbatecola AM, Lattanzio F, Spazzafumo L, Molinari AM, Cioffi M, Canonico R, DiCioccio L, Paolisso G: Adiposity predicts cognitive decline in older persons with diabetes: a 2-year follow-up. *PLoS ONE* 5:e10333, 2010

Ajilore O, Haroon E, Kumaran S, Darwin C, Binesh N, Mintz J, Miller J, Thomas MA, Kumar A: Measurement of brain metabolites in patients with type 2 diabetes and major depression using proton magnetic resonance spectroscopy. *Neuropsychopharmacology* 32:1224–1231, 2007

Akisaki T, Sakurai T, Takata T, Umegaki H, Araki A, Mizuno S, Tanaka S, Ohashi Y, Iguchi A, Yokono K, Ito H: Cognitive dysfunction associates with white matter hyperintensities and subcortical atrophy on magnetic resonance imaging of the elderly diabetes mellitus Japanese Elderly Diabetes Intervention Trial (J-EDIT). *Diabetes/Metabolism Research and Reviews* 22:376–384, 2006

Allen KV, Frier BM, Strachan MWJ: The relationship between type 2 diabetes and cognitive dysfunction: longitudinal studies and their methodological limitations. *European Journal of Pharmacology* 490:169–175, 2004

Araki Y, Nomura M, Tanaka H, Yamamoto H, Yamamoto T, Tsukaguchi I, Nakamura H: MRI of the brain in diabetes mellitus. *Neuroradiology* 36:101–103, 1994

Arvanitakis Z, Wilson RS, Li Y, Aggarwal NT, Bennett DA: Diabetes and function in different cognitive systems in older individuals without dementia. *Diabetes Care* 29:560–565, 2006

Asimakopoulou KG, Hampson SE, Morrish NJ: Neuropsychological functioning in older people with type 2 diabetes: the effect of controlling for confounding factors. *Diabetic Medicine* 19:311–316, 2002

Auer RN: Hypoglycemic brain damage. *Metabolic Brain Disease* 19:169–175, 2004

Auer RN, Hugh J, Cosgrove E, Curry B: Neuropathologic findings in three cases of profound hypoglycemia. *Clinical Neuropathology* 8:63–68, 1989

Auer RN, Wieloch T, Olsson Y, Siesjo BK: The distribution of hypoglycemic brain damage. *Acta Neuropathologica* 64:177–191, 1984

Awad N, Gagnon M, Messier C: The relationship between impaired glucose tolerance, type 2 diabetes, and cognitive function. *Journal of Clinical and Experimental Neuropsychology* 26:1044–1080, 2004

Biessels GJ, Deary IJ, Ryan CM: Cognition and diabetes: a lifespan perspective. *Lancet: Neurology* 7:184–190, 2008

Biessels G-J, Staekenborg S, Brunner E, Scheltens P: Risk of dementia in diabetes mellitus: a systematic review. *Lancet: Neurology* 5:64–74, 2006

Brands AMA, Biessels GJ, Kappelle LJ, de Haan EHF, de Valk HW, Algra A, Kessels RPC, Utrecht Diabetic Encephalopathy Study Group: Cognitive functioning and brain MRI in patients with type 1 and type 2 diabetes mellitus: a comparative study. *Dementia and Geriatric Cognitive Disorders* 23:343–350, 2007

Brands AMA, Kessels RPC, Biessels GJ, Hoogma RPLM, Henselmans JML, van der Beek Boter JW, Kappelle LJ, de Haan EHF: Cognitive performance, psychological well-being, and brain magnetic resonance imaging in older patients with type 1 diabetes. *Diabetes* 55:1800–1806, 2006

Brands AMA, Biessels G-J, de Haan EHF, Kappelle LJ, Kessels RPC: The effects of type 1 diabetes on cognitive performance: a meta-analysis. *Diabetes Care* 28:726–735, 2005

Brismar T, Hyllienmark L, Ekberg K, Johansson B-L: Loss of temporal lobe beta power in young adults with type 1 diabetes mellitus. *Neuroreport* 13:2469–2473, 2002

Bruehl H, Sweat V, Hassenstab J, Polyakov V, Convit A: Cognitive impairment in nondiabetic middle-aged and older adults is associated with insulin resistance. *Journal of Clinical and Experimental Neuropsychology* 32:487–493, 2010

Cardoso S, Correia S, Santos RX, Carvalho C, Santos MS, Oliveira CR, Perry G, Smith MA, Zhu X, Moreira PI: Insulin is a two-edged knife on the brain. *Journal of Alzheimer's Disease* 18:483–507, 2009

Cavalieri M, Ropele S, Petrovic K, Pluta-Fuerst A, Homayoon N, Enzinger C, Grazer A, Katschnig P, Schwingenschuh P, Berghold A, Schmidt R: Metabolic syndrome, brain magnetic resonance imaging, and cognition. *Diabetes Care* 33:2489–2495, 2010

Chalmers J, Risk MTA, Kean DM, Grant R, Ashworth B, Campbell IW: Severe amnesia after hypoglycemia. *Diabetes Care* 14:922–925, 1991

Cicerone KD, Dahlberg C, Malec JF, Langenbahn DM, Felicetti T, Kneipp S, Ellmo W, Kalmar K, Giacino JT, Harley JP, Laatsch L, Morse PA, Catanese J: Evidence-based cognitive rehabilitation: updated review of the literature from 1998 through 2002. *Archives of Physical Medicine and Rehabilitation* 86:1681–1692, 2005

Cole AR, Astell A, Green C, Sutherland C: Molecular connexions between dementia and diabetes. *Neuroscience and Biobehavioral Review* 31:1046–1063, 2007

Convit A: Links between cognitive impairment in insulin resistance: an explanatory model. *Neurobiology of Aging* 26(Suppl. 1):S31–S35, 2005

Convit A, Wolf OT, Tarshish C, de Leon MJ: Reduced glucose tolerance is associated with poor memory performance and hippocampal atrophy among normal elderly. *Pro Nat Acad Sci* 100:2019–2022, 2003

Cooper LS, Wong TY, Klein R, Sharrett AR, Bryan N, Hubbard LD, Couper DJ, Heiss G, Sorlie PD: Retinal microvascular abnormalities and MRI-defined subclinical cerebral infarction: the Atherosclerosis Risk in Communities Study. *Stroke* 37:82–86, 2006

Craft S, Watson GS: Insulin and neurodegenerative disease: shared and specific mechanisms. *Lancet: Neurology* 3:169–178, 2004

Cukierman T, Gerstein HC, Williamson JD: Cognitive decline and dementia in diabetes: systematic overview of prospective observational studies. *Diabetologia* 48:2460–2469, 2005

Cukierman-Yaffe T, Gerstein HC, Anderson C, Zhao F, Sleight P, Hilbrich L, Jackson SHD, Yusuf S, Teo K, ONTARGET/TRANSCEND Investigators: Glucose intolerance and diabetes as risk factors for cognitive impairment in people at high cardiovascular risk: results from the ONTARGET/TRANSCEND Research Programme. *Diabet Res Clin Prac* 83:387–393, 2009

de Bresser J, Tiehuis AM, van den Berg E, Reijmer YD, Jongen C, Kappelle LJ, Mali WP, Viergever MA, Biessels GJ: Progression of cerebral atrophy and white matter hyperintensities in patients with type 2 diabetes. *Diabetes Care* 33:1309–1314, 2010

de la Torre JC: Alzheimer's disease is a vasocognopathy: a new term to describe its nature. *Neurological Research* 26:517–524, 2004

Deary I, Crawford J, Hepburn DA, Langan SJ, Blackmore LM, Frier BM: Severe hypoglycemia and intelligence in adult patients with insulin-treated diabetes. *Diabetes* 42:341–344, 1993

Dejgaard A, Gade A, Larsson H, Balle V, Parving A, Parving H: Evidence for diabetic encephalopathy. *Diabet Med* 8:162–167, 1991

den Heijer T, Vermeer SE, van Dijk EJ, Prins ND, Koudstaal PJ, Hofman A, Breteler MMB: Type 2 diabetes and atrophy of medial temporal lobe structures on brain MRI. *Diabetologia* 46:1604–1610, 2003

Dey J, Misra A, Desai NG, Mahapatra AK, Padma MV: Cerebral function in a relatively young subset of NIDDM patients. *Diabetologia* 38:251, 1995

Diabetes Control and Complications Trial / Epidemiology of Diabetes Interventions and Complications Study Research Group, Jacobson AM, Musen G, Ryan CM, Silvers N, Cleary P, Waberski B, Burwood A, Weinger K, Bayless M, Dahms W, Harth J: Long-term effects of diabetes and its treatment on cognitive function. *N Engl J Med* 356:1842–1852, 2007

Dik MG, Jonker C, Comijs HC, Deeg DJH, Kok A, Yaffe K, Penninx BW: Contribution of metabolic syndrome to components of cognition in older individuals. *Diabetes Care* 30:2655–2660, 2007

Elderkin-Thompson V, Kumar A, Bilker W, Dunkin JJ, Mintz J, Moberg PJ, Mesholam RI, Gur RE: Neuropsychological deficits among patients with late-onset minor and major depression. *Archives of Clinical Neuropsychology* 18:529–549, 2003

Elias M, Elias P, Sullivan L, Wolf P, Dagostino R: Obesity, diabetes and cognitive deficit: the Framingham Heart Study. *Neurobiology of Aging* 26:11–16, 2005

Ferguson SC, Blane A, Perros P, McCrimmon RJ, Best JJK, Wardlaw JM, Deary IJ, Frier BM: Cognitive ability and brain structure in type 1 diabetes: relation to microangiopathy and preceding severe hypoglycemia. *Diabetes* 52:149–156, 2003

Flory JD, Manuck SB, Ferrell RE, Ryan CM, Muldoon MF: Memory performance and the apolipoprotein E polymorphism in a community sample of middle-aged adults. *American Journal of Medical Genetics (Neuropsychiatric Genetics)* 96:707–711, 2000

Frier BM: How hypoglycaemia can affect the life of a person with diabetes. *Diabetes/Metabolism Research and Reviews* 24:87–92, 2008

Fujioka M, Okuchi K, Hiramatsu K, Sakaki T, Sakaguchi S, Ishii Y: Specific changes in human brain after hypoglycemic injury. *Stroke* 28:584–587, 1997

Fülesdi B, Limburg M, Bereczki D, Michels RPJ, Neuwirth G, Legemate D, Valikoics A, Csiba L: Impairment of cerebrovascular reactivity in long-term type 1 diabetes. *Diabetes* 46:1840–1845, 1997

Gaudieri PA, Chen R, Greer TF, Holmes CS: Cognitive function in children with type 1 diabetes: a meta-analysis. *Diabetes Care* 31:1892–1897, 2008

Geissler A, Fründ R, Schölmerich J, Feuerbach S, Zietz B: Alterations of cerebral metabolism in patients with diabetes mellitus studied by proton magnetic resonance spectroscopy. *Experimental and Clinical Endocrinology and Diabetes* 111:421–427, 2003

Gold AE, Deary IJ, Frier BM: Recurrent severe hypoglycaemia and cognitive function in type 1 diabetes. *Diabet Med* 10:503–508, 1993

Gold SM, Dziobek I, Sweat V, Tirsi A, Rogers K, Bruehl H, Tsui W, Richardson S, Javier E, Convit A: Hippocampal damage and memory impairments as possible early brain complications of type 2 diabetes. *Diabetologia* 50:711–719, 2007

Gunstad J, Lhotsky A, Wendell CR, Ferrucci L, Zonderman AB: Longitudinal examination of obesity and cognitive function: results from the Baltimore Longitudinal Study of Aging. *Neuroepidemiology* 34:222–229, 2010

Haan MN: Therapy insight: type 2 diabetes mellitus and the risk of late-onset Alzheimer's disease. *Nature Clinical Practice: Neurology* 2:159–166, 2006

Hallschmid M, Schultes B: Central nervous insulin resistance: a promising target in the treatment of metabolic and cognitive disorders? *Diabetologia* 52:2264–2269, 2009

Hassing LB, Hofer SM, Nilsson SE, Berg S, Pedersen NL, McClearn G, Johansson B: Comorbid type 2 diabetes mellitus and hypertension exacerbates cognitive decline: evidence from a longitudinal study. *Age and Ageing* 33:355–361, 2004

Hissa MN, D'Almeida JA, Cremasco F, de Bruin VM: Event related P300 potentials in NIDDM patients without cognitive impairment and its relationship with previous hypoglycemic episodes. *Neuroendocrinology Letters* 23:226–230, 2002

Hyllienmark L, Maltez J, Dandenell A, Ludviggson J, Brismar T: EEG abnormalities with and without relation to severe hypoglycaemia in adolescents with type 1 diabetes. *Diabetologia* 48:412–419, 2005

Jacobson AM, Ryan CM, Cleary PA, Waberski BH, Weinger K, Musen G, Dahms W; Diabetes Control and Complications Trial / EDIC Research Group: Biomedical risk factors for decreased cognitive functioning in type 1 diabetes: an 18 year follow-up of the Diabetes Control and Complications Trial (DCCT) cohort. *Diabetologia* 54:245–255, 2011

Jiménez-Bonilla JF, Quirce R, Hernández A, Vallina NK, Guede C, Banzo I, Amado JA, Carril JM: Assessment of cerebral perfusion and cerebrovascular reserve in insulin-dependent diabetic patients without central neurological symptoms by means of 99mTc-HMPAO SPET with acetazolamide. *European Journal of Nuclear Medicine* 28:1647–1655, 2001

Jongen C, Biessels GJ: Structural brain imaging in diabetes: a methodological perspective. *European Journal of Pharmacology* 585:208–218, 2008

Jongen C, van der Grond J, Kappelle LJ, Biessels GJ, Viergever MA, Pluim JPW; Utrecht Diabetic Encephalopathy Study Group: Automated measurement of brain and white matter lesion volume in type 2 diabetes mellitus. *Diabetologia* 50:1509–1516, 2007

Kent S: Is diabetes a form of accelerated aging? *Geriatrics* 31:140–154, 1976

Keymeulen B, Jacobs A, de Metz K, de Sadeleer C, Bossuyt A, Somers G: Regional cerebral hypoperfusion in long-term type 1 (insulin-dependent) diabetic patients: relation to hypoglycaemic events. *Nuclear Medicine Communications* 16:10–16, 1995

Kim J, Basak JM, Holtzman DM: The role of apolipoprotein E in Alzheimer's disease. *Neuron* 63:287–303, 2009

Kloppenborg PR, van den Berg E, Kappelle LJ, Biessels GJ: Diabetes and other vascular risk factors for dementia: what factor matters most? A systematic review. *European Journal of Pharmacology* 585:97–108, 2008

Kodl CT, Franc DT, Rao JP, Anderson FS, Thomas W, Mueller BA, Lim KO, Seaquist ER: Diffusion tensor imaging identifies deficits in white matter microstructure in subjects with type 1 diabetes that correlate with reduced neurocognitive function. *Diabetes* 57:3083–3089, 2008

Korf ESC, White LR, Scheltens P, Launer LJ: Brain aging in very old men with type 2 diabetes. *Diabetes Care* 29:2268–2274, 2006

Kramer L, Fasching P, Madl C, Schneider B, Damjancic P, Waldhäusl W, Irsigler K, Grimm G: Previous episodes of hypoglycemic coma are not associated with permanent cognitive brain dysfunction in IDDM patients on intensive insulin treatment. *Diabetes* 47:1909–1914, 1998

Kreis R, Ross BD: Cerebral metabolic disturbances in patients with subacute and chronic diabetes mellitus: detection with proton MR spectroscopy. *Radiology* 184:123–130, 1992

Kumar A, Haroon E, Darwin C, Pham D, Ajilore O, Rodriguez G, Mintz J: Gray matter prefrontal changes in type 2 diabetes detected using MRI. *Journal of Magnetic Resonance Imaging* 27:14–19, 2008

Kumar R, Anstey KJ, Cherbuin N, Wen W, Sachdev PS: Association of type 2 diabetes with depression, brain atrophy, and reduced fine motor speed in a 60- to 64-year-old community sample. *American Journal of Geriatric Psychiatry* 16:989–998, 2008

Kumari M, Brunner E, Fuhrer R: Minireview: mechanisms by which the metabolic syndrome and diabetes impair memory. *Journal of Gerontology: Biological Sciences* 55:B228–B232, 2000

Kumari M, Marmot M: Diabetes and cognitive function in a middle-aged cohort: findings from the Whitehall II study. *Neurology* 65:1597–1603, 2005

Kurita A, Katayama K, Mochio S: Neurophysiological evidence for altered higher brain functions in NIDDM. *Diabetes Care* 19:361–364, 1996

Last D, Alsop DC, Abduljalil AM, Marquis RP, de Bazelaire C, Hu K, Cavallerano J, Novak V: Global and regional effects of type 2 diabetes on brain tissue volumes and cerebral vasoreactivity. *Diabetes Care* 30:1193–1199, 2007

Lesage SR, Mosley TH, Wong TY, Szklo M, Knopman DS, Catellier DJ, Cole SR, Klein R, Coresh J, Coker LH, Sharrett AR: Retinal microvascular abnormalities and cognitive decline: the ARIC 14-year follow-up. *Neurology* 73:862–868, 2009

Longstreth WT, Marino-Larson EK, Klein R, Wong TY, Sharrett AR, Lefkowitz D, Manolio T: Associations between findings on cranial magnetic resonance imaging and retinal photography in the elderly: the Cardiovascular Health Study. *American Journal of Epidemiology* 165:78–84, 2006

Lyoo IK, Yoon SJ, Musen G, Simonson DC, Weinger K, Ryan CM, Kim JE, Renshaw PF, Jacobson AM: Altered prefrontal glutamate-glutamine-γ-aminobutyric acid levels and relation to low cognitive performance and depressive symptoms in type 1 diabetes mellitus. *Archives of General Psychiatry* 66:879–887, 2009

MacLullich AMJ, Seckl JR: Diabetes and cognitive decline: are steroids the missing link? *Cell Metabolism* 7:286–287, 2008

Mäkimattila S, Malmberg-Cèder K, Häkkinen A-M, Vuori K, Salonen O, Summanen P, Yki-Järvinen H, Kaste M, Heikkinen S, Lundbom N, Roine RO: Brain metabolic alterations in patients with type 1 diabetes-hyperglycemia-induced injury. *Journal of Cerebral Blood Flow and Metabolism* 24:1393–1399, 2004

Manschot SM, Biessels GJ, de Valk HW, Algra A, Rutten GEHM, van der Grond J, Kappelle LJ, Utrecht Diabetic Encephalopathy Study Group: Metabolic and vascular determinants of impaired cognitive performance and abnormalities on brain magnetic resonance imaging in patients with type 2 diabetes. *Diabetologia* 50:2388–2397, 2007

Manschot SM, Brands AMA, van der Grond J, Kessels RPC, Algra A, Kappelle LJ, Biessels GJ, Utrecht Diabetic Encephalopathy Study Group: Brain magnetic resonance imaging correlates of impaired cognition in patients with type 2 diabetes. *Diabetes* 55:1106–1113, 2006

McNay EC: Insulin and ghrelin: peripheral hormones modulating memory and hippocampal function. *Current Opinion in Pharmacology* 7:628–632, 2007

Messier C, Gagnon M: Cognitive decline associated with dementia and type 2 diabetes: the interplay of risk factors. *Diabetologia* 52:2471–2474, 2009

Mooradian AD, Perryman K, Fitten J, Kavonian GD, Morley JE: Cortical function in elderly non-insulin dependent diabetic patients: behavioral and electrophysiologic studies. *Archives of Internal Medicine* 148:2369–2372, 1988

Moreo G, Mariani E, Pizzamiglio G, Colucci GB: Visual evoked potentials in NIDDM: a longitudinal study. *Diabetologia* 38:573–576, 1995

Musen G, Lyoo IK, Sparks CR, Weinger K, Hwang J, Ryan CM, Jimerson DC, Hennen J, Renshaw PF, Jacobson AM: Effects of type 1 diabetes on gray matter density as measured by voxel-based morphometry. *Diabetes* 55:326–333, 2006

Nagamachi S, Nishikawa T, Ono S, Ageta M, Matsuo T, Jinnouchi S, Hoshi H, Ohnishi T, Futami S, Watanabe K: Regional cerebral blood flow in diabetic patients: evaluation by N-isopropyl-123I-IMP with SPECT. *Nuclear Medicine Communications* 15:455–460, 1994

Nakamura Y, Takahashi M, Kitaguti M, Imaoka H, Kono N, Tarui S: Abnormal brainstem evoked potentials in diabetes mellitus: evoked potential testings and magnetic resonance imaging. *Electromyography and Clinical Neurophysiology* 31:243–249, 1991

Northam EA, Rankins D, Lin A, Wellard RM, Pell GS, Finch SJ, Werther GA, Cameron FJ: Central nervous system function in youth with type 1 diabetes 12 years after disease onset. *Diabetes Care* 32:445–450, 2009

Northam EA, Rankins D, Cameron FJ: Therapy insight: the impact of type 1 diabetes on brain development and function. *Nature Clinical Practice: Neurology* 2:78–86, 2006

Northam EA, Anderson PJ, Jacobs R, Hughes M, Warne GL, Werther GA: Neuropsychological profiles of children with type 1 diabetes 6 years after disease onset. *Diabetes Care* 24:1541–1546, 2001

Northam EA, Anderson PJ, Werther GA, Warne GL, Adler RG, Andrewes D: Neuropsychological complications of IDDM in children 2 years after disease onset. *Diabetes Care* 21:379–384, 1998

Obisesan TO, Obisesan OA, Martins S, Alamgir L, Bond V, Maxwell C, Gillum RF: High blood pressure, hypertension, and high pulse pressure are associated with poorer cognitive function in persons aged 60 and older: the Third National Health and Nutrition Examination Survey. *Journal of the American Geriatric Society* 56:501–509, 2008

Patiño-Fernández AM, Delamater AM, Applegate EB, Brady E, Eidson M, Nemery R, Gonzalez-Mendoza L, Richton S: Neurocognitive functioning in preschool-age children with type 1 diabetes mellitus. *Pediatric Diabetes* 11:424–430, 2010

Peila R, Rodriguez BL, Launer LJ: Type 2 diabetes, APOE gene, and the risk for dementia and related pathologies: the Honolulu-Asia Study. *Diabetes* 51:1256–1262, 2002

Perlmuter LC, Hakami MK, Hodgson-Harrington C, Ginsberg J, Katz J, Singer DE, Nathan DM: Decreased cognitive function in aging non-insulin-dependent diabetic patients. *American Journal of Medicine* 77:1043–1048, 1984

Perros P, Deary IJ, Sellar RJ, Best JJK, Frier BM: Brain abnormalities demonstrated by magnetic resonance imaging in adult IDDM patients with and without a history of recurrent severe hypoglycemia. *Diabetes Care* 20:1013–1018, 1997

Petrak F, Herpertz S: Treatment of depression in diabetes: an update. *Current Opinion in Psychiatry* 22:211–217, 2009

Pozzessere G, Rizzo PA, Valle E, Mollica MA, Meccia A, Morano S, Di Mario U, Andreani D, Morocutti C: Early detection of neurological involvement in IDDM and NIDDM: multimodal evoked potentials versus metabolic control. *Diabetes Care* 11:473–480, 1988

Qiu C, Cotch MF, Sigurdsson S, Klein R, Jonasson F, Klein BEK, Garcia M, Jonsson PV, Harris TB, Eiriksdottir G, Kjartansson O, van Buchem MA, Gudnason V, Launer LJ: Microvascular lesions in the brain and retina: the Age, Gene/Environment Susceptibility–Reykjavik Study. *Annals of Neurology* 65:569–576, 2009

Quirce R, Carril JM, Jiménez-Bonilla JF, Amado JA, Gutiérrez-Mendiguchía C, Banzo I, Blanco I, Uriarte I, Montero A: Semi-quantitative assessment of cerebral blood flow with 99mTc-HMPAO SPET in type 1 diabetic patients with no clinical history of cerebrovascular disease. *European Journal of Nuclear Medicine* 24:1507–1513, 1997

Reijmer YD, van den Berg E, Ruis C, Jaap Kappelle L, Biessels GJ: Cognitive dysfunction in patients with type 2 diabetes. *Diab Metab Res Re* 27:195–202, 2010

Reitz C, Tang M-X, Manly J, Mayeux R, Luchsinger JA: Hypertension and the risk of mild cognitive impairment. *Archives of Neurology* 64:1734–1740, 2007

Reske-Nielsen E, Lundbaek K, Rafaelsen OJ: Pathological changes in the central and peripheral nervous system of young long-term diabetics. *Diabetologia* 1:232–241, 1965

Reske-Nielsen E, Lundbaek K: Diabetic encephalopathy: diffuse and focal lesions of the brain in long-term diabetes. *Acta Neurologica Scandinavica* 39:273–290, 1963

Rohling ML, Faust ME, Beverly B, Demakis G: Effectiveness of cognitive rehabilitation following acquired brain injury: a meta-analytic re-examination of Cicerone et al.'s (2000, 2005) systematic reviews. *Neuropsychology* 23:20–39, 2009

Romero JR, Beiser A, Seshadri S, Benjamin EJ, Polak JF, Vasan RS, Au R, DeCarli C, Wolf PA: Carotid artery atherosclerosis, MRI indices of brain ischemia, aging, and cognitive impairment: the Framingham Study. *Stroke* 40:1590–1596, 2009

Ruis C, Biessels GJ, Gorter KJ, van den Donk M, Kappelle LJ, Rutten GEHM: Cognition in the early stage of type 2 diabetes. *Diabetes Care* 32:1261–1265, 2009

Ryan CM: Searching for the origin of brain dysfunction in diabetic children: going back to the beginning. *Pediatric Diabetes* 9:527–530, 2008

Ryan CM: Diabetes and brain damage: more (or less) than meets the eye? *Diabetologia* 49:2229–2233, 2006a

Ryan CM, Freed MI, Rood JA, Cobitz AR, Waterhouse BR, Strachan MWJ: Improving metabolic control leads to better working memory in adults with type 2 diabetes. *Diabetes Care* 29:345–351, 2006b

Ryan CM: Diabetes, aging, and cognitive decline. *Neurobiology of Aging* 26(Suppl. 1):S21–S25, 2005

Ryan CM, Geckle MO, Orchard TJ: Cognitive efficiency declines over time in adults with type 1 diabetes: effects of micro- and macrovascular complications. *Diabetologia* 46:940–948, 2003

Ryan CM, Geckle MO: Circumscribed cognitive dysfunction in middle-aged adults with type 2 diabetes. *Diabetes Care* 23:1486–1493, 2000

Sabri O, Hellwig D, Schreckenberger M, Schneider R, Kaiser H-J, Wagenknecht G, Mull M, Buell U: Influence of diabetes mellitus on regional cerebral glucose metabolism and regional cerebral blood flow. *Nuclear Medicine Communications* 21:19–29, 2000

Sabri O, Ringelstein E-B, Hellwig D, Schneider R, Schreckenberger M, Kaiser H-J, Mull M, Buell U: Neuropsychological impairment correlates with hypoperfusion and hypometabolism but not with severity of white matter lesions on MRI in patients with cerebral microangiopathy. *Stroke* 30:556–566, 1999

Saczynski JS, Jónsdóttir MK, Garcia MF, Jonsson PV, Peila R, Eiriksdottir G, Ólafsdottir E, Harris TB, Gudnason V, Launer LJ: Cognitive impairment: an increasingly important complication of type 2 diabetes: the Age, Gene/Environment Susceptibility-Reykjavik Study. *American Journal of Epidemiology* 168:1132–1139, 2008

Schott JM, Price SL, Frost C, Whitwell JL, Rossor MN, Fox NC: Measuring atrophy in Alzheimer disease: a serial MRI study over 6 and 12 months. *Neurology* 65:119–124, 2005

Seidl R, Birnbacher R, Hauser E, Gernert G, Freilinger M, Schober E: Brainstem auditory evoked potentials and visually evoked potentials in young patients with IDDM. *Diabetes Care* 19:1220–1224, 1996

Shaw J: Epidemiology of childhood type 2 diabetes and obesity. *Pediatric Diabetes* 8:7–15, 2007

Stocco A, Lebiere C, Anderson JR: Conditional routing of information to the cortex: a model of the basal ganglia's role in cognitive coordination. *Psychological Review* 117:541–574, 2010

Strachan MWJ, Reynolds RM, Frier BM, Mitchell RJ, Price JF: The relationship between type 2 diabetes and dementia. *British Medical Bulletin* 88:131–146, 2008

Strachan MWJ, Deary IJ, Ewing FME, Frier BM: Is type II diabetes associated with an increased risk of cognitive dysfunction? A critical review of published studies. *Diabetes Care* 20:438–445, 1997

Tiehuis AM, Mali WPTM, van Raamt AF, Visseren FLJ, Biessels GJ, van Zandvoort MJE, the SMART Study Group: Cognitive dysfunction and its clinical and radiological determinants in patients with symptomatic arterial disease and diabetes. *Journal of the Neurological Sciences* 283:170–174, 2009

Tiehuis AM, Vincken KL, van den Berg E, Hendrikse J, Manschot SM, Mali WPTM, Kappelle LJ, Biessels GJ: Cerebral perfusion in relation to cognitive function and type 2 diabetes. *Diabetologia* 51:1321–1326, 2008

van den Berg E, Reijmer YD, de Bresser J, Kessels RPC, Kappelle LJ, Biessels GJ, Utrecht Diabetic Encephalopathy Study Group: A 4 year follow-up study of cognitive functioning in patients with type 2 diabetes mellitus. *Diabetologia* 53:58–65, 2010

van den Berg E, Kloppenborg RP, Kessels RPC, Kappelle LJ, Biessels GJ: Type 2 diabetes mellitus, hypertension, dyslipidemia and obesity: a systematic comparison of their impact on cognition. *Biochimica et Biophysica Acta* 1792:470–481, 2009

van den Berg E, De Craen AJM, Biessels GJ, Gusselkloo J, Westendorp RGJ: The impact of diabetes mellitus on cognitive decline in the oldest old: a prospective population-based study. *Diabetologia* 49:2015–2023, 2006

van Harten B, Oosterman J, Muslimovic D, van Loon B-J, Scheltens P, Weinstein HC: Cognitive impairments and MRI correlates in the elderly patients with type 2 diabetes mellitus. *Age and Ageing* 36:164–170, 2007

van Harten B, de Leeuw F-E, Weinstein HC, Scheltens P, Biessels GJ: Brain imaging in patients with diabetes: a systematic review. *Diabetes Care* 29:2539–2548, 2006

Várkonyi TT, Petõ T, Dégi R, Keresztes K, Lengyel C, Janáky M, Kempler P, Lonovics J: Impairment of visual evoked potentials: an early central manifestation of diabetic neuropathy? *Diabetes Care* 25:1161–1162, 2002

Vázquez LA, Amado JA, Carcía-Unzueta MT, Quirce R, Jiménez-Bonilla JF, Pazos F, Pesquera C, Carril JM: Decreased plasma endothelin-1 levels in asymptomatic type 1 diabetic patients with regional cerebral hypoperfusion assessed by Spect. *Journal of Diabetes and Its Complications* 13:325–331, 1999

Verhaeghen P, Salthouse TA: Meta-analysis of age-cognition relations in adulthood: estimates of linear and nonlinear age effects and structural models. *Psychological Bulletin* 122:231–249, 1997

Virtaniemi J, Laakso M, Kärjä J, Nuutinen J, Karjalainen S: Auditory brainstem latencies in type 1 (insulin-dependent) diabetic patients. *American Journal of Otolaryngology* 14:413–418, 1993

Waldstein SR: The relation of hypertension to cognitive function. *Current Directions in Psychological Science* 12:9–12, 2003

Warren RE, Frier BM: Hypoglycaemia and cognitive function. *Diabetes, Obesity and Metabolism* 7:493–503, 2005

Watari K, Letamendi A, Elderkin-Thompson V, Haroon E, Miller J, Darwin C, Kumar A: Cognitive function in adults with type 2 diabetes and major depression. *Archives of Clinical Neuropsychology* 21:787–796, 2006

Waters F, Bucks RS: Neuropsychological effects of sleep loss: implications for neuropsychologists. *Journal of the International Neuropsychological Society* 17:571–586, 2011

Wessels AM, Scheltens P, Barkhof F, Heine RJ: Hyperglycaemia as a determinant of cognitive decline in patients with type 1 diabetes. *European Journal of Pharmacology* 585:88–96, 2008

Wessels AM, Simsek S, Remijnse PL, Veltman DJ, Biessels GJ, Barkhof F, Scheltens P, Snoek FJ, Heine RJ, Rombouts SARB: Voxel-based morphometry demonstrates reduced gray matter density on brain MRI in patients with diabetic retinopathy. *Diabetologia* 49:2474–2480, 2006

Whitmer RA, Karter AJ, Yaffe K, Quesenberry CP, Selby JV: Hypoglycemic episodes and risk of dementia in older patients with type 2 diabetes mellitus. *JAMA* 301:1565–1572, 2009

Whitmer RA: Type 2 diabetes and risk of cognitive impairment and dementia. *Current Neurology and Neuroscience Reports* 7:373–380, 2007

Winblad B, Palmer K, Kivipelto M, Jelic V, Fratiglioni L, Wahlund L-O, Nordberg A, Bäckman L, Albert M, Almkvist O, Arai H, Basun H, Blennow K, De Leon M, DeCarli C, Erkinjuntti T, Giacobini E, Graff C, Hardy J, Jack C, Jorm A, Ritchie K, van Juijn C, Visser P, Petersen RC: Mild cognitive impairment—beyond controversies, towards a consensus: report of the International Working Group on Mild Cognitive Impairment. *Journal of Internal Medicine* 256:240–246, 2004

Wong TY, Mosley TH, Klein R, Klein BEK, Sharrett AR, Couper DJ, Hubbard L, for the Atherosclerosis Risk in Communities (ARIC) Study Investigators: Retinal microvascular changes and MRI signs of cerebral atrophy in healthy, middle-aged people. *Neurology* 61:806–811, 2003

Wong TY, Klein R, Sharrett AR, Nieto FJ, Boland LL, Couper DJ, Mosley TH, Klein BEK, Hubbard LD, Szklo M: Retinal microvascular abnormalities and cognitive impairment in middle-aged persons: the Atherosclerosis Risk in Communities Study. *Stroke* 33:1487–1492, 2002

Wong TY, Klein R, Klein BEK, Tielsch JM, Hubbard L, Nieto FJ: Retinal microvascular abnormalities and their relationship with hypertension, cardiovascular disease, and mortality. *Survey of Ophthalmology* 46:59–80, 2001

Yau PL, Javier DC, Ryan CM, Tsui WH, Ardekani BA, Ten S, Convit A: Preliminary evidence for brain complications in obese adolescents with type 2 diabetes mellitus. *Diabetologia* 53:2298–2306, 2010

Zammitt NN, Frier BM: Hypoglycemia in type 2 diabetes: Pathophysiology, frequency, and effects of different treatment modalities. *Diabetes Care* 28:2948–2961, 2005

Ziegler D, Langen K-J, Herzog H, Kuwert T, Mühlen H, Feinendegen LE, Gries AF: Cerebral glucose metabolism in type 1 diabetic patients. *Diabetic Medicine* 11:205–209, 1994

Christopher M. Ryan, PhD, is Professor of Psychiatry at the University of Pittsburgh School of Medicine in Pittsburgh, PA.

Chapter 6

Assessment of Diabetes Knowledge, Self-Care Skills, and Self-Care Behaviors by Questionnaire

Garry Welch, PhD, and Sofija E. Zagarins, PhD

Diabetes is a well-documented example of a high cost, common, chronic illness where a significant quality gap exists. Despite high clinical expenditures ($174 billion in 2007), only 7% of patients are at goal for A1C, blood pressure, and blood lipids (Bojadzievski 2011), and clinicians in primary care face considerable challenges in helping their patients meet these goals. Assessing diabetes knowledge, skills, and self-care behaviors may give clinicians a means to provide more individualized diabetes care and education, but to do this clinicians require assessment batteries that are easy to administer and score in busy clinical settings, are sensitive to change, and produce results that can be directly used in clinical care (Glasgow 2005).

A substantial number of potential assessments have been identified in this review that may potentially be applied in routine care with some modification, as appropriate. The evidence suggests that many available measures may provide useful information for the interested clinician. However, substantial work remains to be done to create a standardized and coherent battery of practical measures that could be applied across a range of clinical settings and patient populations. Two emerging computerized assessment tools (i.e., the AADE7™ and DSCP, which will be described) show promise in terms of usability and early research findings, ability to leverage information technologies, and potential to be integrated into diabetes clinical information systems and care processes in a scalable fashion.

Although the patient assessment strategies reviewed here have the potential to help a wide range of patients, medically high-risk patients or those with poor clinic attendance are examples of patient subgroups that could especially benefit (Glasgow 2002, American Association of Diabetes Educators [AADE] 2007a). Issues of low health literacy, cognitive and visual limitations, cultural and motivational barriers, and patient and provider preferences are important factors to consider in planning the use of any assessments (AADE 2007a, AADE 2007b).

THE NEED FOR SYSTEMATIC AND STANDARDIZED ASSESSMENT METHODS

In the context of this discussion of patient self-management assessments in primary care settings, it is important to note that we are currently witnessing the emergence of the patient-centered medical home (PCMH) and the Accountable Care Organization (ACO) model. This PCMH/ACO approach stresses the central role of the primary care provider in coordinating all aspects of patient care (e.g., primary, specialist, hospital, home health, hospice), seamless data sharing and communication across all providers and care settings, and a focus on prevention, comprehensive care, and patient-centric care. To achieve these goals the PCMH/ACO model would foster the routine, population-based use of diabetes self-management education (DSME) in primary care and by extension the systematic and targeted use of DSME assessments, as discussed here. Scalable and practical questionnaires assessing diabetes knowledge, skills, and behaviors that are accessible across a variety of assessment channels and are configured to fit each clinic's needs and patient populations will be needed. These assessments could be accessed by secure websites, patient portals, interactive voice message services via landline phone, smartphone applications, tablet PCs, or kiosks in shared community areas such as nursing homes or community housing. In electronic rather than traditional paper and pencil format, such patient assessments could eventually fit seamlessly into electronic medical record (EMR) systems for protocol-driven action by the appropriate staff members within the clinical team and be accessible by the patient or (with approval) by caregivers or community health workers through personally controlled health records (PCHRs).

Although numerous patient self-report measures have been developed to assess diabetes knowledge, self-care skills, and self-care behaviors, it is important to note that these measures have principally been designed for diabetes research studies. Despite early expectations (Bradley 1994), they have not generally been used in clinical practice in the U.S., regardless of treatment setting. Research-focused questionnaires are designed to meet specific research goals and are often lengthy and demanding to complete in terms of required literacy/numeracy level, comprehension level, and cultural fit (Rosal 2011). Research studies also typically test behavioral theories or evaluate mechanisms and outcomes associated with behavioral, educational, or clinical interventions. By contrast, practical and relevant assessments suitable for busy diabetes providers working in primary care settings would be used to identify patients who could benefit from interventions, inform the design of interventions, or help evaluate a few key outcomes (Glasgow 2005).

To be useful in clinical care, assessments of diabetes knowledge, skills, and behaviors need to be broadly applicable, self-administrable by patients, and appropriate for a range of age, cultural, socioeconomic status (SES), and literacy groups, and they need to have reasonable reliability and validity, particularly around responsiveness to change (Glasgow 2005, Boren 2009, Rosal 2011). Despite their research heritage, many currently available patient self-report assessments of knowledge, skills, and behaviors have potential as brief clinical tools that could enhance the tailoring (and thus likely success) of diabetes treatment planning by primary care providers (AADE 2007a, AADE 2007b).

USE OF CLINICAL ASSESSMENT TOOLS

Much of the diabetes treatment plan is carried out by the patient on a daily basis, while the face-to-face time spent with the health care team represents only a brief and episodic window of engagement (Anderson 2000). Thus, a profile of each patient's diabetes knowledge, self-management skills, and recent pattern of daily self-management behaviors obtained between clinic visits could help providers tailor DSME efforts and generate a more accurate picture of the patient's preferences, needs, and self-management barriers. Effective use of these assessments could further enhance clinical care by increasing patient engagement and participation in care planning because the obtained information is of likely importance to the patient. When combined with effective communication, this patient profile can foster collaborative goal setting and identification of specific barriers to self-management, encourage direct problem-solving training, and support the planning and implementation of treatment and follow-up (Anderson 2000, Mulcahy 2003, Hill-Briggs 2011).

Before outlining currently available assessment tools for potential adoption by diabetes providers, it is important to discuss the range of existing practical barriers to the routine use of patient assessments in clinical care, as these structural and logistical issues will need to be addressed if wider acceptance of such assessments is to occur. These barriers include: the lack of accreditation and regulatory imperatives for providers to conduct assessments of knowledge, skills, and behaviors (i.e., such assessments are not generally mandated or recommended by recognized organizations or authorities); lack of financial incentives for clinic administrators and providers to conduct assessments; lack of professional training regarding these constructs, their assessment, and their clinical application; and the presence of practical barriers to a clinically integrated assessment program (e.g., need for additional support staff, integration of assessments and data generated into existing clinical databases and electronic medical records, standardization of interpretation and practical use of assessment findings, and alignment with individual clinical staff goals and annual performance metrics).

A further barrier to routine assessments of diabetes knowledge, skills, and behaviors in primary-care settings is the reality that there is a paucity of practical assessment tools, supporting materials, and training programs to help clinicians interpret and use the findings of these assessments. Although repositories of paper-based measures salient to this discussion exist on the Internet (e.g., Resource Centers for Minority Aging Research, Quality of Life Instruments Database [QOLID], Robert Wood Johnson Diabetes Initiative, Michigan and Vanderbilt Diabetes Research Training Centers, Diabetes HealthSense), they may be difficult to access or not routinely updated. Some potentially useful questionnaires can be located only through a systematic literature search followed by informal professional networking (e.g., Behavioral Research In Diabetes Group Exchange [BRIDGE], Society of Behavioral Medicine Diabetes Special Interest Group, American Diabetes Association Interest Group on Behavioral Medicine & Psychology).

Despite these caveats regarding the feasibility of conducting patient assessments in busy clinical settings in the U.S., there are practical strategies available for "adopters" who would like to improve the clinical care of specific patients (e.g., those who are in poor blood metabolic control or who are regular and costly "no shows"); alternatively, these assessments could be incorporated into annual diabetes check-up procedures for all diabetes patients. The latter strategy was used in the large-scale, multinational Monitoring of Individual Needs in Diabetes (MIND) program focusing on quality of life and diabetes (Snoek 2011). MIND provides a free, standardized, and brief CD-ROM assessment battery of diabetes practices that can be incorporated into annual clinical review visits and used to promote patient-centered care.

Assessment of Knowledge, Skills, and Self-Care Behaviors

Many assessments of diabetes knowledge, skills, and self-care behaviors are available, and a discussion of a selection of these follows. This discussion is not based on a systematic database search, so it is not an exhaustive representation of all available tools but rather focuses on a range of common or promising published assessments that have been applied in clinical settings.

The following questionnaires are currently provided in pencil-and-paper versions and could be used in individual visits or group settings. Internet and interactive voice recognition systems are currently being developed for some of these questionnaires to simplify data collection, scoring, and interpretation and enable the assessments to be integrated into routine clinical processes (Jackson 2006, Welch 2006).

Diabetes Knowledge

There are many unpublished and informal diabetes knowledge questionnaires used by individual diabetes education services or specialty medical clinics in the U.S. Though relatively few of these questionnaires have been subjected to empirical scrutiny or published in peer-reviewed journals, there are several available published knowledge assessment tests that have been applied in clinical research studies:

The Diabetes Knowledge Test (DKT). The DKT consists of 23 knowledge questions that provide a test of a patient's general knowledge of diabetes (Fitzgerald 1998). Although the first 14 items are appropriate only for people who do not use insulin, all 23 items can be administered to people who do use insulin. The DKT is scored as the percentage of correct answers, with higher scores indicating greater diabetes knowledge. The DKT content is based on expert opinion and was tested using U.S. community–based patients with type 1 and type 2 diabetes. Empirical findings included sound reliability, positive correlation with A1C, adequate difficulty level (i.e., the percentage of patients who scored each item correctly was not overly high or low), an ability to discriminate groups of differing treatment intensity and exposure to diabetes education, and responsiveness to change after diabetes education programs. These findings suggest that the DKT may be clinically useful and potentially appropriate for a variety of clinical settings and patient populations.

Audit of Diabetes (ADKnowl). The ADKnowl (Bradley 1994) has been recently updated (2009) and is a 138-item measure of diabetes-related knowledge that has been used to identify the nature and extent of both diabetes patient and health professional knowledge deficits (Khamis 2004, Quackenbush 2005). Content validity is based on clinical consensus and ongoing review process among a range of diabetes specialists. ADKnowl responsiveness to change has been supported in both a clinical trial of insulin dose adjustment skills training (Dose Adjustment for Normal Eating [DAFNE] Study Group 2002) and a video-based lifestyle education program for people newly diagnosed with type 2 diabetes (Dyson 2010). Though the ADKnowl is lengthy, specific items and components could be appropriately used in clinical settings. The components include: diabetes treatment and testing, sick day management, insulin use, hypoglycemia management, physical activity, diet and food, alcohol, complications reduction, smoking cessation, foot care, and blood glucose levels.

Diabetes Knowledge Scales (DKN A, B, and C). The DKN Scales (Beeney 1994) consist of three equivalent 15-item questionnaires (A, B, and C) that were developed for use with type 1 and type 2 diabetes patients in settings where general diabetes knowledge needed to be assessed quickly, reliably, and repeatedly. The DKN questionnaires were developed by researchers in Australia using an expert opinion panel and literature review and have been used in diabetes education research studies. Three parallel forms were created to allow for repeated measurements and to eliminate minimal recall bias as a result of using the same form on repeat occasions. The DKN items cover basic physiology and insulin action, hypoglycemia, food groups and substitutions, sick day management, and general diabetes care. The DKN score range is from 0 to 100 with higher scores indicating greater diabetes knowledge. Reliability of the DKN scales is sound and showed responsiveness to change when administered before and after intensive education programs. Findings suggested that the DKN scales are clinically useful, although the original items may require updating and review of specific local (Australian) wording used.

The Diabetes and Cardiovascular Disease Test (DCDT). This 14-item questionnaire assesses awareness of risk for cardiovascular disease in people with diabetes. Items include awareness assessment of "good" and "bad" cholesterol; clinical targets for fasting blood glucose, blood pressure, and low-density lipoprotein (LDL) and high-density lipoprotein (HDL) cholesterol; and knowledge of self-monitoring of blood glucose (SMBG), nutrition, and physical activity. The assessment reflects our more recent awareness that blood glucose, blood pressure, and blood lipids are critical control factors in diabetes complications progression. The DCDT has been used in several studies, including an evaluation of problem solving for diabetes self-management in which knowledge scores improved significantly following condensed and intense education interventions (Hill-Briggs 2008a, Hill-Briggs 2011). Thus, this brief scale may be useful for clinicians wishing to focus on cardiovascular risk reduction among their diabetes patients.

Other Knowledge Questionnaires. Other more specific diabetes knowledge questionnaires that show promise for clinical applications have been developed. For example, the AdultCarbQuiz (Watts 2011) is a 43-item questionnaire that assesses six domains of patient carbohydrate counting knowledge: recognition, counting carbohydrates in single foods, food labels, glycemic targets, preventing and managing hypoglycemia, and counting carbohydrates in meals. The AdultCarbQuiz has demonstrated encouraging discriminant- and criterion-related validity. For example, patients' scores on the AdultCarbQuiz correlated significantly with matched evaluations of patient carbohydrate counting knowledge obtained from registered dietitians.

Most diabetes knowledge assessments are used based on their face validity and reflect local clinical consensus. Generally, diabetes knowledge measurement poses challenges because the questions comprising a given assessment tool may not match the particular educational content provided by the practice or individual educators, or the questions become outdated as the DSME practices or evidence base changes. An evaluation should be conducted first to establish that there is good questionnaire content match for its use in any given setting. Also, patient literacy, language preference, and visual and cognitive deficits should be considered if patient assistance is not available during the assessment process. Currently, diabetes knowledge questionnaires have not been linked to changes in clinical outcomes.

Diabetes Self-Care Skills

Problem solving. Diabetes requires a high level of daily patient engagement and active decision making if the treatment regimen is to be effective. In particular, the patient must learn a variety of self-care skills to effectively carry out the diabetes treatment plan. Specific skills may include effective problem solving to overcome self-management barriers, daily stress management, planning and adaptive coping, and obtaining social support from others. Problem solving skills in particular are critical for effective diabetes self-management but are difficult to teach and challenging for patients to acquire (Schumann 2011). Problem solving has been defined as "a series of cognitive operations used to figure out what to do when the way to reach a goal is not apparent" (Stetson 2010, Schumann 2011). It is mostly taught as a component of a multifaceted DSME intervention but has also been applied as a stand-alone strategy (Schumann 2011). It typically focuses on a sequence of problem awareness, barrier identification, solution generation, implementation planning, implementation, outcome evaluation, and revisiting of the barriers. A recent review found a range of methodological weaknesses in problem-solving intervention studies to date. However, several measures were identified that can be used to assess problem-solving skills, including the Diabetes Problem-Solving Inventory (Glasgow 2004), the Diabetes Problem Solving Scale (Hill-Briggs 2007), and the Health Problem Solving Scale (Hill-Briggs 2008b). These scales have shown some evidence of internal reliability, construct validity, and responsiveness that suggest they may be useful tools in clinical practice.

Self-efficacy. Having a strong perception of diabetes self-efficacy is another key characteristic of effective diabetes self-management that is amenable to strengthening through clinician influence and DSME. Self-efficacy is derived from Bandura's social cognitive theory (SCT) and provides a link between self-perceptions and specific behaviors. Bandura described self-efficacy as a cognitive process involving judgment of one's ability to perform specific behaviors required to produce certain outcomes. The individual's confidence in their ability to perform a task determines those behaviors that they will engage in, how long they persist, and the amount of effort they will expend to achieve their goals (Hurley 1992, Hill-Briggs 2008b). From a practical and theoretical perspective, there are four important sources of information for increasing patient self-efficacy for a specific behavior: performance accomplishments (mastery), vicarious learning (modeling from peers), verbal persuasion, and self-appraisal of emotional and physiological responses. These can be assessed systematically and used to structure patient education and behavior change strategies provided to the patient. A recent review identified a proliferation (i.e., >10) of diabetes self-efficacy measures

(Frei 2009), and many others have been reported, including those that are modifications of earlier scales. Frei et al. (2009) identified significant weaknesses in approach and methodology seen in the development of many of these scales. Moreover, there is an overall lack of clarity concerning the purpose of the assessments and their relationship to SCT. They also differ widely in item content and test characteristics, length, global versus multidimensional focus, and level of evidence for reliability and validity, particularly responsiveness. Despite these concerns, some available self-efficacy scales (Van der Ven 2003, Sarkar 2005) could help to identify patients with low levels of confidence regarding specific self-management tasks under review and to track patient progress over time.

Diabetes Self-Care Behaviors

Assessments of self-care behaviors have been a consistent focus of the diabetes research literature. Typically SMBG, diet, exercise, and medication adherence are the key diabetes self-care activities assessed in patient self-management questionnaires. Other included assessments may relate to cardiovascular risk reduction (e.g., aspirin use and smoking cessation) and/or recommended screenings for feet, eyes, and kidneys. Available published measures to assess diabetes self-care behaviors include the following:

The Summary of Diabetes Self Care Activities (SDSCA). The SDSCA is a brief self-report questionnaire of diabetes self-management behaviors that assesses general diet, specific diet, exercise, blood-glucose testing, foot care, and smoking. The questions focus on patient perceptions of frequency or percentage of time that recommended self-care behaviors were followed over the previous week. Adequate reliability, correlations as expected between the SDSCA subscales and a range of criterion measures, and sensitivity-to-change scores from seven reviewed studies showed that the SDSCA is a brief yet reliable and valid self-report questionnaire of diabetes self-management that is useful for clinical practice (Glasgow 2003).

The Self-Care Inventory-Revised (SCI-R). Like the SDSCA, the SCI-R was also designed for self-care behavior assessment in busy clinical practices and research (Weinger 2005). It is a measure of perceived adherence to diabetes self-care recommendations and is administered to the patient by the provider. Empirical studies have shown it to be adequately reliable and to demonstrate evidence of validity based on its correlations with measures of diabetes-related distress, self-esteem, self-efficacy, depression, anxiety, and blood glucose control (A1C). It has also shown good responsiveness to change based on its use with a range of diabetes educational interventions. There is support, therefore, for the SCI-R as a brief, reliable, and valid measure of patients' own perceptions of their adherence to recommended diabetes self-care behaviors.

TECHNOLOGY-BASED ASSESSMENTS OF KNOWLEDGE, SKILLS, AND BEHAVIORS

Several CD-ROM, Internet, and telephone-based self-care behavior and barriers assessment tools have been developed and published (Piette 2001, Welch 2002, Glasgow 2003, AADE 2008, Quinn 2008, Quinn 2009, Welch 2009). Although some of these are in early stages of development and do not have outcomes data available (AADE 2008, Quinn 2009), others have been associated with significant improvements in A1C (Piette 2001, Quinn 2008, Welch 2009).

Two of these assessments are currently available for dissemination to health care providers and will be discussed in more detail (AADE 2008, Welch 2009). These assessments are both embedded in broader diabetes self-management education care systems, but they are also useful as stand-alone tools to provide clinicians and other care providers with a tailored profile of patient goals, skills, and barriers.

The American Association of Diabetes Educators' AADE7™ Self-Care Behaviors Tool

The National Diabetes Education Outcomes System (NDEOS) was developed by the AADE to improve diabetes education and outcomes tracking (Peeples 2001). This system and its components, including the original Diabetes Self-Management Assessment Report Tool (D-SMART), have been incorporated into the development of the AADE7™ Self-Care Behaviors tool, which provides a conceptual framework for standardized diabetes self-management training.

The AADE7™ framework provides a structured format for patient diabetes education and care and provides information about seven targeted diabetes self-care behaviors (i.e., physical activity, healthy eating, medication, blood glucose monitoring, problem solving, risk reduction activities, and psychosocial adaptation) (AADE 2008). The AADE7™ System measurement tools include the original D-SMART, which is a more comprehensive tool than the SDSCA and the SCI-R questionnaires in that it not only assesses behaviors but also assesses patient behavior change intentions and barriers to self-care. It is used to guide the development of the clinical plan and to focus on areas that are important to the patient, thus potentially enhancing patient engagement in treatment as well as motivation for behavior change. It is designed to be used in a wide range of clinical settings and for repeated patient measurements to assess change over time. The Diabetes Educator Tool (D-ET) is also included in the AADE7™ Self-Care Behaviors tool and is a complementary educator-completed tool that is designed to document patient knowledge, skills, confidence, and barriers.

Although the AADE7™ Self-Care Behaviors tool is still in an early phase of evaluation, some preliminary research has been done with the D-SMART. The D-SMART has been functionally integrated in a recent study into computer and telephonic systems at five diabetes self-management programs to test its feasibility and patient acceptability (Charron-Prochownik 2007). A process evaluation was conducted involving diabetes patients who completed the questions at home by telephone or computer. The development of automated technologies to implement the D-SMART assessment strengthens its clinical potential, as questionnaire assessments are typically difficult to complete at the point of care because of professional time, space, and resource constraints. Results of the D-SMART study showed that 76% of patients felt the questions were easy to understand, and only 12% needed assistance to complete the questions. Overall, the D-SMART was reported to be easily completed at home in a single attempt, and patients were generally satisfied with the wording of the questions, the selection of answers, and its ease of use.

A second analysis of both the D-SMART and D-ET was conducted in which the AADE7™ Outcome System was integrated into web-based, touch screen, and telephone-based systems at eight different diabetes self-management programs (Zgibor 2007). Of 954 patients with diabetes who were included in the study, 527 patients identified goals that were also recommended by their diabetes educator, including healthy eating (94%), being active (59%), and glucose monitoring (49%).

Computer-based and telephonic D-SMART versions thus appear to be feasible assessment methods for use in clinical practice. These findings suggest that the D-SMART has good face validity based on its careful development by an expert panel, is acceptable and feasible to patients, and has the advantage of being available in automated formats that may overcome barriers to assessment faced by the SDSCA and SCI-R pencil-and-paper assessment tools. Also, its integration within the AADE7™ Self-Care Behaviors tool and its link with a clinical site registration form suggest that over time the D-SMART has considerable potential to consistently measure diabetes care and outcomes in a variety of clinical settings.

The Diabetes Self-Care Profile (DSCP)

The DSCP is part of the Comprehensive Diabetes Management Program (CDMP), an interactive, web-based, diabetes management tool based on American Diabetes Association (ADA) practice guidelines (ADA 2011, Welch 2011). The CDMP focuses on clinical management, lifestyle modification, and psychosocial health, and it provides chronic care managers with a set of clinical and behavioral alerts that guide treatment decisions and structure the medical care and diabetes education plan (Fonda 2008, Welch 2011).

The DSCP, formerly called the Accu-Chek Interview in a CD-ROM version, is a web-based patient assessment tool designed to support provider-patient communication and assist patients and providers in working together to improve the patient's blood glucose control and quality of life (Fisher 2006, Barnard 2007, Welch 2009, Welch 2011). The DSCP identifies current self-care behaviors and psychosocial problems that can undermine diabetes self-care and elevate blood glucose levels and gives the patient visual feedback on A1C, blood pressure, and blood lipid control. The goal of the DSCP is to capture key patient self-management information in a systematic, brief, and user-friendly manner. This approach allows the diabetes educator to spend less time assessing DSME needs and potentially more time developing rapport with the patient and providing diabetes education and skills training based on the patient's needs and interests.

The DSCP assesses diet, exercise, medication, and physical activity behaviors that impact blood glucose control, highlighting one of these behaviors selected by the patient for discussion. In addition, the DSCP assesses attitudes and barriers to commencing insulin therapy (if on oral agents only) and documents psychosocial problems that can impede optimal self-management, including depression, diabetes distress, hypoglycemia, low social support, binge eating, alcohol abuse, and negative attitudes toward insulin therapy. When the patient has completed the DSCP assessment, a one-page report identifying the patient's current self-care problems and issues is generated for printout. This report can therefore help focus the conversation between the patient and clinician about potential behavior change areas and strategies for making those changes.

An analysis of the original Accu-Chek Interview system (the precursor of the current DSCP web tool) found that patients who completed the assessments prior to an outpatient consultation with a health care professional were more engaged during the consultation (Barnard 2007). These patients asked twice as many questions during the consultation ($P < 0.01$), and over half of patients completing the Accu-Chek Interview assessment reported that it had positive benefits for their consultation.

In a pre–post analysis of 59 patients with type 2 diabetes, all patients completed the DSCP at baseline and following a four-session, six-month diabetes education intervention (Welch 2009). Of the four self-care topics included in the DSCP, meal plan was selected as the top priority for the majority of patients (76.3%), and low social support (49.2%), depression (42.4%), and emotional distress (42.9%) were selected as the major life challenges. A1C improved significantly over the course of the six months when the DSCP was applied in DSME (mean difference: $-1 \pm 1.3\%$, $P < 0.01$). Overall, these early findings suggest the DSCP has considerable potential to focus diabetes care on modifiable diabetes-specific issues and regimen behaviors that are known to affect glycemic control.

SUMMARY

Our U.S. health care delivery system is currently incentivized through its system of fee-for-service, billing codes, and reimbursement schedules to focus on acute medical problems or the provision of specialty or heroic care for late-stage or complex medical conditions. Often these efforts are needed for the management of chronic disease–related medical complications that could have been prevented. There is a weak current focus in our health care system on the critical preventive aspects of medical care including the provision of comprehensive, patient-centric self-management support for individuals with chronic conditions such as diabetes. Comprehensive hospital-based diabetes programs that support local primary care clinics often face an ongoing struggle to generate sufficient revenue to meet program overheads and are subject to budget cuts and staffing adjustments that stress clinically effective programs. The fruits of meaningful system-wide reform to improve patient self-management support for patients seen in primary care with diabetes and other chronic conditions will include improved patient access and satisfaction with care, enhanced care quality and clinical outcomes, and reduced total health care costs.

Assessing diabetes knowledge, skills, and self-care behaviors as discussed in this chapter may provide clinicians a means to provide more individualized diabetes care and education in a busy clinical setting. Although there has been a notable expansion in the number, type, and quality of measures assessing diabetes knowledge, skills, and self-care behaviors after the major review of diabetes questionnaires conducted in 1994 (Bradley 1994), it is interesting that we have witnessed little or no subsequent adoption of these measures into clinical practice. Despite this lack of adoption, the emergence of the PCMH/ACO model of medical care holds great promise to foster a more comprehensive, patient-centered care model for diabetes that would logically include more effective patient self-management education and support (Bojadzievski 2011) and stimulate wider use of patient DSME and its assessments. Support of the national diabetes research and care community for initiatives such as the emergent PCMH/ACO model and its diabetes pilot demonstration projects and National Committee for Quality Assurance (NCQA) certification program currently underway across the U.S. may increase the use of research-based patient assessments discussed in this chapter.

A variety of research-based diabetes measures currently exist that could potentially be applied to clinical practice. However, more study is needed to determine their ability to fit into primary care practice. Specifically, they must be broadly applicable, self-administered by patients, appropriate for a range of age, cultural, SES, and literacy groups, and have reasonable reliability and validity, particularly around responsiveness to change (Glasgow 2005).

There is a lack of coherence and standardization among available measures of diabetes knowledge, skills, and behaviors that hampers systematic progress in the field both in terms of research insights and effective clinical practice. There has been little national consensus around key psychometric, theoretical, and practical issues, including agreement on "best-in-class assessments."

RECOMMENDATIONS FOR CLINICAL CARE

In summary, several recommendations are offered regarding the use of assessments of knowledge, skills, and behaviors in current diabetes clinical practice:

1. Where knowledge is an issue, formal instruments should be used for assessment. Brief knowledge measures are available to obtain a qualitative assessment of a patient's knowledge level, and longer measures are available to obtain relatively detailed and comprehensive assessments of knowledge. These instruments can guide a detailed assessment of specific knowledge gaps and educational efforts.
2. Assessment of self-care skills should be used when self-care behaviors and outcomes are less than optimal. Instruments to assess factors such as problem-solving skills, health literacy, and self-efficacy may be superior to unsystematic assessments by clinicians.
3. Assessment of patient self-care behaviors is the key to identifying self-care gaps, and assessment tools should be used when clinicians do not have the time to perform a comprehensive, detailed assessment of these behaviors.
4. Electronic systems for obtaining and storing patient self-care assessments are available and can be used to reduce provider burden while enhancing the tracking of self-care over time.

BIBLIOGRAPHY

American Association of Diabetes Educators (AADE): AADE7™ Self-Care Behaviors. *Diabetes Educ* 34:445–449, 2008

American Association of Diabetes Educators: AADE position statement: cultural sensitivity and diabetes education: recommendations for diabetes educators. *Diabetes Educ* 33:41–44, 2007a

American Association of Diabetes Educators: AADE position statement: individualization of diabetes self management education. *Diabetes Educ* 33:45–49, 2007b

American Diabetes Association: Executive summary: standards of medical care in diabetes—2011. *Diabetes Care* 34 (Suppl. 1):S4–S10, 2011

Anderson RM, Funnell MM: *The Art of Empowerment: Stories and Strategies for Diabetes Educators.* Alexandria, VA, American Diabetes Association, 2000

Barnard KD, Cradock S, Parkin T, Skinner TC: Effectiveness of a computerised assessment tool to prompt individuals with diabetes to be more active in consultations. *Pract Int Diab* 24:36–41, 2007

Beeney LJ, Dunn SM, Welch GW: Measurement of diabetes knowledge: the development of the DKN scales. In *Handbook of Psychology and Diabetes: A Guide to Psychological Measurement in Diabetes Research and Practice.* Bradley C, Ed. London, Harwood Academic Publishers, 1994, p. 159–190

Bojadzievski T, Gabbay RA: Patient-centered medical home and diabetes. *Diabetes Care* 34:1047–1053, 2011

Boren SA: A review of health literacy and diabetes: opportunities for technology. *J Diabetes Sci Technol* 3:202–209, 2009

Bradley C: *Handbook of Psychology and Diabetes: A Guide to Psychological Measurement in Diabetes Research and Practice.* 1st ed. Chur, Switzerland, Harwood Academic Publishers, 1994

Charron-Prochownik D, Zgibor JC, Peyrot M, Peeples M, McWilliams J, Koshinsky J, et al.: The diabetes self-management assessment report tool (D-SMART): process evaluation and patient satisfaction. *Diabetes Educ* 33:833–838, 2007

Dose Adjustment For Normal Eating (DAFNE) Study Group: Training in flexible, intensive insulin management to enable dietary freedom in people with type 1 diabetes: dose adjustment for normal eating (DAFNE) randomised controlled trial. *BMJ* 325:746, 2002

Dyson PA, Beatty S, Matthews DR: An assessment of lifestyle video education for people newly diagnosed with type 2 diabetes. *J Hum Nutr Diet* 23:353–359, 2010

Fisher KL: Assessing psychosocial variables: a tool for diabetes educators. *Diabetes Educ* 32:51–58, 2006

Fitzgerald JT, Funnell MM, Hess GE, Barr PA, Anderson RM, Hiss RG, Davis WK: The reliability and validity of a brief diabetes knowledge test. *Diabetes Care* 21:706–710, 1998

Fonda SJ, Paulsen CA, Perkins J, Kedziora RJ, Rodbard D, Bursell SE: Usability test of an internet-based informatics tool for diabetes care providers: the comprehensive diabetes management program. *Diabetes Technol Ther* 10:16–24, 2008

Frei A, Svarin A, Steurer-Stey C, Puhan MA: Self-efficacy instruments for patients with chronic diseases suffer from methodological limitations: a systematic review. *Health Qual Life Outcomes* 7:86, 2009

Glasgow RE, Ory MG, Klesges LM, Cifuentes M, Fernald DH, Green LA: Practical and relevant self-report measures of patient health behaviors for primary care research. *Ann Fam Med* 3:73–81, 2005

Glasgow RE, Toobert DJ, Barrera M Jr, Strycker LA: Assessment of problem-solving: a key to successful diabetes self-management. *J Behav Med* 27:477–490, 2004

Glasgow RE, Boles SM, McKay HG, Feil EG, Barrera M Jr: The D-Net diabetes self-management program: long-term implementation, outcomes, and generalization results. *Prev Med* 36:410–419, 2003

Glasgow RE, Toobert DJ, Hampson SE, Strycker LA: Implementation, generalization and long-term results of the "choosing well" diabetes self-management intervention. *Patient Educ Couns* 48:115–122, 2002

Hill-Briggs F, Lazo M, Peyrot M, Doswell A, Chang YT, Hill MN, et al.: Effect of problem-solving-based diabetes self-management training on diabetes control in a low income patient sample. *J Gen Intern Med* 26:972–978, 2011

Hill-Briggs F, Lazo M, Renosky R, Ewing C: Usability of a diabetes and cardiovascular education module in an African American, diabetic sample with physical, visual, and cognitive impairment. *Rehab Psychol* 53:1–8, 2008a

Hill-Briggs F, Smith AS: Evaluation of diabetes and cardiovascular disease print patient education materials for use with low-health literate populations. *Diabetes Care* 31:667–671, 2008b

Hill-Briggs F, Gemmell L, Kulkarni B, Klick B, Brancati FL: Associations of patient health-related problem solving with disease control, emergency department visits, and hospitalizations in HIV and diabetes clinic samples. *J Gen Intern Med* 22:649–654, 2007

Hurley AC, Shea CA: Self-efficacy: strategy for enhancing diabetes self-care. *Diabetes Educ* 18:146–150, 1992

Jackson CL, Bolen S, Brancati FL, Batts-Turner ML, Gary TL: A systematic review of interactive computer-assisted technology in diabetes care: interactive information technology in diabetes care. *J Gen Intern Med* 21:105–110, 2006

Khamis A, Hoashi S, Duffy SG, Forde R, Vizzard N, Keenan P, et al.: Diabetes knowledge deficits in adolescents and young adults with type 1 diabetes mellitus. *Endocrine Abstracts* 7:P71, 2004

Martin C, Daly A, McWhorter LS, Shwide-Slavin C, Kushion W, American Association of Diabetes Educators: The scope of practice, standards of practice, and standards of professional performance for diabetes educators. *Diabetes Educ* 31:487–488, 490, 492 passim, 2005

Mulcahy K, Maryniuk M, Peeples M, Peyrot M, Tomky D, Weaver T, Yarborough P: Diabetes self-management education core outcomes measures. *Diabetes Educ* 29:768–770, 773–784, 787–788 passim, 2003

Peeples M, Mulcahy K, Tomky D, Weaver T, National Diabetes Education Outcomes System (NDEOS): The conceptual framework of the National Diabetes Education Outcomes System (NDEOS). *Diabetes Educ* 27:547–562, 2001

Piette JD, Weinberger M, Kraemer FB, McPhee SJ: Impact of automated calls with nurse follow-up on diabetes treatment outcomes in a Department of Veterans Affairs health care system: a randomized controlled trial. *Diabetes Care* 24:202–208, 2001

Quackenbush PA: Physiologic and psychosocial stage-based differences for dietary fat consumption in women with type 2 diabetes. Texas Medical Center Dissertations (via ProQuest), 2005

Quinn CC, Gruber-Baldini AL, Shardell M, Weed K, Clough SS, Peeples M, et al.: Mobile diabetes intervention study: testing a personalized treatment/ behavioral communication intervention for blood glucose control. *Contemp Clin Trials* 30:334–346, 2009

Quinn CC, Clough SS, Minor JM, Lender D, Okafor MC, Gruber-Baldini A: WellDoc mobile diabetes management randomized controlled trial: change in clinical and behavioral outcomes and patient and physician satisfaction. *Diabetes Technol Ther* 10:160–168, 2008

Rosal MC, Ockene IS, Restrepo A, White MJ, Borg A, Olendzki B, et al.: Randomized trial of a literacy-sensitive, culturally tailored diabetes self-management intervention for low-income Latinos: Latinos en Control. *Diabetes Care* 34:838–844, 2011

Sarkar U, Fisher L, Schillinger D: Is self-efficacy associated with diabetes self-management across race/ethnicity and health literacy? *Diabetes Care* 29:823–829, 2005

Schumann KP, Sutherland JA, Majid HM, Hill-Briggs F: Evidence-based behavioral treatments for diabetes: problem-solving therapy. *Diabetes Spectrum* 24:64–69, 2011

Snoek FJ, Kersch NY, Eldrup E, Harman-Boehm I, Hermanns N, Kokoszka A, et al.: Monitoring of Individual Needs in Diabetes (MIND): baseline data from the Cross-National Diabetes Attitudes, Wishes, and Needs (DAWN) MIND study. *Diabetes Care* 34:601–603, 2011

Stetson B, Boren S, Leventhal H, Schlundt D, Glasgow R, Fisher EB, et al.: Embracing the evidence on problem solving in diabetes self management education and support. *Self Care* 1:83–99, 2010

Van der Ven NCW, Ader H, Weinger K, Van der Ploeg HM, Yi J, Pouwer F, Snoek FJ: The confidence in diabetes self-care scale: psychometric properties or a new measure of diabetes-specific self-efficacy in Dutch and US patients with type 1 diabetes. *Diabetes Care* 26:713–718, 2003

Watts SA, Anselmo JM, Ker E: Validating the AdultCarbQuiz: a test of carbohydrate counting knowledge for adults with diabetes. *Diabetes Spectrum* 24:154–160, 2011

Weinger K, Butler HA, Welch GW, La Greca AM: Measuring diabetes self-care: a psychometric analysis of the Self-Care Inventory-Revised with adults. *Diabetes Care* 28:1346–1352, 2005

Welch G, Allen NA, Zagarins SE, Stamp KD, Bursell SE, Kedziora RJ: Comprehensive diabetes management program for poorly controlled Hispanic type 2 patients at a community health center. *Diabetes Educ* 37:680–688, 2011

Welch G, Shayne R, Zagarins S, Garb J: A web-based self-management assessment tool that improves HbA1c. *J Diab Nursing* 13:319, 2009

Welch G, Shayne R: Interactive behavioral technologies and diabetes self-management support: recent research findings from clinical trials. *Curr Diab Rep* 6:130–136, 2006

Welch GW, Guthrie DW: Supporting lifestyle change with a computerized psychosocial assessment tool. *Diabetes Spectrum* 15:203–207, 2002

Zgibor JC, Peyrot M, Ruppert K, Noullet W, Siminerio LM, Peeples M, et al.: Using the American Association of Diabetes Educators Outcomes System to identify patient behavior change goals and diabetes educator responses. *Diabetes Educ* 33:839–842, 2007

Garry Welch, PhD, is Director of Behavioral Medicine Research at Baystate Medical Center in Springfield, MA, and Research Associate Professor at Tufts University School of Medicine in Boston, MA.

Sofija E. Zagarins, PhD, is a Postdoctoral Research Fellow in the Department of Behavioral Medicine Research at Baystate Medical Center in Springfield, MA, and a Visiting Assistant Professor in the Department of Public Health at the University of Massachusetts, Amherst, MA.

Chapter 7
Adherence to Medical Regimens

SUZANNE BENNETT JOHNSON, PHD

DEFINING ADHERENCE

More than 30 years ago, Haynes (1979) defined medical regimen compliance as "the extent to which a person's behavior (in terms of taking medications, following diets, or executing lifestyle changes) coincides with medical advice." This definition remains useful today (World Health Organization 2003) although the term "compliance" has fallen out of favor because it connotes passive patient acceptance of provider recommendations. The term "adherence" is now more commonly used, providing recognition of the patient's active role in accepting the provider's recommendations. Failure to follow medical advice can be a purposeful act in which the patient knowingly refuses the medical advice (willful or volitional or intentional nonadherence) or it can result despite the patient's effort to follow medical advice (inadvertent, accidental, or unintentional nonadherence). Inadvertent nonadherence may be a product of a patient's failure to understand the medical advice and/or lack of the necessary skills to carry out the medical advice correctly (e.g., draws up insulin incorrectly, has poor insulin injection technique), forgetting, or inability to overcome barriers to implementing tasks that are within the patient's competence (Johnson 1992). Over 25 years ago, Glasgow et al. (1985) argued that since diabetes is essentially a patient-managed disease, "diabetes self-management behavior" is a better way to refer to diabetes management tasks that are patient controlled. "Self-management" is now accepted terminology with National Standards for Diabetes Self-Management Education (Funnell 2011).

PREVALENCE OF NONADHERENCE

Diabetes is a complex and costly disease to manage, and patient difficulties adhering to the daily medication, blood glucose testing, diet, and exercise recommendations are common (Cramer 2004, Lerman 2005, Odegard 2007, Patton 2011). In the U.S., over $116 billion were spent on the medical care of patients with diabetes in 2007; these costs are escalating with one in three Americans born today expected to develop diabetes in their lifetime (Herman 2011). Costs appear to be higher for those who fail to adhere to their diabetes care regimen (Balkrishnan 2003, Breitscheidel 2010).

Prevalence studies typically do not distinguish between willful and inadvertent nonadherence. However, there is substantial literature showing that poor comprehension or recall of the treatment regimen and lack of the necessary skills to carry out the regimen correctly are substantial components of the problem. Multiple studies indicate that patients often fail to understand or accurately recall provider recommendations (Page 1981, Heisler 2005, Rubin 2005), fail to administer medications or conduct glucose tests accurately (Johnson 1982, Harkavy 1983, Newman 1994, Thompson 1995, Perwien 2000, Alto 2002), fail to understand the meaning of a "healthy diet," or lack the skills to count carbohydrates correctly (Patton 2011). Children and the elderly are particularly likely to exhibit skill deficits. Children often lack the cognitive maturity and dexterity to carry out complex disease management tasks (Silverstein 2005). The elderly may have visual problems or cognitive deficits that interfere with their diabetes self-care (Cooke 2001, Messier 2005, Reijmer 2010).

A variety of other factors have been associated with poor diabetes regimen adherence: higher medication copayments or cost sharing, increased treatment complexity, elevated patient depression, and adolescence have been most consistently associated with less than ideal diabetes self-care (Cramer 2004, Lerman 2005, Wysocki 2006, Goldman 2007, Odegard 2007). Other factors linked to poor adherence include low socioeconomic status, low health literacy, family conflict or lack of family support, inordinate child responsibility for treatment tasks, and concerns about hypoglycemia (Lerman 2005, Fu 2009, Peeters 2011).

ADHERENCE AND GLYCEMIC CONTROL

Although better diabetes regimen adherence is presumed to result in better glycemic control, empirical evidence for this association is strongest for patients with type 1 diabetes (T1D) (Hood 2009), with more frequent blood glucose testing showing a consistent relationship to lower levels of glycosylated hemoglobin A1C (Anderson 1997, Levine 2001, Stewart 2003, Haller 2004, Moreland 2004, Helgeson 2011, Ziegler 2011). In type 2 diabetic populations, study results have been mixed, with some studies documenting an association between increased blood glucose testing and better glycemic control and other studies showing no clinical benefit. Most patients with type 2 diabetes (T2D) are on oral medications, and some studies have suggested that glucose testing may be more important for regulating dose adjustment in insulin-treated patients (Fontbonne 1989, Faas 1997, Davis 2006, Polonsky 2011a).

Cramer (2004) attempted to assess the link between adherence with diabetes medications and glycemic control in her systematic review but was unable to find sufficient studies that included adequate measures of both medication adherence and glycemic control in the same investigation. This study design and measurement problem has been highlighted again in a recent Cochrane review of the impact of interventions designed to improve adherence in patients with T2D (Vermeire 2009).

Although adequate measurement of both adherence and glycemic control is critical to demonstrating any link between the two, the relationship between diabetes regimen adherence and glycemic control is complex and dependent on factors other than patient behavior per se. Most importantly, the impact of patient adherence is entirely dependent on the effectiveness of the prescribed treatment regimen. Even perfect adherence with inappropriate treatment recommendations—or recommendations that can only have a weak effect on glycemic control—will have little or no impact on patient health outcomes (Johnson 1994).

Even the best available treatments are not always as powerful as we would like them to be. Perhaps of greater concern is the fact that many providers do not make appropriate treatment recommendations to their patients.

PROVIDER ADHERENCE

We began this chapter by quoting the Haynes (1979) definition of adherence that has been in use for more than 30 years: "the extent to which a person's behavior (in terms of taking medications, following diets, or executing lifestyle changes) coincides with medical advice." When discussing adherence, there is a strong tendency to think only about patient behavior. However, the "medical advice" component of the definition is equally important; the recommendations the provider gives to the patient are as critical to health outcomes as the patient's ability and willingness to follow a provider's "medical advice." Although standards of care are published annually by the American Diabetes Association (ADA), there is ample evidence that many providers do not adhere to these recommendations (Zoorob 1996, Lawler 1997, Centers of Disease Control and Prevention 2001, Renders 2001, Bouldin 2002, Coon 2002, Kirkman 2002, Peek 2007, Krane 2008). Improving provider adherence to ADA standards of care is as important as enhancing patient adherence with provider recommendations.

ASSESSING PATIENT ADHERENCE

Diabetes self-management involves multiple behaviors including medication taking, blood glucose monitoring, attention to diet, and regular exercise. Many patients vary in their adherence across diabetes care tasks; some patients may carefully take all of their medications but rarely monitor blood glucose or follow their diet. Others may religiously avoid sweets but fail to exercise regularly (Johnson 1992). This variability in patient self-care behaviors presents real challenges to adherence assessment.

Blood glucose meters from which data can be downloaded provide an objective measure of blood glucose testing, a self-care behavior consistently linked to glycemic control in patients with T1D (Hood 2009); however, this adherence behavior may be less important when assessing patients with T2D on oral medication (Davis 2006). For those on the insulin pump, the data can be downloaded to provide a measure of medication adherence, but this is available for only the limited number of patients who have selected insulin pump therapy as their treatment of choice. Medication Event Monitoring Systems (e.g., MEMS caps) have been successfully used to assess oral medication adherence in a number of studies (Quittner 2008) but have not been widely used as an indicator of oral medication adherence in patients with T2D.

Self-report measures of diabetes regimen adherence have been developed with good psychometric properties, including the Self-Care Inventory and the Diabetes Regimen Adherence Questionnaire (Quittner 2008). Generally self-report measures provide higher estimates of adherence compared with other assessment strategies (Johnson 2008, Quittner 2008) and serve as an overall indicator of adherence rather than providing information about specific diabetes care behaviors. However, self-report instruments can be adapted to focus on individual behaviors in addition to providing an estimate of overall adherence.

Some consider the use of multiple 24-hour recall interviews as the gold standard for adherence assessment because this strategy permits assessment of all behaviors relevant to diabetes care; the strategy also compares favorably with objective data from downloaded data or from direct observation and generally yields lower adherence estimates than self-report data (Johnson 2008, Quittner 2008). Interviews are typically conducted by telephone by trained interviewers and usually focus on both week- and weekend-day behaviors. As a consequence, the approach is time-consuming and can present a number of data management and analysis challenges. To date, this approach has been predominantly used in research studies and has not been developed for easy application in the clinical setting.

Selection of an adherence assessment strategy will depend on the focus of the adherence assessment (for example, medication taking versus glucose testing), whether a single behavior is of interest or a broad picture of the patient's diabetes care activities is the focus, and the psychometric quality of the measurement strategy, as well as practical issues. The use of A1C levels as an index of patient adherence is not recommended. Although a patient's A1C level provides an important index of glycemic control, it provides no information about what the patient is or is not doing to manage diabetes on a daily basis. A high-quality adherence assessment should use measurement tools developed explicitly for this purpose. The absence of data derived from good-quality diabetes-specific adherence measures—in addition to measures of glycemic control—in the extant literature has seriously handicapped our understanding of the relationship between adherence and glycemic control in patients with diabetes (Cramer 2004, Vermeire 2009).

STRATEGIES TO IMPROVE PATIENT ADHERENCE

Medication adherence, as measured by prescription refills, appears to be very price-sensitive. A number of studies have documented increased medication adherence with reduction or elimination of patient copays or cost-sharing (Mahoney 2005, Roblin 2005, Berger 2007, Goldman 2007, Gu 2010, Maciejewski 2010, Athanasakis 2011). Several of these studies also report associated reductions in total health care costs when patient adherence improves in response to lowering patient copays or cost-sharing for diabetes medications (Mahoney 2005, Berger 2007). From a health systems perspective, reducing patient costs for medication and glucose testing may be one of the most effective ways to increase patient adherence with these components of the treatment regimen.

Systematic reviews of other types of interventions targeting medical regimen adherence have separately addressed studies of patients with type 1 and type 2 diabetes. This is understandable given that the patient age and medical recommendations differ substantially between these two populations. Nevertheless, most of the relevant literature for patients with both type 1 and type 2 diabetes suffers from a "black box" approach, testing the impact of an adherence intervention on A1C with no measure of change in patient adherence behaviors (Vermeire 2009).

The systematic reviews of adherence interventions with patients who have T1D suggest that education alone is unlikely to impact adherence or glycemic control (Savage 2010). Reviews that focus on psychological (as opposed to educational) interventions suggest that behavioral and multicomponent interventions can produce substantive change in patient adherence (Kahana 2008). However, the effect of these interventions on glycemic control was much more modest, with multicomponent interventions focusing on family processes more effective than interventions addressing a single adherence behavior (Winkley 2006, Hood 2010, Savage 2010).

In populations of patients with T2D, systematic reviews again suggest that education alone does not have substantive effects on adherence or glycemic control (Wens 2008, Vermeire 2009). However, there is good evidence that medication adherence can be improved by reducing the frequency of doses and by the use of simple reminders, like the use of calendar blister packs (Norris 2001, Norris 2002b, Gary 2003, Ismail 2004, Moore 2004, Deakin 2005, Lindenmeyer 2006, Magione 2006, Thomas 2006, Kavookjian 2007, Roumen 2009, Vermeire 2009, Misono 2010). Psychological interventions and those that focus on self-management training have shown positive effects on glycemic control, at least in the short term (Centers for Disease Control and Prevention 2001, Norris 2001, Gary 2003, Ismail 2004, Moore 2004, Deakin 2005, Thomas 2006). Interventions that increase exercise in patients with T2D also have had consistent positive effects on glycemic control and cardiovascular health (Kavookjian 2007); this finding was not replicated in patients with T1D. Further, lifestyle interventions that have an exercise component have been consistently associated with the prevention of T2D in at-risk populations (Roumen 2009). Given the high prevalence of T2D in African-American, Latino, and Native American groups, the importance of culturally tailored intervention programs is receiving increased attention; the use of nurse case managers and community health workers appears particularly promising (Peek 2007).

STRATEGIES TO IMPROVE PROVIDER ADHERENCE

Didactic instruction alone does not appear to be a sufficient method to improve provider adherence to practice guidelines, such as monitoring glycosylated hemoglobin, urine protein, and lipid assays and foot and dilated eye exams. However, provider adherence behaviors can be further enhanced through organizational interventions that prompt the target behavior through computerized tracking systems, standardized patient-care flow sheets, medical record audits, and feedback (Centers for Disease Control and Prevention 2001, Renders 2001, Norris 2002b, Magione 2006, Lin 2007). Evidence for the impact of these interventions on patient glycemic control is less clear (Norris 2002a, Magione 2006).

Although implementing structures to assure appropriate physician monitoring is an important first step, it appears insufficient to guarantee improvements in patient glycemic control. The patient must be engaged in constructive ways to assure meaningful daily diabetes self-care behaviors. Toward that end, there has been increased interest in collaborative patient-provider approaches that encourage joint definition of treatment goals and management strategies. Studies have reported poor patient–provider agreement on treatment goals but improved diabetes self-management when patient and provider goals are in accord (Heisler 2003). A systematic review of interventions to enhance patient-provider interactions found little evidence that counseling providers on their communication style is a successful approach to enhancing patient-provider interactions; instead, interventions aimed at empowering patients to ask questions and engage the provider in treatment and diabetes-management goals was substantially more effective (van Dam 2003). The Structured Testing Program (STeP) is one example; both patients with T2D and primary care physicians participate in a collaborative program in which the patient records and plots a seven-point profile of blood glucose testing results for 3 consecutive days before a clinic visit and the primary physician uses an algorithm to make changes to the patient's regimen. This approach has resulted in both an increase in physician modifications of treatment recommendations and improved glycemic control (Polonsky 2011a, Polonsky 2011b).

RECOMMENDATIONS FOR CLINICAL CARE

Medical regimen adherence is a complex phenomenon that occurs within a broad context that includes the patient, the patient's family, the health care system, and the larger community. Fisher et al. (2005) have described one such ecological model that provides a useful structure for those interested in designing effective adherence intervention programs. The model includes individualized patient assessment, patient-provider collaborative goal-setting, patient skills enhancement, follow-up and support, increased access to resources in the patient's daily life, and continuity of quality clinical care.

From a health care system perspective, the evidence suggests that reducing the cost to the patient of medications and blood glucose testing strips will enhance patient adherence. Health care providers must also take responsibility for assuring that their "medical advice" is consistent with ADA standards of care. Organizational systems—such as computerized tracking systems, provider audits, and feedback to providers—can be put in place to enhance the likelihood that providers deliver appropriate and effective medical advice.

The patient's knowledge of the treatment plan and skills to carry it out should be carefully assessed. Inadvertent nonadherence is extremely common and can be eliminated by direct observation of patient behavior. Knowledge and skills assessment will frequently identify difficulties or misunderstandings that were not readily apparent during the clinic visit (e.g., cognitive, hearing, vision, or manual dexterity problems in an older person; manual dexterity or misunderstandings in a child). This assessment provides an opportunity for corrective feedback or modification of the regimen.

Knowledge and skills should be assessed in all those who have a primary role in carrying out daily diabetes care tasks. This is particularly important when a child has diabetes, since other family members are involved in the child's diabetes care. Determining who has responsibility for each component of the regimen should be part of the assessment because there is considerable evidence that increasing parental involvement may improve the child's glycemic control (Fonagy 1987, Follansbee 1989, Grey 1998, Holmes 2006).

Diabetes knowledge and skill assessments should be repeated on an annual basis or more frequently as circumstances indicate. Patients live in families and communities, and as a consequence, they are receiving "medical advice" from many different sources, some of which may conflict with the provider's recommendations. Children grow older, and responsibilities for diabetes care shift. Adult patients may develop cognitive, vision, or manual dexterity problems that interfere with their ability to carry out their regimen correctly. Without repeated knowledge and skills assessments, inadvertent nonadherence can easily reoccur.

Successfully addressing inadvertent nonadherence does not assure that the patient will successfully follow the treatment regimen: diabetes knowledge and skills are a necessary—but not sufficient—condition for good adherence and good glycemic control. Consequently, patient adherence assessments should be incorporated as part of usual care. There are a number of reliable and valid assessment strategies available; selection should be dependent on whether the focus is on a specific diabetes management behavior (e.g., downloaded meter data to assess blood glucose testing, MEMS caps to assess oral medication taking, 24-hour recall interviews to assess dietary behavior) or on the broad array of behaviors required for diabetes care (e.g., Self-Care Inventory, Diabetes Regimen Adherence Questionnaire, 24-hour recall interview). A1C should not be used as a measure of adherence, although it remains the gold standard for assessing glycemic control. Adherence behaviors, like diabetes knowledge and skills, may change over time. Children grow and develop, the circumstances of patients' lives change, and adherence behaviors may change accordingly. Consequently, repeated adherence assessments—annually or more frequently if circumstances warrant—should become part of standard care.

A good adherence assessment will help the provider identify what behaviors are problematic for the patient and should be targeted for intervention. There is ample evidence that diabetes self-care behaviors can be improved. For medication taking, reducing medication costs, simplifying the medication regimen, or providing the medication in ways that successfully cue the behavior (e.g., providing the medication in calendar blister packs) can enhance adherence. For more complex diabetes care behaviors, behavioral and multicomponent interventions have proved successful for patients with both type 1 and type 2 diabetes. Because most studies have not included adequate measures of both adherence and glycemic control in the same investigation, it remains unclear which adherence behaviors are most strongly linked to improved glycemic control. Although medication taking is presumed essential, the available data suggest that frequent blood glucose testing is consistently linked to good glycemic control in patients with T1D, and exercise is linked to good glycemic control in patients with T2D. As the quality of the diabetes adherence intervention research improves, clinicians will be able to provide better guidance as to what treatments work best for whom. Interventions specifically tailored to ethnic minority populations—who suffer the greatest burden from T2D—are particularly needed.

SUMMARY OF RECOMMENDATIONS

1. Medical advice must be provided using clear communications. Health care systems that empower the patient to ask questions and that emphasize

treatment goals and diabetes management plans that are collaboratively developed between the patient and provider are particularly effective.

2. Knowledge and skills should be assessed in all those who have a primary role in carrying out daily diabetes care tasks.

3. Diabetes knowledge and skill assessments should be repeated on an annual basis or more frequently if poor glucose control is unexplained, at the onset of complications, or if there is a major change in treatment regimen.

4. Adherence assessments should include evaluation of perceived barriers to care as well as knowledge and skills.

BIBLIOGRAPHY

Alto WA, Meyer D, Schneid J, Bryson P, Kindig J: Assuring the accuracy of home glucose monitoring. *J Am Board Fam Pract* 15:1–6, 2002

Anderson B, Ho J, Brackett J, Finkelstein D, Laffel L: Parental involvement in diabetes management tasks: relationships to blood glucose monitoring adherence and metabolic control in young adolescents with insulin-dependent diabetes mellitus. *J Pediatr* 130:257–265, 1997

Athanasakis K, Skroumpelos AG, Tsiantou V, Milona K, Kyriopoulos J: Abolishing coinsurance for oral antihyperglycemic agents: effects on social insurance budgets. *American Journal of Managed Care* 17:130–135, 2011

Balkrishnan R, Rajagopalan R, Camacho F, Huston S, Murray F, Anderson R: Predictors of medication adherence and associated health care costs in an older population with type 2 diabetes mellitus: a longitudinal cohort study. *Clinical Therapeutics* 25:2958–2971, 2003

Berger J: Economic and clinical impact of innovative pharmacy benefit designs in the management of diabetes pharmacotherapy. *American Journal of Managed Care* 13 (Suppl. 2):S55–S58, 2007

Bouldin MJ, Low AK, Blackston JW, Duddleston DN, Holman HE, Hicks GS, Brown CA: Quality of care in diabetes: understanding the guidelines. *Am J Med Sci* 324:196–206, 2002

Breitscheidel L, Stamenitis S, Dippel FW, Schoffski O: Economic impact of compliance to treatment with antidiabetes medication in type 2 diabetes mellitus: a review paper. *Journal of Medical Economics* 13:8–15, 2010

Centers for Disease Control and Prevention: Strategies for reducing morbidity and mortality from diabetes through health-care system interventions and diabetes self-management education in community settings: a report on recommendations of the Task Force on Community Preventive Strategies. *Morbidity and Mortality Weekly Report* 50 (RR–16):1–15, 2001

Cooke JB: A practical guide to low vision management of patients with diabetes. *Clin Exp Optom* 84:155–161, 2001

Coon P, Zulkowski K: Adherence to American Diabetes Association standards of care by rural health care providers. *Diabetes Care* 25:2224–2229, 2002

Cramer J: A systematic review of adherence with medications for diabetes. *Diabetes Care* 27:1218–1224, 2004

Davis WA, Bruce DG, Davis TM: Is self-monitoring of blood glucose appropriate for all type 2 patients? The Fremantle Diabetes Study. *Diabetes Care* 29:1764–1770, 2006

Deakin T, McShane CE, Cade JE, Williams RD: Group based training for self-management strategies in people with type 2 diabetes mellitus. *Cochrane Database Syst Rev* CD003417, 2005

Faas A, Schellevis F, van Eijk J: The efficacy of self-monitoring of blood glucose in NIDDM subjects: a criteria-based review. *Diabetes Care* 20:1482–1486, 1997

Fisher EB, Brownson CA, O'Toole ML, Shetty G, Anwuri VV, Glasgow RE: Ecological approaches to self-management: the case of diabetes. *Am J Public Health* 95:1523–1535, 2005

Follansbee DS: Assuming responsibility for diabetes management: what age? what price? *Diabetes Educ* 15:347–353, 1989

Fonagy P, Moran GS, Lindsay MK, Kurtz AB, Brown R: Psychological adjustment and diabetic control. *Arch Dis Child* 62:1009–1013, 1987

Fontbonne A, Billault B, Acosta M, Percheron C, Varenne P, Besse A, Eschwege I, Monnier L, Slama G, Passa P: Is glucose self-monitoring beneficial to non-insulin-treated patients? Results of a randomized comparative trial. *Diabete Metab* 15:255–260, 1989

Fu AZ Qui Y, Radican L: Impact of fear of insulin or fear of injection on treatment outcomes of patients with diabetes. *Current Medical Research Opinion* 25:1413–1420, 2009

Funnell MM, Brown TL, Childs BP, Haas LB, Hosey GM, Jensen B, Maryniuk M, Peyrot M, Piette JD, Reader D, Siminerio LM, Weinger K, Weiss M: National Standards for Diabetes Self-Management Education. *Diabetes Care* 34 (Suppl. 1):S89–S96, 2011

Gary TL, Genkinger JM, Guallar E, Peyrot M, Brancati FL: Meta-analysis of randomized educational and behavioral interventions in type 2 diabetes. *Diabetes Educ* 29:488–501, 2003

Glasgow R, Wilson W, McCaul D: Regimen adherence: a problematic construct for diabetes research. *Diabetes Care* 8:300–301, 1985

Goldman DP, Joyce GF, Zheng Y: Prescription drug cost sharing: association with medication and medical utilization and spending and health. *JAMA* 298:61–69, 2007

Grey M, Boland EA, Yu C, Sullivan-Bolyai S, Tamborlane WV: Personal and family factors associated with quality of life in adolescents with diabetes. *Diabetes Care* 21:909–914, 1998

Gu Q, Zeng F, Patel BV, Tripoli LC: Part D coverage gap and adherence to diabetes medications. *American Journal of Managed Care* 16:911–918, 2010

Haller MJ, Stalvey MS, Silverstein JH: Predictors of control of diabetes: monitoring may be the key. *J Pediatr* 144:660–661, 2004

Harkavy J, Johnson SB, Silverstein J, Spillar R, McCallum M, Rosenbloom A: Who learns what at diabetes camp. *Journal of Pediatric Psychology* 8:143–153, 1983

Haynes R: Introduction. In *Compliance in Health Care*. Haynes R, Taylor D, Sackett D, Eds. Baltimore, MD, Johns Hopkins Press, 1979, p. 2–3

Heisler M, Piette JD, Spencer M, Kieffer E, Vijan S: The relationship between knowledge of recent HbA1c values and diabetes care understanding and self-management. *Diabetes Care* 28:816–822, 2005

Heisler M, Vijan S, Anderson RM, Ubel PA, Bernstein SJ, Hofer TP: When do patients and their physicians agree on diabetes treatment goals and strategies, and what difference does it make? *Journal of General Internal Medicine* 18:893–902, 2003

Helgeson VS, Honcharuk E, Becker D, Escobar O, Siminerio L: A focus on blood glucose monitoring: relation to glycemic control and determinants of frequency. *Pediatr Diabetes* 12:25–30, 2011

Herman M: The economics of diabetes prevention. *Medical Clinics of North America* 95:373–384, 2011

Holmes CS, Chen R, Streisand R, Marschall DE, Souter S, Swift EE, Peterson CC: Predictors of youth diabetes care behaviors and metabolic control: a structural equation modeling approach. *J Pediatr Psychol* 31:770–784, 2006

Hood KK, Rohan JM, Peterson CM, Drotar D: Interventions with adherence-promoting components in pediatric type 1 diabetes. *Diabetes Care* 33:1658–1664, 2010

Hood KK, Peterson CM, Rohan JM, Drotar D: Association between adherence and glycemic control in pediatric type 1 diabetes: a meta-analysis. *Pediatrics* 124:e1171–1179, 2009

Ismail K, Winkley K, Rabe-Hesketh S: Systematic review and meta-analysis of randomised controlled trials of psychological interventions to improve glycaemic control in patients with type 2 diabetes. *Lancet* 363:1589–1597, 2004

Johnson SB: Measuring adherence to medical regimens. Invited address, NIH Conference on Non-Adherence in Adolescents with Chronic Illness, Bethesda MD, September 2008

Johnson SB: Health behavior and health status: concepts, methods and applications. *Journal of Pediatric Psychology* 19:129–141, 1994

Johnson SB: Methodological issues in diabetes research: measuring adherence. *Diabetes Care* 15:1658–1672, 1992

Johnson SB, Pollak RT, Silverstein J, Rosenbloom A, Spillar RP, McCallum M, Harkavy J: Cognitive and behavioral knowledge about insulin-dependent diabetes among children and parents. *Pediatrics* 69:708–713, 1982

Kahana S, Drotar D, Frazier T: Meta-analysis of psychological interventions to promote adherence to treatment in pediatric chronic health conditions. *Journal of Pediatric Psychology* 33:590–611, 2008

Kavookjian J, Elswick BM, Whetsel T: Interventions for being active among individuals with diabetes: a systematic review of the literature. *Diabetes Educ* 33:962–988, 2007

Kirkman MS, Williams SR, Caffrey HH, Marrero DG: Impact of a program to improve adherence to diabetes guidelines by primary care physicians. *Diabetes Care* 25:1946–1951, 2002

Krane NK, Anderson D, Lazarus CJ, Termini M, Bowdish B, Chauvin S, Fonseca V: Physician practice behavior and practice guidelines: using unannounced standardized patients to gather data. *J Gen Intern Med* 24:53–56, 2008

Lawler FH, Viviani N: Patient and physician perspectives regarding treatment of diabetes: compliance with practice guidelines. *J Fam Pract* 44:369–373, 1997

Lerman I: Adherence to treatment: the key to avoiding the long-term complications of diabetes. *Archives of Medical Research* 36:300–306, 2005

Levine BS, Anderson BJ, Butler DA, Antisdel JE, Brackett J, Laffel LM: Predictors of glycemic control and short-term adverse outcomes in youth with type 1 diabetes. *J Pediatr* 139:197–203, 2001

Lin D, Hale S, Kirby E: Improving diabetes management. *Canadian Family Physician* 53:73–77, 2007

Lindenmeyer A, Hearnshaw H, Vermeire E, Van Royen P, Wens J, Biot Y: Interventions to improve adherence to medication in people with type 2 diabetes mellitus: a review of the literature on the role of pharmacists. *Journal of Clinical Pharmacy and Therapeutics* 31:409–419, 2006

Maciejewski ML, Farley JF, Parker J, Wansink D: Copayment reductions generate greater medication adherence in targeted populations. *Health Affairs* 29:2002–2008, 2010

Magione CM, Gerzoff RB, Williamson DF, Steers WN, Kerr EA, Brown AF, Waitzfelder BE, Marrero DG, Dudley A, Kim C, Herman W, Thompson TJ, Safford MM, Selby JV: The association between quality of care and the intensity of diabetes disease management programs. *Annals of Internal Medicine* 145:107–116, 2006

Mahoney JJ: Reducing patient drug acquisition costs can lower diabetes health claims. *American Journal of Managed Care* 11 (Suppl. 5):S170–S176, 2005

Messier C: Impact of impaired glucose tolerance and type 2 diabetes on cognitive aging. *Neurobiol Aging* 26 (Suppl. 1):26–30, 2005

Misono AS, Cutrona SL, Choudhry NK, Fischer MA, Stedman MR, Liberman JN, Brennan TA, Jain SH, Shrank WH: Healthcare information technology interventions to improve cardiovascular and diabetes medication adherence. *American Journal of Managed Care* 16 (Suppl. 12 HIT):SP82–SP92, 2010

Moore H, Summerbell C, Hooper L, Cruickshank K, Vyas A, Johnstone P, Ashton V, Kopelman P: Dietary advice for treatment of type 2 diabetes mellitus in adults. *Cochrane Database Syst Rev* CD004097, 2004

Moreland EC, Tovar A, Zuehlke JB, Butler DA, Milaszewski K, Laffel LM: The impact of physiological, therapeutic and psychosocial variables on glycemic control in youth with type 1 diabetes mellitus. *J Pediatr Endocrinol Metab* 17:1533–1544, 2004

Newman KD, Weaver MT: Insulin measurement and preparation among diabetic patients at a county hospital. *Nurse Practitioner* 19:44–45, 48, 1994

Norris SL, Lau J, Smith SJ, Schmid CH, Engelgau MM: Self-management education for adults with type 2 diabetes: a meta-analysis of the effect on glycemic control. *Diabetes Care* 25:1159–1171, 2002a

Norris SL, Nichos PJ, Caspersen CJ, Glasglow RE, Engelgau MM, Jack L, Isham G, Snyder SR, Carnade-Kulis VG, Garfield S, Briss P, McCulloch D: The effectiveness of disease and case management for people with diabetes: a systematic review. *American Journal of Preventive Medicine* 22 (Suppl. 4):15–38, 2002b

Norris SL, Engelgau MM, Naryan KMV: Effectiveness of self-management training in type 2 diabetes: a systematic review of randomized controlled trials. *Diabetes Care* 24:561–587, 2001

Odegard PS, Cappocia K: Medication taking and diabetes: a systematic review of the literature. *Diabetes Educ* 33:1014–1029, 2007

Page P, Verstraete DG, Robb JR, Etzwiler DD: Patient recall of self-care recommendations in diabetes. *Diabetes Care* 4:96–98, 1981

Patton SR: Adherence to diet in youth with type 1 diabetes. *Journal of the American Dietetic Association* 111:550–553, 2011

Peek ME, Cargill A, Huang ES: Diabetes health disparities: a systematic review of health care interventions. *Med Care Res Rev* 64 (Suppl. 5):S101–S156, 2007

Peeters B, Van Tongelen I, Boussery K, Mehys E, Remon JP, Willems S: Factors associated with medication adherence to oral hypoglycaemic agents in different ethnic groups suffering from type 2 diabetes: a systematic literature review and suggestions for further research. *Diabet Med* 28:262–275, 2011

Perwien A, Johnson SB, Dymtrow D, Silverstein J: Blood glucose monitoring skills in children with type 1 diabetes. *Clinical Pediatrics* 39:351–357, 2000

Polonsky WH, Fisher L, Schikman CH, Hinnen DA, Parkin CG, Jelsovsky Z, Axel-Schweitzer M, Petersen, B, Wagner RS: A structured self-monitoring of blood glucose approach to type 2 diabetes encourages more frequent, intensive, and effective physician interventions: results from the STeP Study. *Diabetes Technology and Therapeutics* 13:797–802, 2011a

Polonsky WH, Fisher J, Schikman CH, Hinnen DA, Parkin CG, Jelsovsky Z, Petersen B, Schweitzer M, Wagner RS: Structured self-monitoring of blood glucose significantly reduces A1C levels in poorly controlled noninsulin-treated diabetes: results from the Structured Testing Program study. *Diabetes Care* 34:262–267, 2011b

Quittner AL, Modi AC, Lermanek KL, Ievers-Landis CE, Rapoff MA: Evidence-based assessment of adherence to medical treatments in pediatric psychology. *Journal of Pediatric Psychology* 33:916–936, 2008

Reijmer YD, van den Berg E, Ruis C, Kappelle LJ, Biessels GJ: Cognitive dysfunction in patients with type 2 diabetes. *Diabetes Metab Res Rev* 26:507–519, 2010

Renders CM, Valk GD, Griffin S, Wagner EH, Eijk Van JT, Assendelft WJ: Interventions to improve the management of diabetes mellitus in primary care, outpatient and community settings: a systematic review. *Diabetes Care* 24:1821–1833, 2001

Roblin DW, Platt R, Goodman MJ, et al.: Effect of increased cost sharing on oral hypoglycemic use in five managed care organizations: how much is too much? *Medical Care* 43:951–959, 2005

Roumen C, Blaak EE, Corpeleijn E: Lifestyle intervention for prevention of diabetes: determinants of success for future implementation. *Nutrition Reviews* 67:132–146, 2009

Rubin RR: Adherence to pharmacologic therapy in patients with type 2 diabetes mellitus. *Am J Med* 118 (Suppl. 5A):S27–S34, 2005

Savage E, Farrell D, McManus V, Grey M: The science of intervention development for type 1 diabetes in children: systemic review. *Journal of Advanced Nursing* 66:2604–2619, 2010

Silverstein J, Klingensmith G, Copeland K, Plotnick L, Kaufman F, Laffel L, Deeb L, Grey M, Anderson B, Holzmeister LA, Clark N: Care of children and adolescents with type 1 diabetes: a statement of the American Diabetes Association. *Diabetes Care* 28:186–212, 2005

Stewart SM, Lee PW, Waller D, Hughes CW, Low LC, Kennard BD, Cheng A, Huen KF: A follow-up study of adherence and glycemic control among Hong Kong youths with diabetes. *Journal of Pediatric Psychology* 28:67–79, 2003

Thomas DE, Elliott EJ, Naughton GA: Exercise for type 2 diabetes mellitus. *Cochrane Database Syst Rev* CD002968, 2006

Thompson CJ, Cummings F, Chalmers J, Newton RW: Abnormal insulin treatment behaviour: a major cause of ketoacidosis in the young adult. *Diabet Med* 12:429–432, 1995 van Dam HA, van der Horst F, van den Borne B, Ryckman R, Crebolder H: Provider-patient interaction in diabetes care: effects on patient self-care and outcomes: a systematic review. *Patient Education and Counseling* 51:17–28, 2003

Vermeire E, Wens J, Van Royen P, Biot Y, Hearnshaw H, Lindenmeyer A: Interventions for improving adherence to treatment recommendations in people with type 2 diabetes mellitus. *Cochrane Database Syst Rev* CD003638, 2009

Wens J, Vermeire E, Hearnshaw H, Lindenmeyer A, Biot Y, Van Royen: Educational interventions aiming at improving adherence to treatment recommendations in type 2 diabetes: a sub-analysis of a systematic review of randomised controlled trials. *Diabet Res Clin Pract* 79:377–388, 2008

Winkley K, Landau S, Eisler I, Ismail K: Psychological interventions to improve glycaemic control in patients with type 1 diabetes: systematic review and meta-analysis of randomised controlled trials. *BMJ* 333:65, 2006

World Health Organization. *Report on Medication Adherence*. Geneva, WHO, 2003

Wysocki T: Behavioral assessment and intervention in pediatric diabetes. *Behavior Modification* 30:72–92, 2006

Ziegler R, Heidtmann B, Hilgard D, Hofer S, Rosenbauer J, Holl R: Frequency of SMBG correlates with HbA1c and acute complications in children and adolescents with type 1 diabetes. *Pediatr Diabetes* 12:11–17, 2011

Zoorob RJ, Mainous AG: Practice patterns of rural family physicians based on the American Diabetes Association standards of care. *J Community Health* 21:175–182, 1996

Suzanne Bennett Johnson, PhD, is Distinguished Research Professor at Florida State University College of Medicine in Tallahassee, FL, and President of the American Psychological Association.

Chapter 8
Lifestyle Modification: Nutrition

Judith Wylie-Rosett, EdD, RD
Linda M. Delahanty, MSRD

MEDICAL NUTRITION THERAPY

Nutrition is defined as the provision of the materials necessary (in the form of food) to support life. Psychosocial and nutrition assessments are intertwined, with consideration of psychosocial factors in a nutrition assessment, and consideration of nutrition intervention on psychosocial outcomes, including physical and psychological well-being. The nutrition statement from the American Diabetes Association (ADA) *"provides evidence-based recommendations and interventions for diabetes medical nutrition therapy (MNT). The goal of the nutrition component of diabetes treatment is preventing, or at least slowing, the rate of development of diabetes complications"* (Bantle 2008). The Academy of Nutrition and Dietetics (formerly known as the American Dietetic Association) defines MNT as "the development and provision of a nutritional treatment or therapy based on a detailed assessment of a person's medical history, psychosocial history, physical examination, and dietary history" (Acad Nutr Diet 1999a, Acad Nutr Diet 1999b, Acad Nutr Diet 1999c). The MNT psychosocial assessment includes evaluation of an individual's economic status, ethnic and cultural background, health literacy, living situation, education level, occupation, mental status, and access to adequate food sources to maintain good health. Although the long-term goals of MNT are to reduce diabetes-related morbidity, shorter-term goals focus on achieving weight-related goals for overweight or obese patients (usually 7–10% loss) and achieving goals for metabolic control (blood glucose, blood pressure, and lipids) consistent with the ADA recommendations. Dietary assessment methods include 24-hour recall, food records, and questionnaires that vary in length and complexity (Wylie-Rosett 1990). A comparison of dietary assessment methods is available at www.p3gobservatory. org/repository/nutritionComparisonChart.htm.

SOCIAL ECOLOGICAL PERSPECTIVE

This chapter focuses on behavioral strategies for diabetes MNT and on the rationale and strategies for addressing environmental issues. The discussion of MNT addresses how motivational interviewing and enhancement techniques are used to develop collaborative goal setting. Using motivational interviewing, which includes open-ended questions, reflective listening, affirmation, and summarization, helps individuals address their concerns about making lifestyle changes (Miller 2010). For those willing to make changes, motivational interviewing provides an opportunity for coaching, including helping individuals set goals and arriving at a change plan (Miller 2010). Consideration of motivation is followed by a review of instruments to assess barriers relevant to implementing diabetes MNT as well as a review of the evidence related to the ADA nutrition recommendations. The rationale and strategies for addressing environmental issues are discussed using the social ecological model as recommended in the *Dietary Guidelines for Americans, 2010*, for translating evidence into action plans (available at www. dietaryguidelines.gov). The chapter concludes with consideration of recommendations specific to diabetes from the social ecological perspective.

FACTORS INFLUENCING ADOPTION OF MEDICAL NUTRITION THERAPY

Assessment of motivation provides a framework for collaborative goal setting to enhance participant motivation in MNT based on the principles of motivational interviewing (Mossavar-Rahmani 2007). The assessment used in motivational interviewing and enhancement involves exploring ambivalence about behavioral change; it examines discrepancies between individuals' current behavior and their core values or personal goals (Mossavar-Rahmani 2007). Motivational interviewing, whether targeting weight loss or improved glycemia, includes reflective listening to clarify goals and concerns as well as eliciting reasons for change in the individual's own words (Miller 2012). Clinicians can use motivational interviewing to "meet in the middle" in harmony with patients rather than wrestling over lifestyle recommendations. Learning how to use motivational interviewing requires training and should not be considered a technique taught using the "see one, do one, teach one" approach often used in training health professionals. However, motivational interviewing can be incorporated into brief counseling sessions based on training procedures developed by the Motivational Interviewing Network of Trainers (MINT). Information regarding motivational interviewing training is available from MINT at http://www.motivationalinterview.net/training/trainers.html. Although motivational interviewing can be used in combination with various behavioral theories, common misperceptions about motivational interviewing include thinking it is the transtheoretical model of behavioral change, a method for tricking people to make changes, cognitive-behavioral therapy, or client-centered therapy (Miller 2009). Objective feedback about weight or glycemic control is presented without judgment to facilitate discussion about personal goals and to address discrepancy between current behavior and personal aspirations.

Few instruments exist to assess the role of psychosocial factors in the nutritional management of diabetes. A search of diabetes and obesity literature yielded the following such instruments: *1*) an instrument to assess barriers to dietary change (formatively evaluated in a sample of African American women with type 2 diabetes [T2D]) (Galasso 2005); *2*) instruments to assess self-efficacy and outcome expectations regarding the quantity and quality of carbohydrate intake and the self-monitoring of blood glucose (psychometric evaluation for internal consistency of instruments and subscales) (Miller 2007); *3*) Veteran Survey of Weight Management, which has a patient and provider version to assess barriers to weight management (Ruelaz 2007); and *4*) instruments to evaluate diabetes-specific quality of life that are related to the impact of diet (e.g., hassles related to choosing or preparing food, preventing and treating symptoms of hypoglycemia, and hyperglycemia) (Polonsky 1995, Diabetes Control and Complications Trial Research Group 1996).

Assessment of community and environmental factors (e.g., increased availability of high-calorie foods in food markets and fast food outlets), which parallel the increase in diabetes and obesity prevalence, has focused on changes associated with increases in caloric consumption in the U.S. (Heini 1997, Duffey 2007, Bleich 2008, Lenz 2008, Wang 2008). Dietary factors that are closely associated with the increase in obesity-diabetes include larger portion sizes, greater food quantity and calories per meal, and increased consumption of sugar-sweetened beverages, snacks, commercially prepared (especially fast food) meals, and energy-dense foods (Nielsen 2003, Kant 2005, Kant 2006, Kant 2007a, Kant 2007b).

Diabetes-related health disparities are associated with economic disparities. Residents in low-income neighborhoods are more likely to live farther away from markets with healthy food options, spend a higher proportion of income on food, and have greater exposure to energy-dense low-nutrient-value foods (Horowitz 2004). Analysis of food insecurity in the National Health and Nutrition Examination Survey (NHANES) found a relationship between food insecurity and increased relative risk of diabetes, which appeared to be accounted for by income and educational level (Seligman 2007, Seligman 2010). NHANES data analysis has indicated that American family expenditure for food was 9.8% of disposable income, but the share of disposable income spent on food increased as absolute income levels declined (Nielsen 2003). Little is known about the effects of the recent economic downturn on nutrition-related diabetes disparities. The Consumer Price Index (CPI) for all food increased to 5.5% in 2008 and slowed to a 1.8% increase in 2009 and 0.8% in 2010. *The forecasted increase is 3.0-4.0% for 2011* (Schnepf 2011). An estimated 14.7% of American households suffered food insecurity (had no money to buy food) at some point during 2009 (Schnepf 2011).

A multilevel or socioecological assessment approach provides a framework for examining the complex interaction of nature (genetic and other biological determinants of appetite and satiety) and nurture (societal, cultural, psychological, economic, and other environmental determinants) that regulate food intake (Hanni 2007). Community-based diabetes interventions, which target structural changes to address nutritional problems, have used mixed-methods assessment. Changes in dietary intake and quality of life are assessed using quantitative surveys and qualitative methods such as focus groups and semistructured interviews. A variety of assessment tools that address obesity and nutritional barriers in diabetes management are available from the Centers for Disease Control and Prevention's (CDC's) Diabetes Prevention and Control Program at http://cdc.gov/diabetes/projects/index.htm and the Robert Wood Johnson Diabetes Initiative at http://diabetesnpo.im.wustl.edu/resources/type/programTraining.html (Hanni 2007, Albright 2008, McCormack 2008). The mixed-methods approach can evaluate how dietary intake relates to psychosocial, community, and economic environments and assess diabetes-related health disparities in relation to nutritional status and how nutrition interrelates with diabetes treatment.

KNOWN (AND PROVEN) TREATMENT METHODS

The ADA addresses the evidence regarding the benefits of MNT in its care standards (ADA 2012). The Academy of Nutrition and Dietetics has developed an Evidence Analysis Library (EAL) (http://adaevidencelibrary.com) that addresses the expected health and psychosocial outcomes for MNT interventions provided by registered dietitians, as the foundation of its type 1 and type 2 diabetes nutrition practice guidelines for adults (Franz 2008). Clinical trials/outcome studies of MNT have reported decreases in A1C of ~1% in individuals with type 1 diabetes (T1D) and 1–2% in individuals with type 2 diabetes (T2D), depending on the duration of diabetes (Pastors 2002, Pastors 2003). Nutrition intervention was integral to the intensive treatment of T1D in the multicenter Diabetes Control and Complications Trial (DCCT). Participants were randomized to conventional or intensive diabetes therapy. Intensive therapy, which used multiple daily injections (MDI) of insulin (three or more injections/day) or continuous subcutaneous insulin infusion (CSII), self-monitoring of blood glucose (SMBG), and a variety of nutrition strategies (e.g., menu plans, algorithm for adjusting insulin based on carbohydrate intake and physical activity, and a protocol for managing hypoglycemia) were used to help achieve the treatment goal of maintaining close to normal blood glucose levels (Anderson 1993, Delahanty 1993a, Delahanty 1993b). Self-reported diet behaviors associated with better A1C levels in the intensive treatment group included adherence to the prescribed meal plan, adjusting food and/or insulin in response to hyperglycemia, and, to a lesser degree, adjusting insulin dose for meal size and content, as well as consistent consumption of an evening snack. Overtreating hypoglycemia and consuming extra snacks beyond the meal plan were associated with higher A1C levels (Delahanty 1993a). Moreover, in the DCCT, there was no difference in diabetes-specific quality of life between those who received standard diabetes treatment compared with those who received intensive treatment. Despite the increased self-care demands related to diet, SMBG, and insulin administration with intensive diabetes treatment, there was no reported deterioration in quality of life (Diabetes Control and Complications Trial Research Group 1996). The Dose Adjustment for Normal Eating (DAFNE) randomized clinical trial, which used a 6-month delayed intervention, demonstrated that training people with T1D in flexible, intensive insulin management to allow freedom in food intake improved A1C level, overall quality of life, general well-being, and treatment satisfaction, but severe hypoglycemia, weight, and lipids remained unchanged (DAFNE Study Group 2002). Weight-loss intervention for people with T2D is being examined in the Look AHEAD (Action for Health in Diabetes) study, which is a multicenter, randomized controlled trial designed to determine whether intentional weight loss reduces cardiovascular morbidity and mortality in overweight individuals with T2D. The study began in 2001 and is scheduled to conclude in 2014 (Look AHEAD Research Group 2006). The evidence base for the Look AHEAD intervention is randomized control trials, including the Diabetes Prevention Program that achieved a 7 to 10% weight loss in 16 to 26 weeks using a combination of diet (i.e., establishing goals for fat and caloric intake to create an energy deficit), exercise (i.e., 150 min of moderate-intensity activity per week), and behavior therapy (Wing 1994, Guare 1995, Pascale 1995, Knowler 2002, Delahanty 2008b). Studies have demonstrated that a

7–10% weight loss results in improved glycemic control in patients with type 2 diabetes (Wing 1987), as well as improved blood pressure (Appel 1995, Appel 2003a, Appel 2003b) and lipids (Dattilo 1992). Evidence also supports providing meal replacements, structured menus that focused on portion control with a shopping list, and use of a low-energy-density diet (Jeffery 1995, Wing 1996, Rolls 2000, Bell 2001, Wing 2001, Ello-Martin 2007). In addition, a meta-analysis of six randomized controlled trials (RCTs) showed that liquid meal replacements resulted in a 3-kg greater weight loss than that produced by conventional dietary instruction (Heymsfield 2003). Observational data indicate that obese individuals underestimated their calorie intake by 40 to 50% when consuming a diet of conventional foods (Lichtman 1992), which was related to problems in estimating portion sizes, macronutrient composition, and calorie content and in remembering all foods consumed. Baseline Look AHEAD data indicate that the behavioral weight-control strategies of regular self-weighing and breakfast consumption, along with infrequent consumption of fast food, were related to lower BMI in the study population, and these variables accounted for 24% of the variance in BMI (Raynor 2008). In an RCT conducted in overweight women with T2D, West et al. (2007) evaluated the effects of motivational interviewing to help tailor intervention goals. In this study, the motivational interviewing approach achieved greater long-term (2 years) weight loss and short-term (6 months) glycemic control than an attention control. The potential use of meta-analysis and systemic reviews in assessing the relationship between nutrition interventions and psychosocial variables is limited by the small number of trials, the failure to include quality of life or other psychosocial variables as endpoints, and issues related to design and research methods (Norris 2004, Norris 2005a, Norris 2005b, Zhang 2007).

In overweight and obese insulin-resistant individuals, modest weight loss has been shown to improve insulin resistance. Thus, weight loss is recommended for all such individuals who have or are at risk for diabetes. The results of the Diabetes Prevention Program and the Look AHEAD trials indicate that a core weekly program of 14–16 weeks achieves a mean weight loss of 7–9%, along with metabolic improvements (Delahanty 2008b). Furthermore, the reach of the Intensive Lifestyle Intervention (ILI) behavioral weight-loss treatment for people with T2D in the first year of the Look AHEAD trial extended to spouses, who lost 2.7% of body weight compared with 0.2% weight loss in spouses of participants who were randomized to an enhanced usual-care program (DSE; Diabetes Support and Education) (Gorin 2008). The ILI participants met weekly for 6 months and monthly for the next 6 months to develop core behavioral skills, such as self-monitoring, problem solving, goal setting, and relapse prevention. Although spouses were not required or expected to attend group meetings, ILI participants were taught ways to enhance social support for their weight-loss efforts (e.g., how to communicate assertively with family members about desired recipe modifications, how to involve friends and family members in their exercise routines). DSE participants were offered three informational group meetings per year that provided basic information on diabetes, nutrition, and physical activity. Spouses were not required or expected to attend meetings, and strategies for enlisting social support were not discussed.

Spouse weight loss was associated with participant weight loss and decreases in high-fat foods in the home, suggesting that social networks can be utilized to promote the spread of weight loss, thus creating a ripple effect (Gorin 2008). In the management of T2D, the effects of weight-loss interventions on physical function and psychosocial outcomes including health-related quality of life (HRQOL) have been assessed. Look AHEAD participants in the ILI experienced significant reductions in body image dissatisfaction, physical function, and knee pain compared with those who received DSE (Foy 2011). Weight loss mediated the effect of the lifestyle intervention on knee pain and physical function (Foy 2011). HRQOL measures also significantly improved after 1 year of weight loss (Norris 2004, Williamson 2009). The improvements in HRQOL were partially mediated by weight loss, improved fitness, and reductions in complaints related to physical problems. Moreover, those with the lowest HRQOL derived the greatest benefit from participation in the lifestyle intervention program (Williamson 2009). After 4 years of follow-up, the weight-loss intervention group had a 48% risk reduction in loss of mobility compared with the support group. Weight loss and improved fitness were also significant mediators of this effect. For every relative reduction of 1% in weight and relative improvement of 1% in fitness, the risk of the loss of mobility was reduced by 7.3 and 1.4%, respectively (Rejeski 2012). These results underscore how the risk of increasing age, obesity, and T2D prevalence can combine to reduce physical function and mobility, which affects quality of life, and the important role of nutrition and lifestyle interventions in preserving a healthy body weight, fitness, physical function, and health-related quality of life.

In patients with type 2 diabetes, diabetes-specific emotional distress is associated with younger age, female gender, higher A1C levels, lesser adherence to diet, exercise, and medication regimens, and greater adherence to blood glucose testing, which was more commonly used in association with insulin therapy and greater severity of diabetes. In addition, even mild depressive symptoms seem to negatively affect adherence to self-care behaviors including diet, exercise, and administration of medication in patients with T2D (Polonsky 2005, Delahanty 2007). A Cochrane Database Systematic Review (Moore 2004) has indicated an urgent need for well-designed studies of dietary advice that examine a range of interventions and MNT approaches in individuals with T2D with follow-up at various time intervals.

ADA NUTRITION-RELATED RECOMMENDATIONS FOR CARE

Based on a systematic review of nutrition care in extended care facilities, the Academy of Nutrition and Dietetics recommended that MNT balance medical needs and individual desires and maintain quality of life (Niedert 2005).

1. Individuals who have diabetes should receive individualized MNT; such therapy is best provided by a registered dietitian familiar with the components of evidence-based diabetes MNT. Medicare and many other third-party payers include MNT coverage for diabetes with benefit basic coverage (year 1) = 3 hours. An episode of care typically includes 1 hour of initial assessment and four 30-min follow-up interventions during the first year. Additional hours are considered to be medically necessary and covered if the treating physician determines there is a change in medical con-

dition, diagnosis, or treatment regimen that requires a change in MNT and orders additional hours during that episode of care. Follow-up (year 2) = 2 hours. For more information see http://www.diabetesarchive.net/for-health-professionals-and-scientists/recognition/mnt-guide.jsp. The National Diabetes Information Clearinghouse provides information about assisting people with diabetes who have no access to MNT and other resources. For more information, see http://diabetes.niddk.nih.gov/dm/pubs/financialhelp/.

2. Nutrition counseling should be sensitive to the personal needs, willingness to change, and ability to make changes of the individual with diabetes.

PSYCHOSOCIAL RECOMMENDATIONS FOR CLINICAL CARE

1. **Develop Patient/Client MNT Self-Management Skills and Support Plan.** To be maximally effective, the provision of evidence-based MNT requires attention to psychosocial factors such as depression or dysthymia, diabetes-specific distress, readiness to change, competing life priorities, and self-efficacy that may represent barriers to implementing MNT recommendations. Thus, dietitians who deliver MNT need to be skilled in attentive and empathic listening, sensitive verbal inquiry, and use of thoughtful and reflective comments—skills that are the hallmarks of good clinical care (Gonzalez 2011). The nutrition assessment process that considers baseline knowledge and skills, past experiences (successes and failures) with behavior change, and current barriers to change is the basis for determining how the nutrition priorities will be translated into a plan that the patient can follow. For example, patients reporting distress due to frustration about unpredictable hyperglycemic episodes or fear of complications (i.e., diabetes-related distress) will likely need different interventions than patients who report being distressed because of life circumstances unrelated to diabetes.

   The use of motivational interviewing and cognitive behavioral strategies such as goal setting, problem solving, self-monitoring, and relapse prevention are important to facilitate the process of behavior change. In addition, the use of strategies that improve self-efficacy for behavior change is critical to the successful implementation of MNT. For example, the process of setting nutrition and behavioral goals is based on both their potential to significantly lower A1C levels and on the participant's self-report of at least 80% confidence in ability to achieve the goals (Delahanty 2008a).

2. **Use Environmental Strategies to Improve Access to Healthier Food Choices and Promote Physical Activity.** The 2010 Dietary Guidelines from the U.S. Department of Health and Human Services and the U.S. Department of Agriculture used the social ecological model (see Figure 8.1) as a multilevel framework for translating the evidence-based review into recommendations (USDA 2010, Rowe 2011, Spahn 2011). The guiding principles for the 2010 Guidelines are to: *1)* ensure access to nutritious foods and opportunities for physical activity; *2)* facilitate individual behavioral change through environmental strategies; and *3)* set the stage for life-

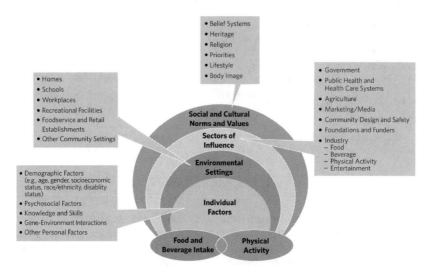

Figure 8.1: A Social Ecological Framework for Nutrition and Physical Activity Decisions.
Source: Adapted from: (1) Centers for Disease Control and Prevention. Division of Nutrition, Physical Activity, and Obesity. State Nutrition, Physical Activity and Obesity (NPAO) Program: Technical Assistance Manual. January 2008, page 36. Accessed April 21, 2010. http://www.cdc.gov/obesity/ downloads/TA_Manual_1_31_08.pdf. (2) Institute of Medicine. Preventing Childhood Obesity: Health in the Balance, Washington, DC: The National Academies Press; 2005, page 85. (3) Story M, Kaphingst KM, Robinson-O'Brien R, Glanz K. Creating healthy food and eating environments: Policy and environmental approaches. Annu Rev Public Health 2008;29:253-272. From USDA 2010.

long healthy eating, physical activity, and weight-management behaviors. Although this "call to action" acknowledges that Americans make their own food and physical activity choices at the individual or family level, emphasis is on providing community-based opportunities to make such choices. A multilevel framework provides a foundation for integrating psychosocial/behavioral issues into recommendations ranging from implementing diabetes MNT at the individual level to societal and policy recommendations relevant to lifestyle and diabetes (Wylie-Rosett 2009). Health profession training in diabetes management needs to include communication skills–related helping of patients/clients with diabetes to make informed nutrition decisions and take charge of their diabetes using counseling techniques such as motivation enhancement (Mossavar-Rahmani 2007).

3. **Optimize Resource with Evidence-Based Policies and Collaborations for Preventing and Controlling Diabetes.** Collaborations and partnerships between public and private organizations are needed to address food intake and obesity trends with regard to diabetes prevalence. Potential collaborators may include health departments, community garden and farmers' market initiatives, food pantries, schools, recreational facilities, hospitals, voluntary health agencies, and businesses.

Institutions need to develop policies or plans to support a healthier body weight. School-based and worksite initiatives to promote healthier weight include environmental changes and counseling support (Hersey 2008). Diabetes prevention strategies need to address obesity. Although third-party coverage includes MNT in situations of overt diabetes (Daly 2009), evaluation of third-party coverage and services for obesity is needed (Katz 2006) to address diabetes disparities including implicit bias (see Project Implicit at https://implicit.harvard.edu/implicit/demo/selectatest.html) related to weight or ethnic/racial stereotyping. Research is needed to address how the recommendation of metformin at the time of diabetes diagnosis is related to attitudes about and availability of diabetes MNT.

BIBLIOGRAPHY

Academy of Nutrition and Dietetics (formerly American Dietetic Association): Medical nutrition therapy protocols: an introduction. *J Am Diet Assoc* 99:351, 1999a

Academy of Nutrition and Dietetics (formerly American Dietetic Association): Medicare Medical Nutrition Therapy Act of 1999: Effort to secure MNT coverage still popular with lawmakers (Public Policy News). *J Am Diet Assoc* 99:796, 1999b

Academy of Nutrition and Dietetics (formerly American Dietetic Association): Position of the American Dietetic Association: Medical nutrition therapy and pharmacotherapy. *J Am Diet Assoc* 99:227–230, 1999c

Albright A: What is public health practice telling us about diabetes? *Journal of the American Dietetic Association* 108 (Suppl. 1):S12–S18, 2008

American Diabetes Association: Standards of medical care in diabetes—2012. *Diabetes Care* 35 (Suppl. 1):S11–S63, 2012

Anderson EJ, Richardson M, Castle G, Cercone S, Delahanty L, Lyon R, Mueller D, Snetselaar L: Nutrition interventions for intensive therapy in the Diabetes Control and Complications Trial: the DCCT Research Group. *J Am Diet Assoc* 93:768–772, 1993

Appel LJ: Lifestyle modification as a means to prevent and treat high blood pressure. *J Am Soc Nephrol* 14 (Suppl. 2):S99–S102, 2003a

Appel LJ, Champagne CM, Harsha DW, Cooper LS, Obarzanek E, Elmer PJ, Stevens VJ, Vollmer WM, Lin PH, Svetkey LP, Stedman SW, Young DR: Effects of comprehensive lifestyle modification on blood pressure control: main results of the PREMIER clinical trial. *JAMA* 289:2083–2093, 2003b

Appel LJ, Espeland M, Whelton PK, Dolecek T, Kumanyika S, Applegate WB, Ettinger WH Jr, Kostis JB, Wilson AC, Lacy C, et al.: Trial of nonpharmacologic intervention in the elderly (TONE): design and rationale of a blood pressure control trial. *Annals of Epidemiology* 5:119–129, 1995

Bantle JP, Wylie-Rosett J, Albright AL, Apovian CM, Clark NG, Franz MJ, Hoog-werf BJ, Lichtenstein AH, Mayer-Davis E, Mooradian AD, Wheeler ML: Nutrition recommendations and interventions for diabetes: a position statement of the American Diabetes Association. *Diabetes Care* 31 (Suppl. 1):S61–78, 2008

Bell EA, Rolls BJ: Energy density of foods affects energy intake across multiple levels of fat content in lean and obese women. *American Journal of Clinical Nutrition* 73:1010–1018, 2001

Bleich S, Cutler D, Murray C, Adams A: Why is the developed world obese? *Annual Review of Public Health* 29:273–295, 2008

DAFNE Stufy Group: Training in flexible, intensive insulin management to enable dietary freedom in people with type 1 diabetes: Dose Adjustment for Normal Eating (DAFNE) randomised controlled trial. *BMJ* 325:746, 2002

Daly A, Michael P, Johnson EQ, Harrington CC, Patrick S, Bender T: Diabetes white paper: defining the delivery of nutrition services in Medicare medical nutrition therapy vs Medicare diabetes self-management training programs. *Journal of the American Dietetic Association* 109:528–539, 2009

Dattilo AM, Kris-Etherton PM: Effects of weight reduction on blood lipids and lipoproteins: a meta-analysis. *Am J Clin Nutr* 56:320–328, 1992

Delahanty L, Heinz, J: Tools and techniques to facilitate nutrition intervention. In *Nutrition in the Prevention and Treatment of Disease*. 2nd Ed. Coulston A, Boushey CJ, Eds. San Diego, CA, Academic Press, 2008a, p. 149–167

Delahanty LM, Nathan DM: Implications of the diabetes prevention program and Look AHEAD clinical trials for lifestyle interventions. *Journal of the American Dietetic Association* 108 (Suppl. 1):S66–S72, 2008b

Delahanty LM, Grant RW, Wittenberg E, Bosch JL, Wexler DJ, Cagliero E, Meigs JB: Association of diabetes-related emotional distress with diabetes treatment in primary care patients with type 2 diabetes. *Diabet Med* 24:48–54, 2007

Delahanty LM, Halford BN: The role of diet behaviors in achieving improved glycemic control in intensively treated patients in the Diabetes Control and Complications Trial. *Diabetes Care* 16:1453–1458, 1993a

Delahanty L, Simkins SW, Camelon K: Expanded role of the dietitian in the Diabetes Control and Complications Trial: implications for clinical practice: the DCCT Research Group. *J Am Diet Assoc* 93:758–764, 767, 1993b

Diabetes Control and Complications Trial Research Group: Influence of intensive diabetes treatment on quality-of-life outcomes in the diabetes control and complications trial. *Diabetes Care* 19:195–203, 1996

Duffey KJ, Popkin BM: Shifts in patterns and consumption of beverages between 1965 and 2002. *Obesity (Silver Spring)* 15:2739–2747, 2007

Ello-Martin JA, Roe LS, Ledikwe JH, Beach AM, Rolls BJ: Dietary energy density in the treatment of obesity: a year-long trial comparing 2 weight-loss diets. *American Journal of Clinical Nutrition* 85:1465–1477, 2007

Foy CG, Lewis CE, Hairston KG, Miller GD, Lang W, Jakicic JM, Rejeski WJ, Ribisl PM, Walkup MP, Wagenknecht LE: Intensive lifestyle intervention improves physical function among obese adults with knee pain: findings from the Look AHEAD trial. *Obesity (Silver Spring)* 19:83–93, 2011

Franz MJ, Boucher JL, Green-Pastors J, Powers MA: Evidence-based nutrition practice guidelines for diabetes and scope and standards of practice. *J Am Diet Assoc* 108:S52–S58, 2008

Galasso P, Amend A, Melkus GD, Nelson GT: Barriers to medical nutrition therapy in black women with type 2 diabetes mellitus. *Diabetes Educ* 31:719–725, 2005

Gonzalez JS, Fisher L, Polonsky WH: Depression in diabetes: have we been missing something important? *Diabetes Care* 34:236–239, 2011

Gorin AA, Wing RR, Fava JL, Jakicic JM, Jeffery R, West DS, Brelje K, Dilillo VG: Weight loss treatment influences untreated spouses and the home environment: evidence of a ripple effect. *Int J Obes (Lond)* 32:1678–1684, 2008

Guare JC, Wing RR, Grant A: Comparison of obese NIDDM and nondiabetic women: short- and long-term weight loss. *Obesity Research* 3:329–335, 1995

Hanni KD, Mendoza E, Snider J, Winkleby MA: A methodology for evaluating organizational change in community-based chronic disease interventions. *Preventing Chronic Disease* 4:A105, 2007

Heini AF, Weinsier RL: Divergent trends in obesity and fat intake patterns: the American paradox. *American Journal of Medicine* 102:259–264, 1997

Hersey J, Williams-Piehota P, Sparling PB, Alexander J, Hill MD, Isenberg KB, Rooks A, Dunet DO: Promising practices in promotion of healthy weight at small and medium-sized US worksites. *Prev Chronic Dis* 5:A122, 2008

Heymsfield SB, van Mierlo CA, van der Knaap HC, Heo M, Frier HI: Weight management using a meal replacement strategy: meta and pooling analysis from six studies. *Int J Obes Relat Metab Disord* 27:537–549, 2003

Horowitz CR, Colson KA, Hebert PL, Lancaster K: Barriers to buying healthy foods for people with diabetes: evidence of environmental disparities. *American Journal of Public Health* 94:1549–1554, 2004

Jeffery RW, Wing RR: Long-term effects of interventions for weight loss using food provision and monetary incentives. *Journal of Consulting and Clinical Psychology* 63:793–796, 1995

Kant AK, Graubard BI: Secular trends in the association of socio-economic position with self-reported dietary attributes and biomarkers in the US population: National Health and Nutrition Examination Survey (NHANES)

1971–1975 to NHANES 1999–2002. *Public Health Nutrition* 10:158–167, 2007a

Kant AK, Graubard BI, Kumanyika SK: Trends in black-white differentials in dietary intakes of U.S. adults, 1971-2002. *American Journal of Preventive Medicine* 32:264–272, 2007b

Kant AK, Graubard BI: Secular trends in patterns of self-reported food consumption of adult americans: NHANES 1971–1975 to NHANES 1999–2002. *American Journal of Clinical Nutrition* 84:1215–1223, 2006

Kant AK, Graubard BI: Energy density of diets reported by American adults: association with food group intake, nutrient intake, and body weight. *Int J Obes (Lond)* 29:950–956, 2005

Katz T: Shaping the marketplace for medical nutrition therapy: advocating for coverage. *Journal of the American Dietetic Association* 106:1027–1028, 2006

Knowler WC, Barrett-Connor E, Fowler SE, Hamman RF, Lachin JM, Walker EA, Nathan DM: Reduction in the incidence of type 2 diabetes with lifestyle intervention or metformin. *N Engl J Med* 346:393–403, 2002

Lenz A, Diamond FB Jr: Obesity: the hormonal milieu. *Current Opinion in Endocrinology, Diabetes, and Obesity* 15:9–20, 2008

Lichtman SW, Pisarska K, Berman ER, Pestone M, Dowling H, Offenbacher E, Weisel H, Heshka S, Matthews DE, Heymsfield SB: Discrepancy between self-reported and actual caloric intake and exercise in obese subjects. *N Engl J Med* 327:1893–1898, 1992

Look AHEAD Research Group, Wadden TA, West DS, Delahanty L, Jakicic J, Rejeski J, Williamson D, Berkowitz RI, Kelley DE, Tomchee C, Hill JO, Kumanyika S: The Look AHEAD study: a description of the lifestyle intervention and the evidence supporting it. *Obesity (Silver Spring)* 14:737–752, 2006

McCormack LA, Williams-Piehota PA, Bann CM, Burton J, Kamerow DB, Squire C, Fisher E, Brownson CA, Glasgow RE: Development and validation of an instrument to measure resources and support for chronic illness self-management: a model using diabetes. *Diabetes Educ* 34:707–718, 2008

Miller CK, Gutschall MD, Lawrence F: The development of self-efficacy and outcome expectation measures regarding glycaemic load and the nutritional management of type 2 diabetes. *Public Health Nutr* 10:628–634, 2007

Miller NH: Motivational interviewing as a prelude to coaching in healthcare settings. *Journal of Cardiovascular Nursing* 25:247–251, 2010

Miller WR, Rollnick S: Meeting in the middle: motivational interviewing and self-determination theory. *International Journal of Behavioral Nutrition and Physical Activity* 9:25, 2012

Miller WR, Rollnick S: Ten things that motivational interviewing is not. *Behavioural and Cognitive Psychotherapy* 37:129–140, 2009

Moore H, Summerbell C, Hooper L, Cruickshank K, Vyas A, Johnstone P, Ashton V, Kopelman P: Dietary advice for treatment of type 2 diabetes mellitus in adults. *Cochrane Database Syst Rev* CD004097, 2004

Mossavar-Rahmani Y: Applying motivational enhancement to diverse populations. *Journal of the American Dietetic Association* 107:918–921, 2007

Niedert KC: Position of the American Dietetic Association: liberalization of the diet prescription improves quality of life for older adults in long-term care. *Journal of the American Dietetic Association* 105:1955–1965, 2005

Nielsen SJ, Popkin BM: Patterns and trends in food portion sizes, 1977–1998. *JAMA* 289:450–453, 2003

Norris SL, Zhang X, Avenell A, Gregg E, Brown TJ, Schmid CH, Lau J: Long-term non-pharmacologic weight loss interventions for adults with type 2 diabetes. *Cochrane Database Syst Rev* CD004095, 2005a

Norris SL, Zhang X, Avenell A, Gregg E, Schmid CH, Lau J: Long-term non-pharmacological weight loss interventions for adults with prediabetes. *Cochrane Database Syst Rev* CD005270, 2005b

Norris SL, Zhang X, Avenell A, Gregg E, Bowman B, Serdula M, Brown TJ, Schmid CH, Lau J: Long-term effectiveness of lifestyle and behavioral weight loss interventions in adults with type 2 diabetes: a meta-analysis. *American Journal of Medicine* 117:762–774, 2004

Pascale RW, Wing RR, Butler BA, Mullen M, Bononi P: Effects of a behavioral weight loss program stressing calorie restriction versus calorie plus fat restriction in obese individuals with NIDDM or a family history of diabetes. *Diabetes Care* 18:1241–1248, 1995

Pastors JG, Franz MJ, Warshaw H, Daly A, Arnold MS: How effective is medical nutrition therapy in diabetes care? *J Am Diet Assoc* 103:827–831, 2003

Pastors JG, Warshaw H, Daly A, Franz M, Kulkarni K: The evidence for the effectiveness of medical nutrition therapy in diabetes management. *Diabetes Care* 25:608–613, 2002

Polonsky WH, Fisher L, Earles J, Dudl RJ, Lees J, Mullan J, Jackson RA: Assessing psychosocial distress in diabetes: development of the diabetes distress scale. *Diabetes Care* 28:626–631, 2005

Polonsky WH, Anderson BJ, Lohrer PA, Welch G, Jacobson AM, Aponte JE, Schwartz CE: Assessment of diabetes-related distress. *Diabetes Care* 18:754–760, 1995

Raynor HA, Jeffery RW, Ruggiero AM, Clark JM, Delahanty LM: Weight loss strategies associated with BMI in overweight adults with type 2 diabetes at entry into the Look AHEAD (Action for Health in Diabetes) trial. *Diabetes Care* 31:1299–1304, 2008

Rejeski WJ, Ip EH, Bertoni AG, Bray GA, Evans G, Gregg EW, Zhang Q: Lifestyle change and mobility in obese adults with type 2 diabetes. *N Engl J Med* 366:1209–1217, 2012

Rolls BJ, Bell EA, Waugh BA: Increasing the volume of a food by incorporating air affects satiety in men. *American Journal of Clinical Nutrition* 72:361–368, 2000

Rowe S, Alexander N, Almeida NG, Black R, Burns R, Bush L, Crawford P, Keim N, Kris-Etherton P, Weaver C: Translating the Dietary Guidelines for Americans 2010 to bring about real behavior change. *Journal of the American Dietetic Association* 111:28–39, 2011

Ruelaz AR, Diefenbach P, Simon B, Lanto A, Arterburn D, Shekelle PG: Perceived barriers to weight management in primary care: perspectives of patients and providers. *J Gen Intern Med* 22:518–522, 2007

Schnepf R, Richardson J: Consumer and food price inflation. Congressional Research Service Report for Congress. R40545. April 14, 2011. Available at www.crs.gov.

Seligman HK, Laraia BA, Kushel MB: Food insecurity is associated with chronic disease among low-income NHANES participants. *J Nutr* 140:304–310, 2010

Seligman HK, Bindman AB, Vittinghoff E, Kanaya AM, Kushel MB: Food insecurity is associated with diabetes mellitus: results from the National Health Examination and Nutrition Examination Survey (NHANES) 1999–2002. *Journal of General Internal Medicine* 22:1018–1023, 2007

Spahn JM, Lyon JM, Altman JM, Blum-Kemelor DM, Essery EV, Fungwe TV, Macneil PC, McGrane MM, Obbagy JE, Wong YP: The systematic review methodology used to support the 2010 Dietary Guidelines Advisory Committee. *Journal of the American Dietetic Association* 111:520–523, 2011

U.S. Department of Agriculture, U.S. Department of Health and Human Services: *Dietary Guidelines for Americans, 2010*. 7th ed. Washington, DC, U.S. Government Printing Office, 2010

Wang YC, Bleich SN, Gortmaker SL: Increasing caloric contribution from sugar-sweetened beverages and 100% fruit juices among US children and adolescents, 1988–2004. *Pediatrics* 121:e1604–1614, 2008

West DS, DiLillo V, Bursac Z, Gore SA, Greene PG: Motivational interviewing improves weight loss in women with type 2 diabetes. *Diabetes Care* 30:1081–1087, 2007

Wildman RP, Muntner P, Reynolds K, McGinn AP, Rajpathak S, Wylie-Rosett J, Sowers MR: The obese without cardiometabolic risk factor clustering and the normal weight with cardiometabolic risk factor clustering: prevalence and correlates of 2 phenotypes among the US population (NHANES 1999–2004). *Arch Intern Med* 168:1617–1624, 2008

Williamson DA, Rejeski J, Lang W, Van Dorsten B, Fabricatore AN, Toledo K: Impact of a weight management program on health-related quality of life in overweight adults with type 2 diabetes. *Archives of Internal Medicine* 169:163–171, 2009

Wing RR, Jeffery RW: Food provision as a strategy to promote weight loss. *Obesity Research* 9 (Suppl. 4):S271–S275, 2001

Wing RR, Jeffery RW, Burton LR, Thorson C, Nissinoff KS, Baxter JE: Food provision vs structured meal plans in the behavioral treatment of obesity. *Int J Obes Relat Metab Disord* 20:56–62, 1996

Wing RR, Blair E, Marcus M, Epstein LH, Harvey J: Year-long weight loss treatment for obese patients with type II diabetes: does including an intermittent very-low-calorie diet improve outcome? *Am J Med* 97:354–362, 1994

Wing RR, Koeske R, Epstein LH, Nowalk MP, Gooding W, Becker D: Long-term effects of modest weight loss in type II diabetic patients. *Archives of Internal Medicine* 147:1749–1753, 1987

Wylie-Rosett J. The diabetes epidemic: what can we do? *Journal of the American Dietetic Association* 109:1160–1162, 2009

Wylie-Rosett J, Elmer P: Cardiovascular risk factor reduction: evaluating dietary intake in assessing nutrition education. *Journal of Patient Education and Counseling* 15:217–227, 1990

Zhang X, Norris SL, Chowdhury FM, Gregg EW, Zhang P: The effects of interventions on health-related quality of life among persons with diabetes: a systematic review. *Medical Care* 45:820–834, 2007

Judith Wylie-Rosett, EdD, RD, is Professor and Head of the Division of Health Promotion and Nutrition Research in the Department of Epidemiology and Population Health at Albert Einstein College of Medicine of Yeshiva University in Bronx, NY.

Linda M. Delahanty, MSRD, is Chief Dietitian and Director of Nutrition and Behavioral Research at Massachusetts General Hospital Diabetes Center in Boston, MA.

Chapter 9
Lifestyle Modification: Exercise

David G. Marrero, PhD
Paula M. Trief, PhD

Exercise is defined as "physical activity and movement, especially when intended to keep a person...fit and healthy" (Casperson 1985), which is reflective of the role it plays in helping to treat diabetes. When considering the role that obesity plays in type 2 diabetes, a second definition is perhaps more useful: "exercise refers to increased physical activity that exceeds normal daily energy expenditures" (Casperson 1985). In this context, exercise can result in calorie consumption, thereby contributing to weight loss and weight maintenance.

In 1953, Joslin wrote, "exercise in the days before insulin we regarded as useful, but by no means did we appreciate it as vital to the care of diabetes.... We should return to it to help us in the treatment of all our cases" (Joslin 1953). Over 40 years of research has proven Joslin's observation to be prophetic: regular physical exercise has many benefits for people with both type 1 and type 2 diabetes. It is well accepted, based on studies with high levels of evidence, that regular participation in physical activity has direct health benefits, especially for patients with diabetes (Sigal 2006). Physical activity is associated with improved insulin action, glycemic control, and weight loss, as well as decreased body fat, blood pressure, cholesterol, and lipids that lead to reduction of cardiovascular risk (Grundy 2004, Waxman 2005, Haskell 2007). Physical activity has also been part of the lifestyle change interventions that have prevented, delayed, or slowed the progression of some diabetes-related complications (Boulé 2001). Moreover, exercise has been shown to help with the maintenance of weight loss, which contributes to the prevention of type 2 diabetes (T2D) in people with increased risk factors (Knowler 2002, Ratner 2005).

Exercise also has been demonstrated to help with the treatment of depression, which is a comorbid condition associated with diabetes (Anderson 2001, de Groot 2001). Meta-analyses demonstrated that exercise reduced depression in community populations (Craft 2004, Sjosten 2006). In the Look AHEAD trial, people with T2D who participated in the intensive lifestyle intervention experienced improvements in quality of life and depression that were mediated by improved physical fitness (Williamson 2009).

UNDERUTILIZATION OF BEHAVIORAL INTERVENTIONS TO INCREASE DAILY ACTIVITY

Based on psychological benefits as well as weight-related improvements in metabolic efficiency (Grundy 2004, Waxman 2005, Haskell 2007), the initiation of leisure time activities that include physical activity is strongly recommended

(American Diabetes Association [ADA] 2004, Hayes 2008). Yet, some data show that diabetes patients are less active than those without diabetes. A survey of inhabitants of South Carolina found that 42% of adults with diabetes (both type 1 and type 2) were "physically inactive," as compared with 27% of adults without diabetes (Van Vrancken 2004). Similarly, in a large survey of Mexican-Americans with diabetes (both type 1 and type 2), only 61% reported that they exercised (Wood 2004), with gardening (33.7%) and walking (31.5%) being the leisure time activities they engaged in most frequently. In another study that explored racial/ethnic differences in physical activity, 32,440 American adults were surveyed, of whom 1,850 had diabetes (both type 1 and type 2). Overall, only 25% engaged in moderate/vigorous physical activity daily, with blacks (16%) less active than Hispanics (23%) or whites (27%) (Egede 2004). More detailed analyses found that the significant racial differences identified were due almost totally to the low level of physical activity of black women. Since physical activity in occupations and housework was not included, findings need to be replicated and expanded. However, these results underscore the fact that the general population of U.S. adults tends to be sedentary; that minority adults—who are at greater risk for T2D—have lower rates of physical activity; and that targeting physical activity to improve health status is indicated in a significant portion of the U.S. population.

For diabetes patients, the presence and severity of complications is likely to affect physical activity. Each type of complication has been linked to specific activity recommendations that may limit one's options. Some recommend that resistance or vigorous aerobic exercise be avoided if one has proliferative or severe nonproliferative retinopathy, due to the risk of retinal detachment or vitreous hemorrhage (Aiello 2002). When one is dealing with severe neuropathy, with associated pain and numbness, non-weight-bearing activities (e.g., biking, swimming) are encouraged (Sigal 2004). Autonomic neuropathy may increase the risk of injury related to exercise, and cardiac evaluation is strongly recommended (Sigal 2004). Most studies of exercise with diabetes patients have confirmed the significant health benefits of all forms of exercise, including aerobic exercise, resistance training, and flexibility training (Sigal 2004). Given the health benefits and the limited evidence of increased risk, most studies recommend that one identify ways to increase physical activity while minimizing risk, rather than avoid activity. Systematic incorporation and monitoring of an exercise goal (which should be considered a self-management behavior) as part of routine diabetes care is often not achieved.

INDICATIONS

Regular daily exercise is indicated for all people and in particular for people with diabetes, unless there are specific contraindications. Increasing evidence suggests that regular physical activity should be initiated upon diagnosis (Basevi 2011). Regular sessions of exercise can contribute to reduced mortality and morbidity, having direct effects on glycemic control, maintenance of weight loss, and improvement of psychological well-being (Scully 1998, Wei 2000, Boulé 2001, Boulé 2003, Church 2004). The potential impact of exercise on weight regulation is particularly important for people with T2D who tend to be overweight or obese, a condition that increases insulin resistance and cardiovascular risk (Berlin 1990, Barrett-Connor 1991, Scully 1998, Borghouts 2000, Wei 2000, Boulé 2001, Boulé 2003, Church 2004). There are potential risks associated with exercise for the person with diabetes and some limitations for those with preexisting diabetes-related complications. These include the potential for hypoglycemia and hyperglycemia resulting from exercise and the risk of exacerbating specific diabetes complications (Gordon 2001, Ganda 2002, Sigal 2006, Basevi 2011). Although exercise tends to reduce glucose levels, it is possible for glucose levels to increase with exercise if the glucose level is high at the start of the exercise session.

Before beginning an exercise program, all people with diabetes should have a physical examination to ensure that a safe, individualized program can be developed (Borghouts 2000, Basevi 2011). This examination should emphasize assessing whether macro- and/or microvascular complications are present, which would mean that some forms of exercise are not recommended. These complications include muscle-skeletal injuries or abnormalities, some forms of cardiovascular disease (CVD), and microangiopathic disease that contraindicates Valsalva activity (Borghouts 2000, Basevi 2011). People with microvascular disease, particularly retinopathy, should avoid exercises that increase blood pressure in the microvascular system by Valsalva processes such as weight lifting (Basevi 2011). In such cases, several alternatives (e.g., walking) may be explored to increase levels of physical activity. In addition, people with T2D should have a stress test to evaluate the integrity of their cardiovascular and respiratory systems (Gordon 2001, Fowler-Brown 2004, U.S. Preventive Services Task Force 2004). An advantage of a stress test is that it helps to establish target heart rate limits within which a person with autonomic neuropathy can safely exercise. In addition, exercise-induced hypertension can be identified, which will enable the most appropriate exercise in terms of type, intensity, and duration that will minimize health risks (Fowler-Brown 2004, U.S. Preventive Services Task Force 2004). There is some disagreement about whether exercise electrocardiogram (ECG) stress tests are required for all diabetes patients or only those with other risk factors. However, the presence of complications heightens concerns regarding the relationship of cardiac and respiratory function to exercise intensity and frequency and the need for screening using stress tests (Sigal 2004).

TARGET OF INTERVENTIONS

The exercise prescription should be based on the patient's personal goals and assessment of the ability of the individual to safely and realistically implement a given exercise activity in his or her environment (Marrero 2001). Likely goals include improved glycemic control, reduced cardiovascular risk, weight loss, and increased strength or endurance. Some may want to exercise for general fitness, whereas others have competitive athletic goals. Regardless of the goal chosen, all people with diabetes are candidates for regular exercise unless, as noted, they have physical conditions that contraindicate engaging in physical activity. In cases where weight-bearing activities are contraindicated due to muscle-skeletal injuries or abnormalities, alternatives that reduce weight load such as swimming and water aerobics can be considered.

KNOWN TREATMENT METHODS

The first step in initiating an exercise program is often the recommendation from the patient's physician. Counseling from a health care provider can be a powerful source of motivation and support (Kirk 2004a, Armit 2009).

  Most people will benefit from having an individualized exercise program developed with the assistance of a certified exercise specialist—an exercise physiologist, a certified exercise trainer, or a cardiac rehabilitation specialist. Qualified exercise staff includes people with certification by the American College of Sports Medicine (ASCM), the American Council on Exercise (ACE), the Aerobic and Fitness Association of America (AFFA), or the International Fitness Professionals Association (IFPA). In addition, depending on the form of exercise chosen, a certified instructor who has training in the specific exercise mode should be used (Gordon 2001, Sigal 2006). When these resources are not available, a community center such as the YMCA that can provide some guidance in proper exercise procedures is recommended (Marrero 2001). If no support resources are available, a program of regular walking is recommended. If a person is going to initiate an unsupervised exercise program, it is important that he or she is counseled to pay attention to basic safety procedures. These include a slow and gradual progression in both exercise duration and intensity, the use of proper footwear if walking is the chosen activity, and awareness of any physical sensations that suggest a potential problem, such as acute pain, tightness in the chest, shortness of breath, or confusion. If any such symptoms are experienced, exercise activity should be suspended until a medical evaluation can be conducted (Gordon 2001). Although these recommendations are not specific to patients with diabetes, they represent foundation guidelines that the clinician can present during a medical management visit.

DEVELOPMENT OF A FORMAL EXERCISE PROGRAM

Before initiation of a formal exercise program, an exercise assessment should be carried out to allow prescription of an appropriate program for the individual. Diabetes history should include type of diabetes, duration of diabetes, presence of complications of diabetes, treatment for glucose control, frequency of self-monitoring of blood glucose, frequency of hypoglycemia, including severity and relationship to activity, and current diabetes control. As noted, exercise can both reduce and elevate blood glucose depending on several factors. If an individual begins exercise when his or her glucose is low normal (i.e., 80 mg/dl), the physical activity may cause low blood glucose levels, especially if insulin is used to control the diabetes. Thus, it is important to both assess blood glucose before beginning to exercise and have a form of fast-acting carbohydrate available to counteract low blood glucose levels. Similarly, for patients with type 1 diabetes beginning to exercise when glucose is high (i.e., >250 mg/dl) can elevate blood glucose by stimulating the release of hepatic glucose stores. Thus, for patients with type 1 diabetes (T1D), it is important to assess blood glucose levels prior to exercise and to time exercise to coincide with glucose ranges that are safe: between 80 and 240 mg/dl. In the absence of severe insulin deficiency, such as type 2 diabetic patients early in disease course, light- or moderate-intensity exercise would tend to decrease plasma glucose. Therefore, provided the person with T2D is hydrated, and urine and/or blood ketones are negative, it is not necessary to postpone exercise based solely on hyperglycemia (Sigal 2006).

If the goal of the exercise program is to help with weight regulation, goals need to be established to achieve a caloric expenditure. This requires that exercise activity be prescribed with regard to duration and intensity to achieve a caloric consumption. There are several charts available that provide estimates of caloric consumption for various physical activities that can be used to determine a suitable program (Ainsworth 2011, Dutton 2008).

BEHAVIORAL INTERVENTIONS

A number of studies have identified effective lifestyle interventions (Kirk 2004b, Jackson 2007, Dutton 2008, Liebreich 2009). Large-scale studies such as the Diabetes Prevention Program and Look AHEAD have used multiple interventions, including goal setting, self-monitoring, frequent contact, and stepped-care protocols (Diabetes Prevention Program [DPP] Research Group 2002, Craft 2004, Look AHEAD Research Group 2006, Eakin 2008). Both of these interventions are taught in a sequential series of sessions by a trained facilitator. The facilitators negotiate the weight-loss goal with the client and teach specific strategies to accomplish weight loss, such as methods for tracking food and reducing fat grams. Effective interventions have been delivered in a variety of formats and modes of delivery, including print (Dutton 2008), Internet (Glasgow 2005, Liebreich 2009), phone (Clark 2004, Kirk 2004a, Sacco 2009), and, of course, in person (Keyserling 2002, Jackson 2007). For example, Weight Watchers uses a sophisticated online intervention that assists users in tracking food intake and making food selections that are based on a point system that reflects composition and calorie content. Although the long-term efficacy and cost-effectiveness of many programs have not been assessed, the existing evaluations suggest that these interventions are cost-effective (Jacobs-van der Bruggen 2007, Jacobs-van der Bruggen 2009).

PSYCHOSOCIAL FACTORS IN TREATMENT

Problems with motivation and psychosocial issues often interfere with adherence to an exercise regimen and the level of physical activity. Thus, a clear assessment of personal motivation and supportive resources is essential to select an exercise form that is likely to be adhered to (Marrero 2001). This includes review of personal likes and dislikes, assessment of the availability of supportive resources (i.e., facilities, trainers, equipment), and assessment of potential barriers to regularly performing a chosen activity. In this regard, it is valuable to question patients about past successes and challenges with exercise and to have them identify the time of day most likely to allow consistency of exercise. The critical factor is that individuals need to select a form of activity that is personally meaningful and rewarding, supportable within their environment, and compatible with their social and economic circumstances and physical status (Gordon 2001, Marrero 2001).

Depression, stress, and anxiety may need to be treated to allow the initiation of an exercise routine (Marrero 2001). In this regard, it is noteworthy that exercise has been shown to help reduce depressive symptoms (Aljasem 2001, Craft 2004, Sjosten 2006, McGale 2011). Self-efficacy, which can decrease depression, is an important determinant of physical activity (Delahanty 2006, Dutton 2009, Williamson 2009). A realistic exercise prescription should allow early success, enhancing self-efficacy for future changes (Peyrot 2007). This includes choosing an appropriate mode, duration, frequency, and intensity of exercise. Once the routine is established, increases can be made to reach long-term exercise goals (Gordon 2001, Marrero 2001, Mullooly 2003).

It is also valuable to engage social support systems, especially family, to help people to both initiate and maintain an exercise program. Because family support is instrumental in maximizing the likelihood that a person will both initiate and sustain a regular exercise program, it is important to include family members in the decision-making process (Carron 1996, Mier 2007, Ogilvie 2007, Gleeson-Kreig 2008).

SETTING OF CARE

There are a wide variety of settings that can support exercise programs, and the availability of appropriate settings may be an important factor influencing regular physical activity (Deshpande 2005). Which are chosen depends upon the form of exercise selected. It is not necessary to exercise in a formal facility. There are several options for setting up an exercise program in the home (Fisher 1994, Duncan 1998, Jette 1998). For example, work by Jette et al. (1998) has demonstrated an effective exercise program using common household items such as canned goods for modest resistance while sitting in chairs. There is also ample evidence that simple walking has many exercise benefits, especially for people with diabetes (Hu 1999). The benefit of walking is that it can be done in a variety of settings that do not involve cost, are easily accessible, and can be adapted to variations in weather.

ONGOING MONITORING OF OUTCOMES

There are several forms of monitoring the outcomes associated with a regular exercise program. These include attendance logs and a variety of performance indicators (e.g., increases in time spent exercising; changes in weight, blood pressure, or glucose levels) (Gordon 2001, Marrero 2001). An essential component is to use some form of self-monitoring and to have assistance by the health care team in monitoring physiologic changes associated with the physical activity bouts and over time. Physical activity per se can be measured by questionnaire, pedometer, or accelerometer (methods for assessing physical activity are available at http://www.cdc.gov/physicalactivity/professionals/data/explanation.html). Pedometer-based interventions have been found to be effective for increasing physical activity (Tudor-Locke 2004, Bravata 2007, Ogilvie 2007), in part because increasing awareness by monitoring of activity is itself a powerful intervention.

RECOMMENDATIONS FOR CLINICAL CARE

A recent review of the relevant research and position statements on exercise and diabetes summarizes the current recommendations concerning exercise, physical activity, and diabetes management (ADA 2004). The authors note that the exercise recommendations vary depending on the patient's health goals. In summary, they recommend:

1. At least 150 min/week of moderate intensity aerobic activity and/or 90 min/week of vigorous aerobic exercise if the goals are to improve glycemic control, reduce CVD risk, or maintain weight (ADA 2004)
2. Resistance exercise 3 times per week for T2D patients, if complications do not contraindicate, with initial assessment and periodic reevaluation by an exercise specialist (ADA 2004)
3. Stress testing before vigorous exercise for patients >30 years of age if there are other risk factors, and for all diabetes patients >40 years of age (ADA 2004)
4. Psychosocial assessment to include assessment of depression (using a standardized survey tool such as the nine-item depression scale of the Patient Health Questionnaire [PHQ-9]) and assessment of the client's perception of self-efficacy to engage in exercise (using a standardized measure) (Lee 1994, Kroenke 2001) should be performed before formulating an exercise prescription or implementing an exercise program (Colberg 2010).
5. Behavioral strategies, including but not limited to goal setting and developing programs that implement gradual but increasing intensity and that integrate reinforcement for achieving milestones, should be used to assist patients in initiating and sustaining an exercise program (Colberg 2010).

BIBLIOGRAPHY

Aiello LP, Wong J, Cavallerano JD, Bursell SE, Aiello LM: Retinopathy. In *Handbook of Exercise in Diabetes.* 2nd ed. Ruderman N, Devlin JT, Schneider SH, Kriska A, Eds. Alexandria, VA, American Diabetes Association, 2002, p. 401–413

Ainsworth BE, et al.: 2011 compendium of physical activities: a second update of codes and MET values. *Med Sci Sports Exerc* 43:1575, 2011

Aljasem LI, Peyrot M, Wissow L, Rubin RR: The impact of barriers and self-efficacy on self-care behaviors in type 2 diabetes. *Diabetes Educ* 27:393–404, 2001

American Diabetes Association: Physical activity/exercise and diabetes (Position Statement). *Diabetes Care* 27 (Suppl. 1):S58–S62, 2004

Anderson RJ, Freedland KE, Clouse RE, Lustman PJ: The prevalence of cormorbid depression in adults with diabetes: a meta analysis. *Diabetes Care* 24:1069–1078, 2001

Armit CM, Brown WJ, Marshall AL, Ritchie CB, Trost SG, Green A, Bauman AE: Randomized trial of three strategies to promote physical activity in general practice. *Prev Med* 48:156–163, 2009

Barrett-Connor EL, Wingard DL, Edelstein SL: Why is diabetes a stronger risk factor for fatal ischemic heart disease in women than in men? The Rancho Bernardo Study. *JAMA* 265:627–631, 1991

Basevi V, Di Mario S, Morciano C, Nonino F, Magrini N: Comment on: American Diabetes Association: Standards of Medical Care in Diabetes—2011. *Diabetes Care* 34 (Suppl. 1):S11–S61, 2011

Berlin JA, Colditz GA: A meta-analysis of physical activity in the prevention of coronary heart disease. *American Journal of Epidemiology* 132:612–628, 1990

Borghouts LB, Keizer HA: Exercise and insulin sensitivity: a review. *International Journal of Sports Medicine* 21:1–12, 2000

Boulé NG, Kenny GP, Haddad E, Wells GA, Sigal RJ: Meta-analysis of the effect of structured exercise training on cardiorespiratory fitness in type 2 diabetes mellitus. *Diabetologia* 46:1071–1081, 2003

Boulé NG, Haddad E, Kenny GP, Wells GA, Sigal RJ: Effects of exercise on glycemic control and body mass in type 2 diabetes mellitus: a meta-analysis of controlled clinical trials. *JAMA* 286:1218–1227, 2001

Bravata DM, Smith-Spangler C, Sundaram V, Gienger AL, et al.: Using pedometers to increase physical activity and improve health: a systematic review. *JAMA* 298:2296–2304, 2007

Carron AV, Hausenblas HA, Mack D: Social influence and exercise: a meta-analysis. *J Sport Exercise Psychology* 18:1–16, 1996

Caspersen CJ, Powell KE, Christenson GM: Physical activity, exercise, and physical fitness: definitions and distinctions for health-related research. *Public Health Rep* 100:126–131, 1985

Church TS, Cheng YJ, Earnest CP, Barlow CE, Gibbons LW, Priest EL, Blair SN: Exercise capacity and body composition as predictors of mortality among men with diabetes. *Diabetes Care* 27:83–88, 2004

Clark M, Hampson SE, Avery L, Simpson R: Effects of a tailored lifestyle self-management intervention in patients with type 2 diabetes. *Br J Health Psychol* 9:365–379, 2004

Colberg SR, Sigal RJ, Fernhall B, Regensteiner JG, Blissmer BJ, Rubin RR, Chasan-Taber L, Albright AL, Braun B: Exercise and type 2 diabetes: the American College of Sports Medicine and the American Diabetes Association: joint position statement. *Diabetes Care* 33:e147–e167, 2010

Craft LL, Perna FM: The benefits of exercise for the clinically depressed. *Prim Care Companion J Clin Psychiatry* 6:104–111, 2004

de Groot M, Anderson RJ, Freedland KE, Clouse RE, Lustman PJ: The association of depression and diabetes complications: a meta analysis. *Psychosomatic Medicine* 63:619–630, 2001

Delahanty LM, Conroy MB, Nathan DM: Psychological predictors of physical activity in the Diabetes Prevention Program. *J Am Diet Assoc* 106:698–705, 2006

Deshpande AD, Baker EA, Lovegreen SL, Brownson RC: Environmental correlates of physical activity among individuals with diabetes in the rural midwest. *Diabetes Care* 28:1012–1018, 2005

Diabetes Prevention Program (DPP) Research Group: The Diabetes Prevention Program (DPP): description of lifestyle intervention. *Diabetes Care* 25:2165–2171, 2002

Duncan P, Richards L, Wallace D, Stoker-Yates J, Pohl P, Luchies C, Ogle A, Studenski S: A randomized, controlled pilot study of a home-based exercise program for individuals with mild and moderate stroke. *Stroke* 29:2055–2060, 1998

Dutton GR, Tan F, Provost BC, Sorenson JL, Allen B, Smith D: Relationship between self-efficacy and physical activity among patients with type 2 diabetes. *J Behav Med* 32:270–277, 2009

Dutton GR, Provost BC, Tan F, Smith D: A tailored print-based physical activity intervention for patients with type 2 diabetes. *Preventive Medicine* 47:409–411, 2008

Eakin EG, Reeves MM, Lawler SP, Oldenburg B, et al.: The Logan Healthy Living Program: a cluster randomized trial of a telephone delivered physical activity and dietary behavior intervention for primary care patients with type 2 diabetes or hypertension from a socially disadvantaged community: rationale, design and recruitment. *Contemp Clin Trials* 29:439–454, 2008

Egede LE, Poston ME: Racial/ethnic differences in leisure-time physical activity levels among individuals with diabetes. *Diabetes Care* 27:2493–2494, 2004

Fisher NM, Kame VD Jr, Rouse L, Pendergast DR: Quantitative evaluation of a home exercise program on muscle and functional capacity of patients with osteoarthritis. *Am J Phys Med Rehabil* 73:413–420, 1994

Fowler-Brown A, Pignone M, Pletcher M, Tice JA, Sutton SF, Lohr KN: Exercise tolerance testing to screen for coronary heart disease: a systematic review for the technical support for the U.S. Preventive Services Task Force. *Ann Intern Med* 140:W9–W24, 2004

Ganda OP: Patients on various drug therapies. In *Handbook of Exercise in Diabetes*. 2nd ed. Ruderman N, Devlin JT, Schneider SH, Kriska A, Eds. Alexandria, VA, American Diabetes Association, 2002, p. 587–599

Glasgow RE, Nutting PA, King DK, Nelson CC, et al.: Randomized effectiveness trial of a computer-assisted intervention to improve diabetes care. *Diabetes Care* 28:33–39, 2005

Gleeson-Kreig J: Social support and physical activity in type 2 diabetes: a social-ecologic approach. *Diabetes Educ* 34:1037–1044, 2008

Gordon NF: The exercise prescription. In *Handbook of Exercise in Diabetes*. Ruderman N, Devlin JT, Schneider SH, Eds. Alexandria, VA, American Diabetes Association, 2001, p. 269–288

Grundy SM, Hansen B, Smith SC, Cleeman JI, Kahn RA, et al.: Clinical management of metabolic syndrome: report of the American Heart Association/National Heart, Lung, and Blood Institute/American Diabetes Association conference on scientific issues related to management. *Circulation* 109:551–556, 2004

Haskell WL, Lee IM, Pate RR, Powell KE, Blair SN, Franklin BA, et al.: Physical activity and public health: updated recommendation for adults from the American College of Sports Medicine and the American Heart Association. *Medicine and Science in Sports and Exercise* 39:1423–1434, 2007

Hayes C, Kriska A: Role of physical activity in diabetes management and prevention. *Journal of the American Dietetic Association* 108 (Suppl. 1):S19–S23, 2008

Hu FB, Sigal RJ, Rich-Edwards JW, Colditz GA, Solomon CG, Willet WC, Speizer FE, Manson JE: Walking compared with vigorous physical activity and risk of type 2 diabetes in women. *JAMA* 282:1433–1439, 1999

Jackson R, Asimakopoulou K, Scammell A: Assessment of the transtheoretical model as used by dietitians in promoting physical activity in people with type 2 diabetes. *J Hum Nutr Diet* 20:27–36, 2007

Jacobs-van der Bruggen MA, van Baal PH, Hoogenveen RT, Feenstra TL, et al.: Cost-effectiveness of lifestyle modification in diabetes patients. *Diabetes Care* 32:1453–1458, 2009

Jacobs-van der Bruggen MA, Bos G, Bemelmans WJ, Hoogenveen RT, Vijgen SM, Baan CA: Lifestyle interventions are cost-effective in people with different levels of diabetes risk: results from a modeling study. *Diabetes Care* 30:128–134, 2007

Jette AM, Rooks D, Lachman M, Lin TH, Levenson C, Helstein D, Giorgetti MM, Harris BA: Home-based resistance training predictors of participation and adherence. *Gerontologist* 38:412–421, 1998

Joslin EP: *A Diabetic Manual for Doctor and Patient*. 9th ed. Philadelphia, Lea & Febiger, 1953

Keyserling TC, Samuel-Hodge CD, Ammerman AS, Ainsworth BE, et al.: A randomized trial of an intervention to improve self-care behaviors of African-American women with type 2 diabetes: impact on physical activity. *Diabetes Care* 25:1576–1583, 2002

Kirk A, Mutrie N, MacIntyre P, Fisher M: Effects of a 12-month physical activity counselling intervention on glycaemic control and on the status of cardiovascular risk factors in people with type 2 diabetes. *Diabetologia* 47:821–832, 2004a

Kirk AF, Mutrie N, Macintyre PD, Fisher MB: Promoting and maintaining physical activity in people with type 2 diabetes. *Am J Prev Med* 27:289–296, 2004b

Knowler WC, Barrett-Connor E, Fowler SE, Hamman RF, Lachin JM, Walker EA, Nathan DM, Diabetes Prevention Program Research Group: Reduction in the incidence of type 2 diabetes with lifestyle intervention or metformin. *N Engl J Med* 346:393–403, 2002

Kroenke K, Spitzer RL, Williams, JBW: The PHQ-9 validity of a brief depression severity measure. *Journal of General Internal Medicine* 16:606–613, 2001

Lee C, Bobko P: Self-efficacy beliefs: comparison of five measures. *Journal of Applied Psychology* 79:364–369, 1994

Liebreich T, Plotnikoff RC, Courneya KS, Boule N: Diabetes NetPLAY: a physical activity website and linked email counselling randomized intervention for individuals with type 2 diabetes. *Int J Behav Nutr Phys Act* 6:18, 2009

Look AHEAD Research Group, Wadden TA, West DS, Delahanty L, et al.: The Look AHEAD study: a description of the lifestyle intervention and the evidence supporting it. *Obesity (Silver Spring)* 14:737–752, 2006

Marrero DG: Initiation and maintenance of exercise in patients with diabetes. *Handbook of Exercise in Diabetes.* Ruderman N, Devlin JT, Schneider SH, Eds. Alexandria, VA, American Diabetes Association, 2001, p. 289–309

McGale N, McArdle S, Gaffney P: Exploring the effectiveness of an integrated exercise/CBT intervention for young men's mental health. *Br J Health Psychol* 16:457–471, 2011

Mier N, Medina AA, Ory MG: Mexican Americans with type 2 diabetes: perspectives on definitions, motivators, and programs of physical activity. *Prev Chronic Dis* 4:A24, 2007

Mulloolly CA, Hanson, CK: Physical activity/exercise. In *A Core Curriculum for Diabetes Education.* 5th ed. Franz M, Ed. Chicago, American Association of Diabetes Educators, 2003

Ogilvie D, Foster CE, Rothnie H, Cavill N, et al.: Interventions to promote walking: systematic review. *BMJ* 334:1204, 2007

Peyrot M, Rubin RR: Behavioral and psychosocial interventions in diabetes: a conceptual review. *Diabetes Care* 30:2433–2440, 2007

Ratner R, Goldberg R, Haffner S, Marcovina S, Orchard T, Fowler S, Temprosa M, Diabetes Prevention Program Research Group: Impact of intensive lifestyle and metformin therapy on cardiovascular disease risk factors in the diabetes prevention program. *Diabetes Care* 28:888–894, 2005

Sacco WP, Malone JI, Morrison AD, Friedman A, Wells K: Effect of a brief, regular telephone intervention by paraprofessionals for type 2 diabetes. *J Behav Med* 32:349–359, 2009

Scully D, Kremmer J, Meade MM, Dudgeon K: Physical exercise and psychological well being: a critical review. *British Journal of Sports Medicine* 32:111–120, 1998

Sigal RJ, Kenny GP, Wasserman DH, Castaneda-Sceppa C, White RD: Physical activity/exercise and type 2 diabetes: a consensus statement from the American Diabetes Association. *Diabetes Care* 29:1433–1438, 2006

Sigal RJ, Kenny GP, Wasserman DH, Castaneda-Sceppa C: Physical activity/exercise and type 2 diabetes. *Diabetes Care* 27:2518–2539, 2004

Sjosten N, Kivela SL: The effects of physical exercise on depressive symptoms among the aged: a systematic review. *Int J Geriatr Psychiatry* 21:410–418, 2006

Tudor-Locke C, Bell RC, Myers AM, Harris SB, et al.: Controlled outcome evaluation of the First Step Program: a daily physical activity intervention for individuals with type II diabetes. *Int J Obes Relat Metab Disord* 28:113–119, 2004

U.S. Preventive Services Task Force: Screening for coronary heart disease: recommendation statement. *Ann Intern Med* 140:569–572, 2004

Van Vrancken C, Bopp CM, Reis JP, DuBose KD, Kirtland KA, Ainsworth BE: The prevalence of leisure-time physical activity among diabetics in South Carolina. *Southern Medical Journal* 97:141–144, 2004

Waxman A: Why a global strategy on diet, physical activity and health? *World Review of Nutrition and Dietetics* 95,162–166, 2005

Wei M, Gibbons LW, Kampert JB, Nichaman MZ, Blair SN: Low cardiorespiratory fitness and physical inactivity as predictors of mortality in men with type 2 diabetes. *Ann Intern Med* 132:605–611, 2000

Williamson DA, Rejeski J, Lang W, Van Dorsten B, et al.: Impact of a weight management program on health-related quality of life in overweight adults with type 2 diabetes. *Arch Intern Med* 169:163–171, 2009

Wood FG: Leisure time activity of Mexican Americans with diabetes. *Journal of Advanced Nursing* 45:190–196, 2004

David G. Marrero, PhD, is the J.O. Ritchey Professor of Medicine and Director, Diabetes Translational Research Center at the Indiana University School of Medicine in Indianapolis, IN.

Paula M. Trief, PhD, is a Professor in the departments of Psychiatry and Medicine at SUNY Upstate Medical University in Syracuse, NY, where she also serves as Senior Associate Dean for Faculty Affairs and Faculty Development.

Chapter 10

Subcutaneous Insulin Infusion or Insulin Pump Therapy

JILL WEISSBERG-BENCHELL, PhD, CDE

Data from the Diabetes Control and Complications Trial Research Group (DCCT) (1993, 1995, 2001) and UK Prospective Diabetes Study (UKPDS) Group (1998) highlight the importance of achieving tight metabolic control in improving health outcomes. Intensified regimens have been recommended to optimize diabetes control, using either multiple daily injections (MDI) or continuous subcutaneous insulin infusion (CSII). CSII offers a more precise physiologic method of insulin administration than multiple daily injections. Although intensified regimens are technologically advanced, they also increase the daily burden on the patient and the patient's family. The increase in daily care tasks and the increase in time focused on diabetes care can make the balance between living a well-rounded life and caring for the medically specific needs of the person's diabetes a challenge for all concerned. Researchers have sought to determine if CSII improves not only an individual's medical outcomes, but also an individual's psychosocial outcomes. A summary of these findings is presented in this chapter.

GLYCEMIC CONTROL

The majority of studies assessing the efficacy of CSII therapy looked at the impact of CSII on glycemic control. Over 100 studies assessed glycohemoglobin, and almost all of these studies found lower glycohemoglobin among patients using CSII than among patients using MDI/CT (multiple daily injections/ conventional treatment), with four meta-analyses confirming this finding (Weissberg-Benchell 2003, Jeitler 2008, Pickup 2008, Pankowska 2009). These findings held for school-aged children, adolescents, and adults (Hoogma 2005, Nuboer 2008). The data on preschoolers is less clear, however. Four randomized controlled trials (RCTs) in preschoolers have been conducted. Two (DiMeglio 2004, Nabhan 2009) found improvements in A1C within the first 6 months of CSII use, with a return to baseline A1C by the end of 1 year. The other two RCTs (Wilson 2005, Opipari-Arrigan 2007) found no difference between MDI and CSII in A1C.

Two studies assessed the underlying reasons for suboptimal control among youth using CSII (Burdick 2004, Olinder 2009) and found that missed meal boluses and infrequent blood glucose checks were the likely cause. There have been 4 meta-analyses, 10 RCTs, 5 matched control studies, and >25 longitudinal pre-post studies assessing glycemic control in CSII since 2003. Overall, the data support the statement that metabolic control is better among individuals (except for preschoolers) using CSII than individuals using MDI therapy.

INSULIN REQUIREMENTS

More than 50 studies assessed changes in the amount of insulin used per day, with 16 published after 2003. Almost all of them found that patients required less insulin per day when using CSII, and these findings held regardless of the age of the subjects (preschoolers, school-aged children, adolescents, or adults) and regardless of the duration of diabetes. Three meta-analyses (Weissberg-Benchell 2003, Jeitler 2008, Pankowska 2009), four RCTs, three matched control studies, and nine longitudinal pre-post studies have assessed insulin requirements in CSII use since 2003. Overall, the data support the statement that individuals using CSII require less insulin per day than individuals using MDI therapy.

BODY WEIGHT

Over 30 studies assessed the impact of CSII on body weight. However actual data for weight (the mean and standard deviations) were not reported in the text of the articles. Meta-analyses have not been able to assess BMI changes due to the relatively low rate of documenting weight. For those studies published since 2003, only three RCTs assessed weight, and the findings were inconsistent (Doyle 2004, Hoogma 2005, Weintrob 2006). Similarly, both matched control studies and longitudinal pre-post studies report inconsistent findings. Overall, CSII does not appear to lead to weight loss, and most studies report that CSII is weight-neutral. Nevertheless, the impact of CSII therapy on weight remains inconclusive.

HYPOGLYCEMIA

Over 60 studies reported comparison data between CSII and injection therapies with respect to the frequency of hypoglycemic events. One barrier to assessing rate of hypoglycemia is the difference in how hypoglycemia was defined in the studies. For example, data were reported in various studies as frequency of events for the duration of the study, frequency of events per patient-week, frequency of events per patient-year, and frequency of events per 100 patient-years. Moreover, many studies did not clearly define what "severe hypoglycemia" meant, and often the definition was deferred to the self-report of the patient. The meta-analysis by Pickup (2008) suggests that rates of severe hypoglycemic episodes are lowered on CSII compared with MDI, whereas the meta-analysis by Pankowska (2009) suggests that the rates of hypoglycemic episodes do not differ based on method of insulin delivery. Of the six RCTs published since 2003, two report decreased rates of severe hypoglycemia (Hoogma 2005, Nuboer 2008), and four report no changes in the rate of severe hypoglycemic episodes (DiMeglio 2004, Fox 2005, Weintrob 2006, Skogsberg 2008). The three matched-control studies are similarly inconclusive, with one showing a reduction in severe hypoglycemia (Jakisch 2008) and two reporting no change (Alemzadeh 2004, Johannesen 2008). The longitudinal pre-post studies seem to support the conclusion that rates of severe hypoglycemic episodes are reduced when moving from MDI to CSII therapy; 14 studies since 2003 report such a reduced rate (e.g., Weinzimer 2004, Nimri 2006, Gimenez 2007, Kapellen 2007) and only three report no change (Shehadeh 2004, Sulli 2006, Rabbone 2009). Overall, the risk of hypoglycemic events does not appear to be higher on CSII therapy than on MDI therapy.

DIABETIC KETOACIDOSIS (DKA)

The studies reporting on the rate of DKA among patients using CSII therapy have inconclusive findings, with approximately equal numbers showing increased and decreased rates. The risk of DKA appeared to be higher on CSII prior to the release of the DCCT in 1993 (Mecklenberg 1984, Dusseldorf Study Group 1990, Weissberg-Benchell 2003). Data after the release of the DCCT are inconclusive, with one meta-analysis (Pankowska 2008) showing no change in rate of DKA and another showing too few episodes of DKA to complete a formal meta-analysis (Jeitler 2009). No RCTs since 2003 have reported on episodes of DKA. One matched-control study (Jakisch 2008) found a decreased risk of DKA in youth on CSII therapy, as did one longitudinal pre-post study (Rodriques 2005). Other longitudinal pre-post studies found no change in DKA risk (Nimri 2006, Sulli 2006, Gimenez 2007).

DEPRESSION AND ANXIETY

Relatively few studies have assessed depression and none have assessed anxiety among individuals using CSII therapy. Two pre-post longitudinal studies on children and teenagers report improved depressive symptoms (Shapiro 1984, Boland 1999) and one cross-sectional study of adults (Hislop 2008) on CSII therapy reports worsening depressive symptoms. It is currently unclear what the impact of CSII therapy is on either depressive or anxious symptoms.

QUALITY OF LIFE

There appears to be an increase in studies assessing the quality of life among individuals using CSII, especially over the past five years, with the majority of them finding improved quality of life, regardless of age or study design (e.g., Hoogma 2005, McMahon 2005, Opipari-Arrigan 2007, Nuboer 2008, Muller-Godeffroy 2009). No studies found worsening quality of life, although a few found no differences (Wilson 2005, Weintrob 2006, Cogen 2007, Fox 2007). One concern in assessing quality of life is the definition of the construct (Varni 2003b, Barnard 2007) as well as the variety of measures used to assess the construct.

TREATMENT SATISFACTION

All studies assessing satisfaction with the treatment regimen showed satisfaction with CSII therapy regardless of age of the user or the study design. RCTs (DiMeglio 2005, Skogsberg 2008) found improved satisfaction with the CSII versus the MDI regimen. Similar findings were reported in longitudinal pre-post studies (Shehadeh 2004, Rodrigues 2005, Scheidegger 2007) and cross-sectional studies (Hammon 2007, Nicolucci 2008).

RESPONSIBILITY FOR REGIMEN

Six studies assessed responsibility for the regimen demands. Four assessed pediatric patients (Slijper 1990, Kaufman 2000, Weissberg-Benchell 2007, Muller-

Godeffroy 2009), and two assessed adults (Felsing 1984, Schottenfeld-Naor 1985). Four studies found that subjects were more adherent and accepted more responsibility for their diabetes regimen while on CSII. One study (Muller-Godeffroy 2009) found no change in level of regimen responsibility. The study by Weissberg-Benchell (2007) assessed the developmental trajectory of responsibility for CSII tasks and reported that half of the parents of young adolescents continue to share in the regimen responsibility and one-third continue to share in the regimen demands of their older adolescents.

OTHER PSYCHOSOCIAL OUTCOMES

A few studies have assessed such issues as locus of control, self-esteem, self-efficacy, and family functioning. None found CSII to cause worsening outcomes, but few found improvement in these aspects of psychosocial functioning (Shapiro 1984, Slijper 1990, Floyd 1993, Boland 1999, McMahon 2005).

Two studies assessed parenting stress; one was a RCT and the other was a longitudinal pre-post study (Nabhan 2008, Muller-Godeffroy 2009). Both found a reduction in parenting stress when their children were on CSII as compared with MDI therapy.

Some studies (Slijper 1990, Bruttomesso 2002) asked subjects to describe their perceptions about the advantages of CSII therapy. The most common response was improved flexibility. Other reported advantages included ease of scheduling and timing of meals, flexibility around sleep/wake schedule, greater freedom, decreased sense of physical restrictions, decreased physical complaints, and improved glycemic control.

Three studies assessed reasons for CSII discontinuation. Two were longitudinal pre-post designs, and one was a cross-sectional study. Reasons for discontinuing CSII use included higher A1Cs (Babar 2009), forgetting to bolus (Scrimgeour 2007), and not wanting to be reminded about living with diabetes (Seereimer 2010).

Three studies assessed the socioeconomic characteristics of CSII users. All three assessed children and adolescents and determined that CSII users were more likely to be Caucasian and to live in families with higher incomes and higher levels of education (Springer 2006, Valenzuela 2006, Paris 2009).

Overall, there are relatively few studies assessing these psychosocial factors, and conclusions about the impact of CSII therapy on locus of control, self-efficacy, parenting stress, and CSII use versus discontinuation are premature. Moreover, since most CSII users are Caucasian, well educated, and economically comfortable, future research must assess the reasons for such disparities in access to CSII technology in addition to assessing both the medical and psychosocial impact of CSII use on a less homogeneous group of patients.

SUMMARY OF LITERATURE

The literature provides strong evidence that CSII therapy is associated with significant improvements in glycemic control. The only difference was in the preschool age-range, where improvement in A1C was not seen. With the exception of preschoolers, there were no differences noted between studies whose samples were composed of pediatric or adult patients, in spite of the unique challenges faced in pediatric diabetes management. The literature also suggests that CSII results in decreases in insulin requirements. CSII does not appear to increase the risk of hypoglycemic episodes, and the evidence seems to suggest that CSII decreases the risk of severe hypoglycemia. The impact of CSII on body weight and on the risk of DKA appears inconclusive. Overall, it appears that CSII therapy results in improved medical outcomes.

Although CSII therapy may be the most sophisticated and precise method of insulin delivery, the opportunity for improved glycemic control is only one of many potential factors that need to be considered when initiating CSII therapy. Compared with the more than 100 studies that assessed medical outcomes, relatively few studies have assessed psychosocial outcomes. Only eight RCTs assessed both medical and psychosocial outcomes. Of those, seven assessed children and teenagers (DiMeglio 2004, Fox 2005, Wilson 2005, Weintrob 2006, Opipari-Arrigan 2007, Nuboer 2008, Skogsberg 2008), and only one assessed adults (Hoogma 2005). Six of these studies only assessed quality of life (QOL), and three assessed treatment satisfaction. The longitudinal pre-post studies, the matched-pairs studies, and the cross-sectional studies that also assessed both medical and psychosocial outcomes primarily assessed QOL as well. No studies that assessed medical outcomes included measures of depression or eating disorders, both extremely worrisome psychosocial issues for individuals with diabetes due to their associations with high medical costs, poor adherence, and poor metabolic control (American Diabetes Association 2008, Gonzales 2008).

The literature on psychosocial functioning, therefore, is an area that is begging for more research. The impact of pump therapy on vital outcomes such as depression and anxiety is inconclusive. The data on the impact of pump therapy on QOL are more consistent, suggesting an improvement in this important outcome when a patient moves from injections to pumps. Similarly, it appears that individuals using pump therapy tend to accept more responsibility for the regimen demands than those using injection therapy. However, it appears that even older adolescents still benefit from parent involvement and support. Treatment satisfaction is clearly improved after the transition from injections to pump therapy.

RECOMMENDATIONS FOR CLINICAL CARE

When patients and their families express an interest in moving from injections (multiple daily injections, or MDI) to pump therapy (continuous subcutaneous insulin infusion, or CSII), it is recommended that a discussion of the known risks and benefits ensue. The discussion should include at least the following points, with follow-up discussions as indicated:

1. Pump therapy improves metabolic control (A1C levels) in all groups except for preschoolers (who maintain similar control on pumps and injections).
2. Pump therapy reduces the amount of insulin per day that patients require.
3. Pump therapy reduces the risk of severe hypoglycemia and does not increase the risk of hypoglycemia in general.
4. Potential risks and complications of pump therapy (e.g., weight gain, DKA) must also be reviewed and should be a strong focus of the education and

training during pump starts. The choice between injections or pump therapy does not appear to affect weight gain or the risk for DKA, but questions remain. These medical outcomes should be routinely assessed and discussed at all clinic visits.

5. With respect to the psychosocial risks and benefits of pump therapy, the literature is less clear, and the clinician is faced with more subtle discussions regarding the choice of pump therapy. There is an extensive body of research that indicates that diabetes increases one's risk for depression (Anderson 2001); therefore targeting depression would seem to be a vital psychosocial variable to include in education programs and in clinic-based assessments. Unfortunately, relatively few studies have assessed either depression or anxiety among individuals using pump therapy, and the findings are inconclusive. Therefore, it is recommended that clinicians continue to educate and screen patients about mood-related issues and monitor their patients for changes in these symptoms over time. Any increase in depressive symptomatology would warrant a referral to a mental health professional for a formal evaluation. Two simple questions to screen for depression in the clinic include: "Have you been feeling more sad or down than usual?" and "Have you noticed that things that used to be fun are not so much fun anymore?"

6. When patients seek pump therapy with the goal of improving their quality of life, including flexibility in their schedule, the evidence from the literature is more clear: treatment satisfaction and quality of life are better for those using CSII as opposed to MDI. Simple assessments of quality of life are available for clinic use, such as the Diabetes Quality-of-Life Measure (DQOL) (Jacobson 1994), the Diabetes-Specific Quality-of-Life Scale (DSQOLS) (Bott 1998), the Audit of Diabetes-Dependent Quality of Life (ADDQoL) (Bradley 1999), and the Pediatric Quality of Life Inventory™ (PedsQL) Diabetes Module (Varni 2003b), and busy clinical practices can also merely ask patients if they feel their quality of life has changed since moving to pump therapy, and how. It is likely that the improved treatment satisfaction seen among pump users is a result of the improvements in QOL.

7. Finally, diabetes is not a "do it yourself" disease. Therefore, the studies assessing shared responsibility and adherence behaviors suggest that family members should be actively involved in all aspects of pump care, from infusion site changes to basal rate decisions to monitoring timing of boluses.

BIBLIOGRAPHY

Alemzadeh R, Ellis J, Holzum M, Parton E, Wyatt D: Beneficial effects of continuous subcutaneous insulin infusion and flexible multiple daily insulin regimen using insulin glargine in type 1 diabetes. *Pediatrics* 114:91–95, 2004

American Diabetes Association: Economic costs of diabetes in the U.S. in 2007. *Diabetes Care* 31:596–615, 2008

Anderson RJ, Freedland K, Clouse R, Lustman P: The prevalence of comorbid depression in adults with diabetes: a meta-analysis. *Diabetes Care* 24:1069–1078, 2001

Babar G, Ali O, Parton E, Hoffman R, Alemzadeh R: Factors associated with adherence to continuous subcutaneous insulin infusion in pediatric diabetes. *Diabetes Technology and Therapeutics* 11:131–137, 2009

Barnard K, Lloyd C, Skinner T: Systematic literature review: quality of life associated with insulin pump use in type 1 diabetes. *Diabet Med* 24:607–617, 2007

Boland E, Grey M, Oesterle A, Fredrickson L, Tamborlane W: Continuous subcutaneous insulin infusion: a new way to lower risk of severe hypoglycemia, improve metabolic control, and enhance coping in adolescents with type 1 diabetes. *Diabetes Care* 22:1779–1784, 1999

Bott U, Muhlhauser I, Overmann H, Berger M: Validation of a diabetes-specific quality-of-life scale for patients with type 1 diabetes. *Diabetes Care* 21:757–769, 1998

Bradley C, Todd C, Gorton T, Symonds E, Martin A, Plowright R: The development of an individualized questionnaire measure of perceived impact of diabetes on quality of life: the ADDQoL. *Quality of Life Research* 8:79–91, 1999

Bruttomesso D, Pianta A, Crazzolara D, Scaldaferri E, Lora L, Guarneri G, Mongillo A, Gennaro R, Miola M, Moretti M, Confortin L, Beltramello G, Pais M, Baritussio A, Casiglia E, Tiengo A: Continuous subcutaneous insulin infusion (CSII) in the Veneto region: efficacy, acceptability and quality of life. *Diabet Medi* 19:628–634, 2002

Burdick J, Chase P, Slover R, Knievel K, Scrimgeour L, Maniatis A, Klingensmith G: Missed insulin meal boluses and elevated hemoglobin A1c levels in children receiving insulin pump therapy. *Pediatrics* 113:221–224, 2004

Cogen F, Henderson C, Hansen J, Streisand R: Pediatric quality of life in transitioning to insulin pump: does prior regimen make a difference? *Clinical Pediatrics* 46: 777–779, 2007

Diabetes Control and Complications Trial (DCCT) Research Group: Influence of intensive diabetes treatment on body weight and composition of adults with type 1 diabetes in the Diabetes Control and Complications Trial. *Diabetes Care* 24:1711–1721, 2001

Diabetes Control and Complications Trial (DCCT) Research Group: Adverse events and their association with treatment regimens in the Diabetes Control and Complications Trial. *Diabetes Care* 18:1415–1427, 1995

Diabetes Control and Complications Trial (DCCT) Research Group: The effect of intensive treatment of diabetes on the development and progression of long-term complications in insulin-dependent diabetes mellitus. *N Engl J Med* 329:977–985, 1993

DiMeglio L, Pottorff T, Boyd S, France L, Fineberg N, Eugster E: A randomized, controlled study of insulin pump therapy in diabetic preschoolers. *Journal of Pediatrics* 145:380–384, 2004

Doyle E, Winzimer S, Steffen A, Ahern JA, Vincent M, Tamborlane W: A randomized, prospective trial comparing the efficacy of continuous subcutaneous insulin infusion with multiple daily injections using insulin glargine. *Diabetes Care* 27:1554–1558, 2004

Dusseldorf Study Group, Ziegler D, Dannehl K, Koschinsky T, Toeller M, Gries F: Comparison of continuous subcutaneous insulin infusion and intensified conventional therapy in the treatment of type I diabetes: a two-year randomized study. *Diabetes Nutrition and Metabolism* 3:203–213, 1990

Felsing W, Bibergeil H, Menzel R, Albrecht G, Felsing U, Dabels J, Reichel G, Luder C: Results of treatment with continuous subcutaneous insulin infusion (CSII) in insulin-dependent (type 1) diabetics. *Experimental and Clinical Endocrinology* 83:136–142, 1984

Floyd JC, Cornell RG, Jacober SJ, Griffith LE, Funnell MM, Wolf LL, Wolf FM: A prospective study identifying risk factors for discontinuance of insulin pump therapy. *Diabetes Care* 16:1470–1478, 1993

Fox L, Buckloh L, Smith S, Wysocki T, Mauras N: A randomized controlled trial of insulin pump therapy in young children with type 1 diabetes. *Diabetes Care* 28:1277–1281, 2005

Gimenez M, Congent M, Jansa M, Vidal M, Chiganer G, Levy I: Efficacy of continuous subcutaneous insulin infusion in type 1 diabetes: a 2-year perspective using the established criteria for funding from a National Health Service. *Diabet Med* 24:1419–1423, 2007

Gonzales JS, Peyrot M, McCarl L, Collins EM, et al.: Depression and diabetes treatment nonadherence: a meta-analysis. *Diabetes Care* 31:2398–2403, 2008

Hammon P, Liebl A, Grunder S: International survey of insulin pump users: impact of continuous subcutaneous insulin infusion therapy on glucose control and quality of life. *Primary Care Diabetes* 1:143–146, 2007

Hislop A, Fegan P, Schlaeppi M, Duck M, Yeap B: Prevalence and association of psychological distress in young adults with type 1 diabetes. *Diabet Med* 25:91–96, 2008

Hoogma R, Hammond P, Gomist R, Kerr D, Bruttomesso D, Bouter K, Wiefels K, de la Calle H, Schweitzer D, Pfohl M, Torlone E, Krinelke L, Bolli G: Comparison of the effects of continuous subcutaneous insulin infusion (CSII) and NPH-based multiple daily insulin injections (MDI) on glycaemic control and quality of life: results of the 5-nations trial. *Diabet Med* 23:141–147, 2005

Hoogma R, Spijker A, Van Doorn-Scheele M, Van Doorn T, Michels R, Van Doorn R, Levi M, Hoekstra J: Quality of life and metabolic control in patients with diabetes mellitus type 1 treated by continuous subcutaneous insulin infusion or multiple daily insulin injections. *The Netherlands Journal of Medicine* 62:383–387, 2004

Jacobson AM, the Diabetes Control and Complications Trial (DCCT) Research Group: The diabetes quality of life measure. In *Handbook of Psychology and Diabetes*. Bradley C, Ed. Chur, Switzerland, Harwood Academic Publishers, 1994, p. 65–87

Jakisch BI, Wagner V, Heidtmann B, Lepler R, Holterhust P, Kapellen T, Vogel C, Rosenbauer J, Holl R: Comparison of continuous subcutaneous insulin infusion (CSII) and multiple daily injections (MDI) in paediatric type 1 diabetes: a multicentre matched-pair cohort analysis over three years. *Diabet Med* 25:80–85, 2008

Jeitler K, Horvath K, Berghold A, Gratzer T, Neeser K, Pieber T, Siebenhofer A: Continuous subcutaneous insulin infusion versus multiple daily insulin injections in patients with diabetes mellitus: systematic review and meta-analysis. *Diabetologia* 51:941–951, 2008

Johannesen J, Eising S, Kohlwes S, Riis S, Beck M, Carstensen B, Bendtson I, Nerup J: Treatment of Danish adolescent diabetic patients with CSII: a matched study to MDI. *Pediatric Diabetes* 9:23–28, 2008

Kapellen T, Heidtmann B, Bachmann J, Ziegler R, Grabert M, Holl R: Indications for insulin pump therapy in different age groups: an analysis of 1,567 children and adolescents. *Diabet Med* 24:836–842, 2007

Kaufman FR, Halvorson M, Kim C, Pitukcheewanont P: Use of insulin pump therapy at nighttime only for children 7-10 years of age with type 1 diabetes. *Diabetes Care* 23:579–582, 2000

Lustman P, Anderson R, Freedland K, DeGroot M, Carney R, Clouse R: Depression and poor glycemic control: a meta-analytic review of the literature. *Diabetes Care* 23:934–942, 2000

McMahon S, Airey F, Marangou D, McElwee K, Carne C, Davis E, Jones T: Insulin pump therapy in children and adolescents: improvements in key parameters of diabetes management including quality of life. *Diabet Med* 22:92–96, 2005

Mecklenburg RS, Benson EA, Benson JW, Fredlund P, Guinn T, Metz R, Nielsen R, Sanner C: Acute complications associated with insulin infusion pump therapy: report of experience with 161 patients. *JAMA* 252:3265–3269, 1984

Muller-Godeffroy E, Treichel S, Wagner M: Investigation of quality of life and family burden issues during insulin pump therapy in children with type 1 diabetes mellitus: a large-scale multicenter pilot study. *Diabet Med* 26:493–501, 2009

Nabhan ZM, Kreher N, Greene D, Eugster E, Kronenberger W, DiMeglio L: A randomized prospective study of insulin pump vs. insulin injection therapy in very young children with type 1 diabetes: 12-month glycemic, BMI, and neurocognitive outcomes. *Pediatric Diabetes* 10:202–208, 2009

Nicolucci A, Maione A, Franciosi M, Amoretti R, Busetto E, Capani F, Bruttomesso D, Di Bartolo P, Girelli A, Leonetti F, Morviducci L, Ponzi P, Vitacolonna E: Quality of life and treatment satisfaction in adults with type 1 diabetes: a comparison between continuous subcutaneous insulin infusion and multiple daily injections. *Diabet Med* 25:213–220, 2008

Nimri R, Weintrob N, Benzaquen H, Ofan R, Fayman G, Phillip P: Insulin pump therapy in youth with type 1 diabetes: a retrospective paired study. *Pediatrics* 117:2126–2123, 2006

Nuboer R, Borsboom GJ, Zoethout J, Koot H, Bruining J: Effects of insulin pump vs. injection treatment on quality of life and impact of disease in children with type 1 diabetes mellitus in a randomized, prospective comparison. *Pediatric Diabetes* 9:291–296, 2008

Olinder AL, Kernell A, Smide B: Missed bolus doses: devastating for metabolic control in CSII-treated adolescents with type 1 diabetes. *Pediatric Diabetes* 10:142–148, 2009

Opipari-Arrigan L, Fredericks E, Burhart N, Dale L, Hodge M, Foster C: Continuous subcutaneous insulin infusion benefits quality of life in preschool-age children with type 1 diabetes. *Pediatric Diabetes* 8:377–383, 2007

Pankowska E, Blazik M, Dziechciarz P, Szypowska A, Szajewska H: Continuous subcutaneous insulin infusion vs. multiple daily injections in children with type 1 diabetes: a systematic review and meta-analysis of randomized control trials. *Pediatric Diabetes* 10:52–58, 2009

Paris C, Imperatore G, Klingensmith G, Petitti D, Rodriguez B, Anderson A, Schwartz D, Standiford D, Pihoker C: Predictors of insulin regimens and impact on outcomes in youth with type 1 diabetes: the SEARCH for Diabetes in Youth study. *Journal of Pediatrics* 155:183–189, 2009

Pickup JC, Sutton A: Severe hypoglycaemia and glycaemic control in type 1 diabetes: a meta-analysis of multiple daily insulin injections compared with continuous subcutaneous insulin infusion. *Diabet Med* 25:765–774, 2008

Rabbone I, Scaramuzza A, Bobbio A, Bonfanti R, Iafusco D, Lombardo F, Toni S, Tumini S, Cerutti F: Insulin pump therapy management in very young children with type 1 diabetes using continuous subcutaneous insulin infusion. *Diabetes Technology and Therapeutics* 11:707–709, 2009

Rodrigues I, Reid H, Ismail K, Amiel S: Indications and efficacy of continuous subcutaneous insulin infusion (CSII) therapy in type 1 diabetes mellitus: a clinical audit in a specialist service. *Diabet Med* 22:842–849, 2005

Scheidegger U, Allemann S, Scheidegger K, Diem P: Continuous subcutaneous insulin infusion therapy: effects on quality of life. *Swiss Medicine Weekly* 137:476–482, 2007

Schottenfeld-Naor Y, Galatzer A, Karp M, Josefsberg Z, Laron Z: Comparison of metabolic and psychological parameters during continuous subcutaneous insulin infusion and intensified conventional insulin treatment in type I diabetic patients. *Israeli Journal of Medical Science* 21:822–828, 1985

Scrimgeour L, Cobry E, McFann K, Burdick P, Weimer C, Slover R, Chase P: Improved glycemic control after long-term insulin pump use in pediatric patients with type 1 diabetes. *Diabetes Technology and Therapeutics* 9:421–428, 2007

Seereiner S, Neeser K, Weber C, Schreiber K, Habacher W, Rakovac I, Beck P, Schmidt L, Pieber T: Attitudes towards insulin pump therapy among adolescents and young people. *Diabetes Technology and Therapeutics* 12:89–94, 2010

Shapiro J, Wigg D, Charles M, Perley M: Personality and family profiles of chronic insulin-dependent diabetic patients using portable insulin infusion pump therapy: a preliminary investigation. *Diabetes Care* 7:137–142, 1984

Shehadeh N, Battelino T, Galatzer A, Naveh T, Hadash A, de Vries L, Phillip M: Insulin pump therapy for 1-6 year old children with type 1 diabetes. *Israel Medical Association Journal* 6:284–286, 2004

Skogsberg L, Fors H, Hannas R, Chaplin J, Lindman E, Skogsberg J: Improved treatment satisfaction but no difference in metabolic control when using continuous subcutaneous insulin infusion versus multiple daily injections in children at onset of type 1 diabetes mellitus. *Pediatric Diabetes* 9:472–479, 2008

Slijper FM, deBeaufort CE, Bruining GJ, deVisser J, Aarsen R, Dicken D, vanStrik R: Psychological impact of continuous subcutaneous insulin infusion pump therapy in non-selected newly diagnosed insulin dependent (type 1) diabetic children: evaluation after two years of therapy. *Diabetes & Metabolisme* 16:273–277, 1990

Springer D, Dziura J, Tamborlane W, Steffen A, Ahern J, Vincent M, Weinzimer S: Optimal control of type 1 diabetes mellitus in youth receiving intensive treatment. *Journal of Pediatrics* 149:227–232, 2006

Sulli N, Shashaj B: Long term benefits of continuous subcutaneous insulin infusion in children with type 1 diabetes: a 4-year follow up. *Diabet Med* 23:900–906, 2006

Tsui E, Barnie A, Ross S, Parkes R, Zinman B: Intensive insulin therapy with insulin lispro. *Diabetes Care* 24:1722–1727, 2001

UK Prospective Diabetes Study (UKPDS) Group: Intensive blood glucose control with sulphonylureas or insulin compared with conventional treatment and risk of complications in patients with type 2 diabetes (UKPDS 33). *Lancet* 352:837–853, 1998

Valenzuela J, Patino A, McCullough J, Ring C, Sanchez J, Eidson M, Nemery R, Delameter A: Insulin pump therapy and health related quality of life in children and adolescents with type 1 diabetes. *Journal of Pediatric Psychology* 31:650–660, 2006

Varni JW, Burwinkle TM, Jacobs JR, Gottschalk M, Kaufman F, Jones KL: The PedsQL in type 1 and type 2 diabetes: reliability and validity of the Pediatric

Quality of Life Inventory Generic Core Scales and Type 1 Diabetes Module. *Diabetes Care* 26:631–637, 2003a

Varni JW, Burwinkle TM, Seid M, Skarr D: The PedsQL 4.0 as a pediatric population health measure: feasibility, reliability, and validity. *Ambulatory Pediatrics* 3:329–341, 2003b

Weintrob N, Benzaquen H, Galatzer A, Shalitin S, Lazar L, Fayman G, Lilos P, Dickerman Z, Phillip M: Comparison of continuous subcutaneous insulin infusion and multiple daily injection regimens in children with type 1 diabetes: a randomized open crossover trial. *Pediatrics* 112:559–564, 2006

Weinzimer S, Ahern J, Doyle E, Vincent M, Dziura J, Steffen A, Tamborlane W: Persistence of benefits of continuous subcutaneous insulin infusion in very young children with type 1 diabetes: a follow-up report. *Pediatrics* 114:1601–1605, 2004

Weissberg-Benchell J, Goodman S, Antisdel-Lomaglio J, Zebracki K: The use of continuous subcutaneous insulin infusion (CSII): parental and professional perceptions of self-care mastery and autonomy in children and adolescents. *Journal of Pediatric Psychology* 32:1196–1202, 2007

Weissberg-Benchell J, Antisdel-Lomaglio J, Seshadri R: Insulin pump therapy: a meta-analysis. *Diabetes Care* 26:1079–1087, 2003

Whittemore R, Urban AD, Tamborlane WV, Grey M: Quality of life in school-aged children with type 1 diabetes on intensive treatment and their parents. *Diabetes Educator* 29:847–854, 2003

Wilson D, Buckingham B, Kunselman E, Sullivan M, Paguntalan H, Gitelman S: A two-center randomized controlled feasibility trial of insulin pump therapy in young children with diabetes. *Diabetes Care* 28:15–19, 2005

Jill Weissberg-Benchell, PhD, CDE, is an Associate Professor of Psychiatry at Northwestern University's Feinberg School of Medicine at the Ann and Robert H. Lurie Children's Hospital of Chicago in Chicago, IL.

Chapter 11
Psychosocial Considerations Regarding Adoption of Intensive Management

LORI LAFFEL, MD, MPH

The current era has heralded epidemic rates of type 1 and type 2 diabetes in both pediatric and adult populations. The disease currently affects hundreds of millions of individuals worldwide, and by 2025, these numbers are expected to increase by 50%. The current era has also seen remarkable advances in technology. Technology, in general, has a major impact in our daily lives and, specifically, in our approaches to managing diabetes. Since the first home blood glucose monitoring (BGM) devices and insulin pumps became available 30 years ago in the late 1970s and early 1980s, multidisciplinary diabetes teams have focused their efforts on designing, implementing, and evaluating optimal approaches to patient education and behavioral support for successful use of these tools with the goal of achieving glycemic control targets.

Technology has substantially impacted diabetes management with opportunities to match more carefully antihyperglycemic therapies—either oral agents, insulin, or other injectable medications—to the person's physiologic needs in efforts to achieve optimal glycemic control. Optimal glycemic control is important for patients with either type 1 or type 2 diabetes to reduce their risks of developing chronic diabetes complications.

This chapter will address four common technologies that are fundamental to modern diabetes management: BGM, continuous glucose monitoring (CGM), intensive insulin therapy aided by insulin pen use, and Internet programs or technologies to support diabetes self-management. There is a separate chapter in this volume addressing insulin pump use (see Chapter 10). This chapter is not intended to be a technical review of these diabetes management tools nor an exhaustive appraisal of diabetes technologies, but, rather, it will highlight the psychosocial considerations that come into play with the implementation and ongoing use of these management tools, with a particular focus on BGM and CGM. Psychosocial considerations will include quality of life, diabetes burden, symptoms of depression and anxiety, fear of hypoglycemia, and adherence challenges associated with patients' efforts to achieve diabetes management goals. The discussion will provide examples of salient studies that highlight the psychosocial issues related to these four areas rather than be exhaustive. When available, technical reviews or meta-analyses are referenced.

As with standard approaches to diabetes management, care is individualized according to the patient's needs and delivered by multidisciplinary treatment teams. This chapter provides information to help the practitioner encourage patient adherence to complex, medically prescribed intensive treatment regimens, and it discusses the behaviors necessary for the achievement of intensive management and glycemic goals.

BLOOD GLUCOSE MONITORING (BGM)

BGM remains the cornerstone of diabetes management as it serves as the guidepost for all therapies, whether indicating a need for more insulin to lower elevated blood glucose levels or for carbohydrates to raise low blood glucose (BG) levels. It is the first step to intensification of treatment. Indeed, the Diabetes Control and Complications Trial (DCCT) established the importance of self-monitoring of blood glucose to guide insulin therapy for patients with type 1 diabetes (T1D) (DCCT Research Group 1993). Insulin-treated patients with type 2 diabetes (T2D) also benefit from self-monitoring of BG (UK Prospective Diabetes Study [UKPDS] Group 1998). However, there remains ongoing debate in the literature for non-insulin-treated patients regarding the effectiveness of self-monitoring of BG for self-management (DCCT Research Group 1996, Wen 2004, Blonde 2005, Welschen 2005, Pistrosch 2006, Goyder 2008, Holman 2008, Farmer 2009). Nonetheless, the American Diabetes Association (ADA) recommends self-monitoring of BG for all patients treated with insulin and supports BGM as a central practice for patients using oral medications or medical nutrition therapy to achieve glycemic goals (ADA 2012).

Increased frequency of daily BGM is associated with lower hemoglobin A1C levels (A1C) in patients with type 1 and type 2 diabetes (Nathan 1996, Levine 2001, Laffel 2006, Dailey 2007). A recent study of over 26,000 youth with T1D observed that A1C was 0.2% lower for each additional daily BG check across the entire range of monitoring frequency from 0–10 and was 0.5% lower for each additional daily BG check in the monitoring range of 0–5 (Ziegler 2011). Furthermore, these authors reported that patients experienced a lower rate of diabetic ketoacidosis (DKA) as daily BGM frequency increased. A review of studies of non-insulin-treated patients with T2D also reported a 0.4% reduction in A1C with BGM (Welschen 2005).

The Centers for Disease Control and Prevention (CDC) analyzed data using the Behavioral Risk Factor Surveillance System (BRFSS) from 1997–2006. In 2006, 63% of all adults with diabetes were checking their BG levels daily, up from 41% in 1997 (CDC 2007). In fact, this exceeded by 2% the *Healthy People 2010* national objective of 61% of individuals with diabetes checking BG levels daily. Furthermore, 87% of all adults treated with insulin were monitoring their BG levels daily. A national objective of the *Healthy People 2020* plan includes the need to increase the proportion of adults with diabetes who perform self-monitoring of BG at least once daily by 10 to 70% (objective D-13; http://healthypeople.gov/2020/topicsobjectives2020/objectiveslist.aspx?topicId=8). To achieve this goal, efforts should include ensuring adequate health insurance coverage for blood glucose strips, diabetes education around self-management, and counseling to encourage more-intensive diabetes medical care.

Barriers to BGM and Approaches to Overcoming Barriers

Despite the recognition that the frequency of BGM is linked to glycemic control, many patients resist this behavior. Recognized barriers (see Table 11.1) to monitoring include cost, pain, lack of uniform insurance coverage, requirement for diabetes education to teach proper usage, and need for ongoing counseling to encourage intensive management, self-care practices, and avoidance of diabetes burnout. The recent generations of home BGM devices remove some barriers such as complexity, technique dependency, and even some of the discomfort associated with large sample size or the requirement for fingerstick puncture. Many new devices use microsamples of blood (under 1 microliter) and are approved for alternate-site monitoring (e.g., the arm), which is often considered virtually painless compared with fingerstick checking. These devices often offer memories with an automated logbook and BG averages by time of day, provide automatic downloading capabilities, and do not require sophisticated coding (Wood 2007).

Table 11.1 Barriers to BGM

Pain with fingerstick
Inconvenience checking BG, logging results, or downloading meter
Interruptions to daily routine
Possible difficulty of use involving coding; formatting date and time; placing blood on tip, top, or sides of strip
Education about meaning of BG results and management changes
Cost of monitoring supplies, especially blood glucose strips
Attitudes related to BG results, including shame, frustration, and fear

The act of checking BG values frequently throughout the day for patients with T1D and for many insulin-treated patients with T2D may include monitoring before and after eating; before, during, and after exercise; at bedtime; and often overnight. This frequency demands significant interruption of usual activities and often elicits feelings of inadequacy or failure when BG levels are out-of-range. In a negative feedback cycle, out-of-range BG levels can lead to diminished monitoring since the patient receives no positive reinforcement for this critically important management behavior. The addition of a psycho-educational manual, called the *BG Monitoring Owner's Manual*, as a supplement to standard diabetes education, has been associated with increased frequency of BGM and a reduction of negative affect associated with BGM in adults with type 1 or type 2 diabetes in suboptimal glycemic control (defined as A1C ≥8%) (Moreland 2006). The *BG Monitoring Owner's Manual* provides realistic expectations for monitoring, includes basic education related to when, why, and how to monitor, avoids the shame and blame often associated with out-of-range BG results, and balances the burdens of monitoring against the increased lifestyle flexibility that results from knowledge of BG levels (Lawlor 1997). In addition, the manual offers a new vocabulary that helps to maintain self-care motivation by talking of "checking" rather than "testing" and describing BG results as either "high or low" and not "bad or good."

To further reduce the burden experienced by patients, most BG meters can be interfaced with computers for direct meter downloading. Some devices have used automated data transfer via phone or fax to reduce the effort required for computer connections. To reduce the burden associated with interpretation of the BG data, there are computer-based algorithms to review the data and provide suggested insulin doses, even taking into consideration other factors such as food intake, exercise, stress, and illness (Garg 2008). A recent 12-month, multicenter study involving insulin-naïve adults with T2D in suboptimal control (defined as A1C ≥7.5%) compared an intervention group instructed in structured self-monitoring of BG at quarterly intervals with a usual-care control group (Polonsky 2011). Both groups received quarterly visits focused on diabetes care, free glucose meters and strips, and point-of-care A1C testing. The structured BGM intervention included use of a paper tool that directed the patient to check and interpret 7-point glucose profiles for 3 consecutive days; hence the trial name of STeP (Structured Testing Program). After the 1-year study, the group using structured BGM demonstrated a significantly greater improvement in A1C by 0.3% in the intent to treat analysis and by 0.5% in the per protocol analysis. Notably, both groups demonstrated significant improvements in general well-being, suggesting that active provider support of monitoring activities improves both medical and psychological outcomes.

One relatively simple approach to interpretation of BG data to aid both the health care provider and patient involves the determination of the BG mean by time of day and the variation associated with those means according to time of day (Hirsch 2008). Although target BG levels require individualization, there are data suggesting that the variation in BG levels should be limited such that the standard deviation is less than 50% of the mean or median (Hirsch 2008).

Some BG meters provide integrated electronic logbooks that enable patients to see graphical displays of blood glucose data as well as average BG data by time of day. Use of this technology along with diabetes education has demonstrated both increased frequency of BGM and improved glycemic control that were sustained beyond the clinical trial and up to 1 year later (Laffel 2007). Notably, glycemic benefit was sustained after the end of the clinical trial and termination of extra support.

There have been a number of short-term, randomized studies aimed at encouraging BGM behaviors with the aid of electronic reminders (Kumar 2004) and newer approaches with cell phone text messaging to encourage increased monitoring frequency (Franklin 2006, Franklin 2008, Hanauer 2009). In a study of insulin-treated youth and young adults, text message reminders to check BG levels resulted in greater daily monitoring frequency compared with email reminders during the course of a 3-month pilot. Another study involving cell phone reminders, entitled Sweet Talk, aimed at supporting intensive insulin therapy with BGM, also demonstrated improved adherence to monitoring (Franklin 2003, Franklin 2006, Franklin 2008). It is unclear, however, if increased BGM would be sustainable beyond the period of active intervention in these clinical trials, suggesting that durable behavior change requires a fundamental acceptance of need and an intrinsic motivation to incorporate what is often viewed as unpleasant physical and emotional activities.

Psychological Outcomes Associated with BGM

In addition to self-reported improvements in well-being associated with increased BGM frequency and improved glycemic control in the STeP trial of adults with T2D that have been discussed, the investigators examined changes in depressive symptoms and diabetes distress (Fisher 2011). After 12 months, both intervention and control groups had significant improvements in depression and diabetes distress. However, use of the structured BG self-monitoring tool compared with usual care was associated with significantly greater reductions in both depressive symptoms and diabetes distress among those with *high* baseline levels of depression and distress. Notably, these benefits were independent of improvements in A1C and in BGM frequency, suggesting that the benefits to mood may have resulted from enhanced identification of glycemic patterns and improved self-efficacy. An earlier study also confirmed the positive impact of structured counseling and BGM on well-being, depression, and self-efficacy in non-insulin-treated adults with T2D (Siebolds 2006).

In youth with T1D, diabetes-specific family conflict is inversely associated with BGM frequency (Anderson 2002). Furthermore, BGM and diabetes-specific family conflict independently impact A1C, with lower conflict and more frequent monitoring predicting better glycemic control. In addition, youth practicing frequent BGM and having optimal glycemic control also report high quality of life (Ingerski 2010). Finally, patients occasionally increase their frequency of BGM to excessive levels, suggestive of psychological distress related to fear of hypoglycemia, or possibly to fear of hyperglycemia and complications (Cox 1987). Such individuals should receive referral to trained mental health specialists experienced in diabetes management. Thus, in summary, increasing BGM frequency is unlikely to negatively impact psychological factors and is likely to positively impact glycemic control. However, there are individual cases in which anxiety about disease state may impel the patient to adopt maladaptive levels of BGM.

CONTINUOUS GLUCOSE MONITORING (CGM)

A quest remains for noninvasive approaches to measuring glucose levels free of discomfort and minimizing interruption in daily activities. While the diabetes community awaits such an advance, real-time CGM technologies present opportunities to provide unprecedented availability of nearly continuous glucose data. CGM devices use a disposable glucose sensor placed subcutaneously in the interstitial space for 3 to 7 days. The sensor is connected to a transmitter, which wirelessly transfers the interstitial glucose signals to a nearby receiver that displays the glucose readings continuously while refreshing the result every 5 min (see Figure 11.1 showing the two currently available CGM devices in the U.S.). The receiver displays the glucose data in numeric and graphical form and provides warning alarms when the glucose value exceeds certain preset low or high thresholds or is rapidly rising or falling. The receiver's alarms can be set to provide audio or vibratory alerts. There are two recent publications reviewing CGM clinical guidelines in adult and pediatric patients (Klonoff 2011, Phillip 2012).

There have been a number of recent clinical trials of CGM use in pediatric and adult patients with T1D. The Juvenile Diabetes Research Foundation (JDRF) 6-month CGM Trial compared CGM with traditional episodic BGM in pediatric and adult patients with T1D and baseline A1C values 7–10% (Juvenile Diabetes Research Foundation Continuous Glucose Monitoring [JDRF CGM] Study Group 2008). The study demonstrated that CGM compared with BGM significantly reduced A1C by 0.5% in adults with T1D (JDRF CGM Study Group

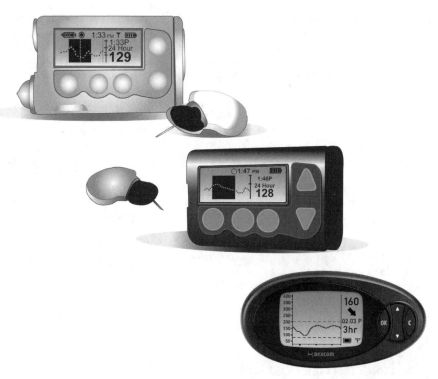

Figure 11.1. Continuous Glucose Monitoring (CGM) Devices consist of three components: the disposable sensor, the transmitter, and the receiver. In the U.S. in 2012, there are currently two available real-time CGM systems produced by Medtronic, Inc. and DexCom, Inc. The Medtronic CGM is available either as a stand-alone CGM device or integrated with an insulin pump. Updated and improved devices may be available outside of the U.S.; ongoing studies and evaluations are awaiting U.S. Food and Drug Administration (FDA) review and approval. Both systems have available software to download the CGM data to allow for retrospective assessment of glucose patterns to help direct insulin adjustments.

2008). On the other hand, CGM compared with BGM did not reduce mean A1C in youth and young adults (age-range 8–24 years) with T1D. Interestingly, although there was no difference in the mean A1C between CGM and BGM groups for the youngest study participants (8–14 years old), a significantly greater proportion of youth (again 8–14 years old) in the CGM group compared with the BGM group did experience a relative improvement in A1C by ≥10% or an absolute A1C improvement of ≥0.5%. Also of note, CGM use varied according to age-group, with 83% of participants aged 25 years and older, 30% of those aged 15–24, and 50% of those aged 8–14 using the technology for ≥6 days per week for the duration of the 6-month clinical trial. Importantly, the improvement in glycemic control was directly related to CGM use. In other words, those participants who used the device most often derived the greatest benefit, with reduction in A1C levels that was independent of age. In addition, the A1C improvement occurred without any increase in severe hypoglycemia (JDRF CGM Study Group 2009a). Interestingly, the factor predictive of CGM use during the first 6 months of the study was the baseline frequency of BGM; those who checked BG levels more frequently were more likely to use CGM more frequently. In a companion study of pediatric and adult patients with T1D and entry A1C values <7%, the CGM group compared with the BGM group maintained optimal target A1C levels without experiencing an increased occurrence of severe hypoglycemia (JDRF CGM Study Group 2009b).

The recently published 12-month Sensor-Augmented Pump Therapy for A1C Reduction (STAR3) clinical study compared sensor-augmented insulin pump therapy against multiple daily injection therapy accompanied by traditional BGM in both pediatric and adult patients with T1D and entry A1C values 7.4–9.5% (Bergenstal 2010). These investigators demonstrated significant improvements in A1C in the sensor-augmented pump group with A1C differences between groups of 0.6% for the adults and 0.5% for the pediatric participants. In addition, there was no significant difference in rates of hypoglycemia or weight gain between the sensor augmented pump group and the injection/BGM study group. Notably, the frequency of CGM use was again associated with the degree of A1C reduction. There have been a number of other short-term, randomized studies that have also reported improvements in A1C levels with CGM use with glycemic benefits accruing when patients wear the CGM device consistently (Deiss 2006, Raccah 2009). Some studies are also using sensor-augmented pump therapy from onset of T1D (Kordonouri 2010), which could possibly maximize use of these technologies across the lifespan of the disease.

Barriers and Psychological Impacts of CGM Use

There are many potential benefits as well as barriers to CGM use (see Table 11.2). The current challenges associated with CGM stem from the additional burdens related to daily sensor wear that are added on top of usual diabetes management tasks. The JDRF CGM trial studied quality of life, fear of hypoglycemia, CGM satisfaction, and barriers to CGM use. The adults in the CGM group compared with the adults in the BGM group reported a slight but significant improvement in fear of hypoglycemia and quality of life according to the physical component subscale of the 12-Item Short Form Health Survey (SF12) quality of life measure (JDRF CGM Study Group 2010b). The pediatric CGM and BGM participants and their parents did not differ with respect to fear of hypoglycemia or quality of life. Notably, the adults, youth, and parents all reported substantial satisfaction with CGM. As expected, CGM satisfaction was significantly correlated with CGM use (JDRF CGM Study Group 2010a).

Table 11.2 Potential Benefits and Barriers of CGM

Benefits:

Continuous glucose data with trend information providing rate and direction of change

Detection of out-of-range glucose levels with high and low alarms

Immediate glucose data to guide insulin dosing, diet, exercise, sick day management, etc.

Improved glycemic control

Reduced frequency of hypoglycemia

Retrospective glucose data to guide treatment changes

Potential need for less frequent fingerstick BGM

Potential for increased stress associated with awareness of out-of-range glucose levels

Barriers:

Pain associated with sensor insertion

Tape to keep the sensor in place on the body

Need to wear the sensor and carry the receiver

Need for frequent calibration of the CGM device

Frequent "nuisance alarms" related to sensor operation or out-of-range glucose levels

Uncertainty as to how to use the extensive amount of sensor glucose data

Concerns about potential disagreement between CGM and BGM values

Potential for reduced anxiety related to fear of hypoglycemia

---

Another publication from the JDRF CGM Study Group reported the perceived barriers and benefits of CGM use as endorsed by the youth, their parents, and the adults in the trial (Tansey 2011). Common benefits were the availability of glucose trend data, opportunities to self-correct out-of-range glucose levels, and the ability to detect hypoglycemia. Frequently reported barriers included pain associated with sensor insertion; system alarms often considered as "nuisance alarms"; and frustration with body issues related to where to place the sensor on the body, skin reactions from the sensor adhesive, and how to carry the receiver on the body. Users of CGM noted that the availability of continuous data, especially after meals and overnight, provided previously unavailable, yet valuable, information regarding how various foods impact BG levels and potential risk for nocturnal hypoglycemia, respectively. Of note, the adults with T1D and the parents of the youth were more likely to report benefits whereas the youth were more likely to report barriers.

A recent publication examined psychosocial correlates of CGM use in an ancillary study of the JDRF CGM trial (Markowitz 2012). Psychological characteristics of youth with T1D, their parents, and adults with T1D were compared between the CGM and BGM groups after 6 months. The youth, their parents, and the diabetic adults appeared to have different psychological responses to CGM use. Youth in the CGM group reported more trait anxiety than youth in the BGM group, whereas adults in the CGM group reported less state and trait anxiety than adults in the BGM group. Parent-proxy report of youth depression was higher in the CGM group than in the BGM group. Both youth in the CGM group and their parents reported more negative affect around BGM than youth and their parents in the BGM group. On the other hand, adults in the CGM group endorsed less diabetes-related burden than adults in the BGM group. Overall, this preliminary study suggests that CGM use in adults tends to have a positive psychosocial impact whereas CGM use in youth tends to have a negative psychosocial impact, suggesting a need for additional research aimed at reducing any negative psychological consequences of CGM use, especially in youth. Another ancillary study involving only adults with T1D in the JDRF CGM trial revealed that effective CGM use likely requires coping skills, frequent retrospective data review, and family support (Ritholz 2010).

Barriers to CGM use likely contribute to the negative psychological responses noted. Additional challenges associated with CGM use include the additional time required to insert the sensor, to perform calibrations, and to react to real or "nuisance" alarms. Currently, CGM users must continue to check their fingerstick blood glucose levels to calibrate the CGM devices and whenever patient-initiated adjustments to diabetes therapies are needed, because the CGM devices are not approved by regulatory agencies as replacement for BGM. Thus, adoption of CGM requires substantially more time and effort from the patient and often triggers feelings of frustration and physical discomfort. Nonetheless, the CGM trials have demonstrated safety as well as substantial efficacy with respect to improved glycemic control without increased hypoglycemia, particularly for adults with T1D. There are ongoing studies in the pediatric population to encourage and sustain CGM use in order for youth with T1D to derive the same benefits afforded to adults. Thus, behavioral interventions are needed to help youth overcome the barriers associated with CGM use.

INTENSIVE INSULIN THERAPY: PEN USE

Since release of the Diabetes Control and Complications Trial (DCCT), intensive insulin therapy has remained the mainstay of treatment for patients with T1D (DCCT Research Group 1993). Further, since the UK Prospective Diabetes Study (UKPDS) released its findings, insulin therapy as a means to optimize glycemic control has been advocated for patients with T2D failing to achieve target A1C levels (UKPDS Group 1998). These approaches became even more salient following recognition of the sustained health benefits of earlier optimization of glycemic control, coined "metabolic memory" or the "legacy effect." These terms refer to the continued protection against the development of chronic diabetes complications a decade following the end of each of these clinical trials that was afforded to those who had been intensively treated (Nathan 2005, Holman 2008, White 2010). Further, intensive insulin treatment in the DCCT trial was not associated with any deterioration in quality of life (DCCT Research Group 1996). Nonetheless, it remains important to offer patients approaches to intensive therapy that are easy to use and incur the fewest burdens.

Insulin pens offer easy insulin administration for patients with T2D transitioning to insulin therapy, particularly for those patients initially resistant to giving injections. On the other hand, for patients with T1D, insulin pens (like insulin pump therapy; see Chapter 10) offer a means to provide physiologic insulin replacement in injection-based basal bolus insulin programs that include long-acting insulin analogs for basal insulin coverage and rapid-acting insulin analogs for bolus insulin delivery at meal or snack times or at times of elevated BG levels.

There are many potential benefits of insulin delivery with the use of pens (see Table 11.3). Approaches to and benefits of physiologic insulin replacement using insulin pump therapy appear in Chapter 10.

Table 11.3 Possible Opportunities with Insulin Pen Use

Avoidance of vial and syringe
Ease of insulin administration
Dosing accuracy
Reduced anxiety
Greater convenience
Social acceptability
Increased flexibility
Availability of insulin dose memory function in some pens
Ease of use for people with impaired vision or manual dexterity
Possible earlier transition to insulin therapy for patients with T2D
Reduction in perceived pain
Potential to improve quality of life
Reduced rates of hypoglycemia
Potential for a favorable impact on health care system use and costs

An insulin pen is a discreet insulin delivery device that comes either as a pre-filled, disposable pen or as a reusable pen case that accepts a small (3-ml) cartridge of insulin. Both types of pens accept single-use, screw-on needle tips that come in various lengths and gauges to match the needs of the individual. The portability and convenience of the pen has led to easier transitions to insulin therapy for patients with T2D and to more rapid adoption of multiple daily injection therapy or basal bolus therapy for patients with T1D. Rapid-acting insulin analogs and basal insulin analogs are all available in insulin pens. Some individuals prefer to use an insulin pen in place of an insulin vial and syringe when they are away from home, either at school or work, or when they are eating out or traveling. Previous research notes improved injection technique in terms of ease of use, dose accuracy, social acceptability, and quality of life (Wood 2007, Dang 2010, Pearson 2010, Williams 2010, Hanas 2011, Magwire 2011). A recent publication of a medication satisfaction rating survey reported that scores for medication convenience and negative events were more favorable among adults with T2D receiving insulin by pen delivery than among those receiving insulin by syringe (Peyrot 2011). In some countries outside of the U.S., more than 90% of people with insulin-treated diabetes use an insulin pen. Recent years have seen an increase in the numbers of pen users in the U.S. because the insulin pen is a good tool for transition to simple insulin therapy or intensive insulin treatment of diabetes. Additionally, insulin pen use may be associated with increased adherence, reduced rates of hypoglycemia, improved quality of life, and a favorable impact on health care system use and costs (Asche 2010, Luijf 2010, Anderson 2011).

INTERNET PROGRAMS AND TECHNOLOGIES

The Internet touches almost everyone's life today. In 2011, 79% of people in North America were Internet users (http://www.internetworldstats.com/stats. htm). There are many Internet sites with social media that focus on diabetes education or support, including sites such as Facebook and YouTube. There are other sites that offer more-focused diabetes information such as Children With Diabetes, Joslin.org, diabetes.org, DLife.com, and the National Diabetes Education Program (Table 11.4). The anonymity, convenience, and expansive surfing options make the Internet and social media potentially valuable sources of diabetes education and support. When "diabetes" is entered into an Internet search engine, there are more than 300,000,000 results. Sites vary with respect to content and expertise, so it is important for health care providers to offer their patients information regarding reputable sites for education and support. There are also many modern interactive technologies that can promote diabetes self-management, such as DVDs, computer applications, smartphone applications, and text messaging reminder systems, which can benefit patients of all ages and be implemented in various settings such as the clinic, workplace, community, or home. There have been a number of recently published reviews on the topic of Internet programs and interactive technologies (Glasgow 2002, Russell-Minda 2009, Kaufman 2010, Misono 2010, Siminerio 2010, Webb 2010, Mulvaney 2011, Harris 2012). A few examples of particular studies follow.

A recent study used a web-based intervention along with usual care in older adults with T2D and demonstrated significant improvements in A1C, weight, cholesterol, and HDL levels after 6 months compared with usual care alone (Bond 2007). The intervention group also had significant improvements on measures of depression, quality of life, social support, and self-efficacy (Bond 2010). The 6-month web-based multicomponent intervention consisted of educational materials, weekly online educational sessions, instant messaging, real-time chat room discussion, bulletin board messaging, and email using goal-setting and problem-solving skills to overcome barriers to improve self-management behaviors and psychosocial well-being. Although the study had limitations related to small sample size ($n = 62$), a homogeneous population, and short duration, the results are encouraging and support additional research using web-based interventions.

A larger 4-month study in over 400 adults with T2D compared an Internet-based diabetes self-management program delivered in English or Spanish with enhanced usual care (Glasgow 2010). Behavioral outcomes related to healthy eating, fat intake, and physical activity were significantly improved with the Internet-based intervention compared with the usual care group although there was no difference in the biologic outcomes of A1C, body mass index, lipids, and blood pressure. After 12 months, the Internet intervention again demonstrated significantly improved health behaviors compared with usual care (Glasgow 2012). The authors suggest, however, that more intensive and tailored interventions are likely needed for meaningful improvements in biologic outcomes. An email intervention, called ALIVE! (A Lifestyle Intervention Via Email) aimed to improve diet and physical activity as well as health-related quality of life and self-efficacy (Block 2008, Sternfeld 2009). Following a 16-week workplace study involving over 700 employees, the email intervention group compared with the control group demonstrated significant improvements in diet, physical activity, quality of life, and self-efficacy. Differences between groups were still present 4 months following the end of the intervention period.

Web-based educational and emotional support discussion boards appear to attract a broad base of patients with diabetes, discussing topics related to nutrition, emotional support, high and low BG levels, and diabetes complications (Zrebiec 2001). In response to a user satisfaction survey, the majority of respondents rated participation on the discussion boards as positive with respect to coping with diabetes and feeling more hopeful (Zrebiec 2005). BG awareness training has also been converted into a web-based intervention (Cox 2008). In an initial pilot study of 40 patients with T1D, users found the web-based intervention to be helpful and easy to use, and they endorsed improved functioning. Another pilot study involving 77 adults with T1D compared a 12-month web-based case management program with usual care in a diabetes specialty clinic (McCarrier 2009). Although there was a only a nonsignificant improvement in A1C with the intervention compared with usual care, diabetes-related self-efficacy significantly increased in the intervention group compared with the usual care group. The authors suggest a need for larger studies.

There are a number of small studies involving youth with T1D that use the Internet or other interactive technologies. Text messaging, in particular, has been used to increase BGM frequency in pediatric patients with T1D, notably because cell phone text messaging appears to be a preferred communication method among teens (Lenhart 2010). Pilot studies, lasting 3–12 months, have used text messaging to enhance adherence, increase self-efficacy, promote behavior change, and improve health outcomes (Franklin 2003, Franklin 2006, Franklin 2008, Hanauer 2009, Nationwide Children's Hospital 2010, Mulvaney 2012). These studies have documented the usability and acceptability of text messaging in the pediatric population along with variable increases in adherence, self-efficacy, and A1C. A few other studies have used wireless transfer of BG data either in the school setting or clinic setting and have demonstrated increased BGM frequency, improved self-care, and/or lower A1C in the intervention compared with the control groups (Kumar 2004, Nguyen 2008, Toscos 2012).

We piloted an automated BGM reminder system using computer-based email compared with cell phone–based text messaging for 12 weeks in 40 adolescents and young adults with T1D, ages 12–25 years (Hanauer 2009). Patients were eager to enter the brief pilot program and preferred the text message reminders to email reminders. During the first month, participants in the cell phone text messaging group sent almost twice as many BG results to the secure central server as did participants in the computer-based email group. However, participant responses to the BG reminders decreased over time in both groups, suggesting that more-intensive, interactive interventions may be needed in the pediatric population with T1D to sustain self-management behaviors. A recent pilot study reports incorporating "gamification," in which routine behaviors are rewarded, for example, with iTunes® and computer or smartphone apps (Cafazzo 2012). Additional studies are needed to determine if such rewards can increase and sustain behavior change and improve health outcomes.

There are additional Internet-based studies in pediatric patients with T1D. For example, following the success of coping skills training at increasing self-efficacy and improving glycemic control in teens with T1D, an Internet coping skills training program has been develop and evaluated in a pilot study (Grey 2000, Whittemore 2010). Additional multicenter studies are underway, aimed at assessing the effectiveness of the Internet coping skills program. An observational study of pediatric patients with T1D treated with insulin pump therapy demonstrated a significant association between use of an Internet-based insulin pump monitoring system and improved glycemic control (Corriveau 2008).

Many of the studies using the Internet and interactive technologies have limitations related to sample size and study duration. Nonetheless, preliminary studies are encouraging with respect to improvements in biologic and psychosocial outcomes in both pediatric and adult populations and in patients with type 1 and type 2 diabetes.

Table 11.4 Diabetes Management Opportunities with the Internet and Interactive Technologies

---

Patient and family education
Patient and family support
Automated reminder systems for appointments, BGM, medications, etc.
Increased adherence to BGM
Increased medication adherence
Automated creation of glucose logs and medication use by date and time
Attention to lifestyle efforts with healthful eating and increased physical activity
Enhanced self-efficacy and empowerment
Improvements in glycemic control and comorbid conditions
Psychosocial well-being
Improved quality of life
Potential for decreased health care system use and cost savings

---

RECOMMENDATIONS FOR CLINICAL CARE

Blood Glucose Monitoring (BGM)

1. Patients with type 1 or type 2 diabetes should receive diabetes self-management education that includes training in BGM and data interpretation.
2. Patients with diabetes should be encouraged to work with their health care team to determine their recommended frequency of daily BGM with the recognition that A1C improves as BGM frequency increases up to 5–10 times each day.
3. Patients with diabetes receiving intensive diabetes management training with frequent BGM should be screened for psychological problems, including diabetes distress, diabetes burnout, symptoms of depression and anxiety, and fear of hypoglycemia (or hyperglycemia), and should be referred to mental health specialists as needed.

Continuous Glucose Monitoring (CGM)

1. Real-time CGM can be used in pediatric and adults patients with T1D in efforts to reduce their A1C levels or maintain target A1C levels without increasing the frequency of hypoglycemia.
2. Patient selection for CGM use should consider the patient's current frequency of BGM, willingness to learn how to insert the sensor and how to set and respond to alarms, and desire to react to glucose trend and downloaded data. When parents want CGM for their child, it is important to make sure attitudes about use are reconciled between parent and child, particularly if the child is old enough to think through whether he or she will actively participate in its use. When spouses, partners, or family members request CGM for patients, it is important to reconcile attitudes about CGM use so that adult patients will not feel unduly pressured to begin CGM without intention to continue use.
3. Current CGM devices are associated with substantial patient burden and require ongoing education and psychological support to help patients sustain CGM use.

Insulin Pen Use

1. Insulin pen use should be considered for patients with T2D transitioning to insulin therapy due to ease of insulin administration, greater convenience, and potential for improved quality of life with pens.
2. Given the ease of insulin pen use, convenience, dosing accuracy, and potential for improved adherence, insulin pen use should be considered for patients with diabetes who are beginning intensive insulin therapy.
3. Cost, ease of use, adherence, and potential psychological barriers, such as hesitation to wear a visible device, should be evaluated when comparing physiologic insulin replacement using injection pen-based basal-bolus intensive insulin therapy with insulin pump therapy.

Internet Program and Interactive Technologies

1. The Internet should be considered as a means for patients with type 1 and type 2 diabetes to receive diabetes education, social support, and problem-solving strategies to improve adherence, self-efficacy, and health outcomes. Public access sites such as libraries and community centers may be helpful for those without home Internet access.
2. Cell phone text messaging automated reminder systems should be considered as a way to increase BGM frequency and to increase adherence and self-efficacy in pediatric and adult patients with T1D.
3. Patients with type 1 or type 2 diabetes should consider transmitting their blood glucose data via the Internet or by text messaging and should consider communicating via the Internet with their health care teams in efforts to improve health outcomes.

BIBLIOGRAPHY

American Diabetes Association: Standards of medical care in diabetes—2012. *Diabetes Care* 35 (Suppl. 1):S11–S63, 2012

Anderson BJ, Redondo MJ: What can we learn from patient-reported outcomes of insulin pen devices? *J Diabetes Sci Technol* 5:1563–1571, 2011

Anderson BJ, Vangsness L, Connell A, Butler D, Goebel-Fabbri A, Laffel LM: Family conflict, adherence, and glycaemic control in youth with short duration type 1 diabetes. *Diabet Med* 19:635–642, 2002

Asche CV, Shane-McWhorter L, Raparla S: Health economics and compliance of vials/syringes versus pen devices: a review of the evidence. *Diabetes Technol Ther* 12 (Suppl. 1):S101–S108, 2010

Bergenstal RM, Tamborlane WV, Ahmann A, Buse JB, Dailey G, Davis SN, et al.: Effectiveness of sensor-augmented insulin-pump therapy in type 1 diabetes. *N Engl J Med* 363:311–320, 2010

Block G, Sternfeld B, Block CH, Block TJ, Norris J, Hopkins D, et al.: Development of Alive! (A Lifestyle Intervention Via Email), and its effect on health-related quality of life, presenteeism, and other behavioral outcomes: randomized controlled trial. *J Med Internet Res* 10:e43, 2008

Blonde L, Karter AJ: Current evidence regarding the value of self-monitored blood glucose testing. *Am J Med* 118 (Suppl. 9A):20S–26S, 2005

Bond GE, Burr RL, Wolf FM, Feldt K: The effects of a web-based intervention on psychosocial well-being among adults aged 60 and older with diabetes: a randomized trial. *Diabetes Educ* 36:446–456, 2010

Bond GE, Burr R, Wolf FM, Price M, McCurry SM, Teri L: The effects of a web-based intervention on the physical outcomes associated with diabetes among adults age 60 and older: a randomized trial. *Diabetes Technol Ther* 9:52–59, 2007

Cafazzo JA, Casselman M, Hamming N, Katzman DK, Palmert MR: Design of an mHealth app for the self-management of adolescent type 1 diabetes: a pilot study. *J Med Internet Res* 14:e70, 2012

Centers for Disease Control and Prevention: Self-monitoring of blood glucose among adults with diabetes: United States, 1997–2006. *MMWR Morb Mortal Wkly Rep* 56:1133–1137, 2007

Corriveau EA, Durso PJ, Kaufman ED, Skipper BJ, Laskaratos LA, Heintzman KB: Effect of Carelink, an internet-based insulin pump monitoring system, on glycemic control in rural and urban children with type 1 diabetes mellitus. *Pediatr Diabetes* 9:360–366, 2008

Cox D, Ritterband L, Magee J, Clarke W, Gonder-Frederick L: Blood glucose awareness training delivered over the Internet. *Diabetes Care* 31:1527–1528, 2008

Cox DJ, Irvine A, Gonder-Frederick L, Nowacek G, Butterfield J: Fear of hypoglycemia: quantification, validation, and utilization. *Diabetes Care* 10:617–621, 1987

Dailey G: Assessing glycemic control with self-monitoring of blood glucose and hemoglobin A(1c) measurements. *Mayo Clin Proc* 82:229–235, 2007

Dang DK, Lee J: Analysis of symposium articles on insulin pen devices and alternative insulin delivery methods. *J Diabetes Sci Technol* 4:558–561, 2010

DCCT Research Group: Influence of intensive diabetes treatment on quality-of-life outcomes in the Diabetes Control and Complications Trial. *Diabetes Care* 19:195–203, 1996

DCCT Research Group: The effect of intensive treatment of diabetes on the development and progression of long-term complications in insulin-dependent diabetes mellitus. *N Engl J Med* 329:977–986, 1993

Deiss D, Bolinder J, Riveline JP, Battelino T, Bosi E, Tubiana-Rufi N, et al.: Improved glycemic control in poorly controlled patients with type 1 diabetes using real-time continuous glucose monitoring. *Diabetes Care* 29:2730–2732, 2006

Farmer AJ, Wade AN, French DP, Simon J, Yudkin P, Gray A, et al.: Blood glucose self-monitoring in type 2 diabetes: a randomised controlled trial. *Health Technol Assess* 13:iii-iv, ix-xi, 1-50, 2009

Fisher L, Polonsky W, Parkin CG, Jelsovsky Z, Amstutz L, Wagner RS: The impact of blood glucose monitoring on depression and distress in insulin-naive patients with type 2 diabetes. *Curr Med Res Opin* 27 (Suppl. 3):39-46, 2011

Franklin VL, Greene A, Waller A, Greene SA, Pagliari C: Patients' engagement with "Sweet Talk": a text messaging support system for young people with diabetes. *J Med Internet Res* 10:e20, 2008

Franklin VL, Waller A, Pagliari C, Greene SA: A randomized controlled trial of Sweet Talk, a text-messaging system to support young people with diabetes. *Diabet Med* 23:1332–1338, 2006

Franklin V, Waller A, Pagliari C, Greene S: "Sweet Talk": text messaging support for intensive insulin therapy for young people with diabetes. *Diabetes Technol Ther* 5:991–996, 2003

Garg SK, Bookout TR, McFann KK, Kelly WC, Beatson C, Ellis SL, et al.: Improved glycemic control in intensively treated adult subjects with type 1 diabetes using insulin guidance software. *Diabetes Technol Ther* 10:369–375, 2008

Glasgow RE, Kurz D, King D, Dickman JM, Faber AJ, Halterman E, et al.: Twelve-month outcomes of an Internet-based diabetes self-management support program. *Patient Educ Couns* 87:81–92, 2012

Glasgow RE, Kurz D, King D, Dickman JM, Faber AJ, Halterman E, et al.: Outcomes of minimal and moderate support versions of an internet-based diabetes self-management support program. *J Gen Intern Med* 25:1315–1322, 2010

Glasgow RE: Using interactive technology in diabetes self-management. In *Practical Psychology for Diabetes Clinicians.* 2nd ed. Anderson BJ, Rubin RR, Eds. Alexandria, VA, American Diabetes Association, 2002, p. 51–62

Goyder E: Should we stop patients with non-insulin treated diabetes using self monitoring of blood glucose? The implications of the Diabetes Glycaemic Education and Monitoring (DiGEM) trial 2. *Prim Care Diabetes* 2:91–93, 2008

Grey M, Boland EA, Davidson M, Li J, Tamborlane WV: Coping skills training for youth with diabetes mellitus has long-lasting effects on metabolic control and quality of life. *J Pediatr* 137:107–113, 2000

Hanas R, de Beaufort C., Hoey H., Anderson B: Insulin delivery by injection in children and adolescents with diabetes. *Pediatr Diabetes* 12:518–526, 2011

Hanauer DA, Wentzell K, Laffel N, Laffel LM: Computerized Automated Reminder Diabetes System (CARDS): e-mail and SMS call phone text messaging reminders to support diabetes management. *Diabetes Technol Ther* 11:99–106, 2009

Harris MA, Hood KK, Mulvaney SA: Pumpers, skypers, surfers and texters: technology to improve the management of diabetes in teenagers. *Diabetes Obes Metab.* doi: 10.1111/j.1463-1326.2012.01599.x.

Hirsch IB, Bode BW, Childs BP, Close KL, Fisher WA, Gavin JR, et al.: Self-Monitoring of Blood Glucose (SMBG) in insulin- and non-insulin-using adults with diabetes: consensus recommendations for improving SMBG accuracy, utilization, and research. *Diabetes Technol Ther* 10:419–439, 2008

Holman RR, Paul SK, Bethel MA, Matthews DR, Neil HA: 10-year follow-up of intensive glucose control in type 2 diabetes. *N Engl J Med* 359:1577–1589, 2008

Ingerski LM, Laffel L, Drotar D, Repaske D, Hood KK: Correlates of glycemic control and quality of life outcomes in adolescents with type 1 diabetes. *Pediatr Diabetes* 11:563–571, 2010

Juvenile Diabetes Research Foundation Continuous Glucose Monitoring Study Group: Validation of measures of satisfaction with and impact of continuous and conventional glucose monitoring. *Diabetes Technol Ther* 12:679–684, 2010a

Juvenile Diabetes Research Foundation Continuous Glucose Monitoring Study Group, Beck RW, Lawrence JM, Laffel L, Wysocki T, Xing D, et al.: Quality-of-life measures in children and adults with type 1 diabetes: Juvenile Diabetes Research Foundation Continuous Glucose Monitoring randomized trial. *Diabetes Care* 33:2175–2177, 2010b

Juvenile Diabetes Research Foundation Continuous Glucose Monitoring Study Group: Factors predictive of use and of benefit from continuous glucose monitoring in type 1 diabetes. *Diabetes Care* 32:1947–1953, 2009a

Juvenile Diabetes Research Foundation Continuous Glucose Monitoring Study Group: The effect of continuous glucose monitoring in well-controlled type 1 diabetes. *Diabetes Care* 32:1378–1383, 2009b

Juvenile Diabetes Research Foundation Continuous Glucose Monitoring Study Group, Tamborlane WV, Beck RW, Bode BW, et al.: Continuous glucose monitoring and intensive treatment of type 1 diabetes. *N Engl J Med* 359:1464–1476, 2008

Kaufman N: Internet and information technology use in treatment of diabetes. *Int J Clin Pract Suppl*, 41–46, 2010

Klonoff DC, Buckingham B, Christiansen JS, Montori VM, Tamborlane WV, Vigersky RA, et al.: Continuous glucose monitoring: an Endocrine Society Clinical Practice Guideline. *J Clin Endocrinol Metab* 96:2968–2979, 2011

Kordonouri O, Pankowska E, Rami B, Kapellen T, Coutant R, Hartmann R, et al.: Sensor-augmented pump therapy from the diagnosis of childhood type 1 diabetes: results of the Paediatric Onset Study (ONSET) after 12 months of treatment. *Diabetologia* 53:2487–2495, 2010

Kumar VS, Wentzell KJ, Mikkelsen T, Pentland A, Laffel LM: The DAILY (Daily Automated Intensive Log for Youth) trial: a wireless, portable system to improve adherence and glycemic control in youth with diabetes. *Diabetes Technol Ther* 6:445–453, 2004

Laffel LM, Hsu WC, McGill JB, Meneghini L, Volkening LK: Continued use of an integrated meter with electronic logbook maintains improvements in glycemic control beyond a randomized, controlled trial. *Diabetes Technol Ther* 9:254–264, 2007

Laffel L, Volkening L, Hood K, Lochrie A, Nansel T, Anderson B, et al.: Optimizing glycemic control in youth with T1DM: importance of BG monitoring and supportive family communication [Abstract]. *Diabetes* 55:A197, 2006

Lawlor MT, Laffel L, Anderson BJ: *Blood Sugar Monitoring Owner's Manual*. Boston, Joslin Diabetes Center, 1997

Lenhart A, Ling R, Campbell S, Purcell K, Pew Internet & American Life Project: Teens and mobile phones, 2010. Available at http://pewinternet.org/reports/2010/teens-and-mobile-phones.aspx. Accessed 21 June 2012

Levine BS, Anderson BJ, Butler DA, Brackett J, Laffel L: Predictors of glycemic control and short-term adverse outcomes in youth with type 1 diabetes. *J Pediatr* 139:197–203, 2001

Luijf YM, DeVries JH: Dosing accuracy of insulin pens versus conventional syringes and vials. *Diabetes Technol Ther* 12 (Suppl. 1):S73–S77, 2010

Magwire ML: Addressing barriers to insulin therapy: the role of insulin pens. *Am J Ther* 18:392–402, 2011

Markowitz JT, Pratt K, Aggarwal J, Volkening LK, Laffel LM: Psychosocial correlates of continuous glucose monitoring use in youth and adults with type 1 diabetes and parents of youth. *Diabetes Technol Ther* 14:523-526, 2012

McCarrier KP, Ralston JD, Hirsch IB, Lewis G, Martin DP, Zimmerman FJ, et al.: Web-based collaborative care for type 1 diabetes: a pilot randomized trial. *Diabetes Technol Ther* 11:211–217, 2009

Misono AS, Cutrona SL, Choudhry NK, Fischer MA, Stedman MR, Liberman JN, et al.: Healthcare information technology interventions to improve cardiovascular and diabetes medication adherence. *Am J Manag Care* 16 (12 Suppl. HIT):SP82–SP92, 2010

Moreland EC, Volkening LK, Lawlor MT, Chalmers KA, Anderson BJ, Laffel LM: Use of a blood glucose monitoring manual to enhance monitoring adherence in adults with diabetes: a randomized controlled trial. *Arch Intern Med* 166:689–695, 2006

Mulvaney SA, Anders S, Smith AK, Pittel EJ, Johnson KB: A pilot test of a tailored mobile and web-based diabetes messaging system for adolescents. *J Telemed Telecare* 18:115–118, 2012

Mulvaney SA, Ritterband LM, Bosslet L: Mobile intervention design in diabetes: review and recommendations. *Curr Diab Rep* 11:486–493, 2011

Nathan DM, Cleary PA, Backlund JY, Genuth SM, Lachin JM, Orchard TJ, et al.: Intensive diabetes treatment and cardiovascular disease in patients with type 1 diabetes. *N Engl J Med* 353:2643–2653, 2005

Nathan DM, McKitrick C, Larkin M, Schaffran R, Singer DE: Glycemic control in diabetes mellitus: have changes in therapy made a difference? *Am J Med* 100:157–163, 1996

Nationwide Children's Hospital: Pilot study supports adolescent diabetes patients through personalized text messages. *ScienceDaily* 10 Aug 2010. Available from http://www.sciencedaily.com/releases/2010/07/100730191628.htm. Accessed 20 July 2012

Nguyen TM, Mason KJ, Sanders CG, Yazdani P, Heptulla RA: Targeting blood glucose management in school improves glycemic control in children with poorly controlled type 1 diabetes mellitus. *J Pediatr* 153:575-578, 2008

Pearson TL: Practical aspects of insulin pen devices. *J Diabetes Sci Technol* 4:522–531, 2010

Peyrot M, Harshaw Q, Shillington AC, Xu Y, Rubin RR: Validation of a tool to assess medication treatment satisfaction in patients with type 2 diabetes: the Diabetes Medication System Rating Questionnaire (DMSRQ). *Diabet Med.* doi: 10.1111/j.1464-5491.2011.03538.x.

Phillip M, Danne T, Shalitin S, Buckingham B, Laffel L, Tamborlane W, et al.: Use of continuous glucose monitoring in children and adolescents (*). *Pediatr Diabetes* 13:215–228, 2012

Pistrosch F, Koehler C, Wildbrett J, Hanefeld M: Relationship between diurnal glucose levels and HbA1c in type 2 diabetes. *Horm Metab Res* 38:455–459, 2006

Polonsky WH, Fisher L, Schikman CH, Hinnen DA, Parkin CG, Jelsovsky Z, et al.: Structured self-monitoring of blood glucose significantly reduces A1C levels in poorly controlled, noninsulin-treated type 2 diabetes: results from the Structured Testing Program study. *Diabetes Care* 34:262–267, 2011

Raccah D, Sulmont V, Reznik Y, Guerci B, Renard E, Hanaire H, et al.: Incremental value of continuous glucose monitoring when starting pump therapy in patients with poorly controlled type 1 diabetes: the RealTrend study. *Diabetes Care* 32:2245–2250, 2009

Ritholz MD, Atakov-Castillo A, Beste M, Beverly EA, Leighton A, Weinger K, et al.: Psychosocial factors associated with use of continuous glucose monitoring. *Diabet Med* 27:1060–1065, 2010

Russell-Minda E, Jutai J, Speechley M, Bradley K, Chudyk A, Petrella R: Health technologies for monitoring and managing diabetes: a systematic review. *J Diabetes Sci Technol* 3:1460–1471, 2009

Siebolds M, Gaedeke O, Schwedes U: Self-monitoring of blood glucose: psychological aspects relevant to changes in HbA1c in type 2 diabetic patients treated with diet or diet plus oral antidiabetic medication. *Patient Educ Couns* 62:104–110, 2006

Siminerio LM: The role of technology and the chronic care model. *J Diabetes Sci Technol* 4:470–475, 2010

Sternfeld B, Block C, Quesenberry CP Jr, Block TJ, Husson G, Norris JC, et al.: Improving diet and physical activity with ALIVE: a worksite randomized trial. *Am J Prev Med* 36:475–483, 2009

Tansey M, Laffel L, Cheng J, Beck R, Coffey J, Huang E, et al.: Satisfaction with continuous glucose monitoring in adults and youths with type 1 diabetes. *Diabet Med* 28:1118–1122, 2011

Toscos TR, Ponder SW, Anderson BJ, Davidson MB, Lee ML, Montemayor-Gonzalez E, et al.: Integrating an automated diabetes management system into the family management of children with type 1 diabetes: results from a 12-month randomized controlled technology trial. *Diabetes Care* 35:498–502, 2012

UK Prospective Diabetes Study (UKPDS) Group: Intensive blood-glucose control with sulphonylureas or insulin compared with conventional treatment and risk of complications in patients with type 2 diabetes (UKPDS 33). *Lancet* 352:837–853, 1998

Webb TL, Joseph J, Yardley L, Michie S: Using the internet to promote health behavior change: a systematic review and meta-analysis of the impact of theoretical basis, use of behavior change techniques, and mode of delivery on efficacy. *J Med Internet Res* 12:e4, 2010

Welschen LM, Bloemendal E, Nijpels G, Dekker JM, Heine RJ, Stalman WA, et al.: Self-monitoring of blood glucose in patients with type 2 diabetes who are not using insulin: a systematic review. *Diabetes Care* 28:1510–1517, 2005

Wen L, Parchman ML, Linn WD, Lee S: Association between self-monitoring of blood glucose and glycemic control in patients with type 2 diabetes mellitus. *Am J Health Syst Pharm* 61:2401–2405, 2004

White NH, Sun W, Cleary PA, Tamborlane WV, Danis RP, Hainsworth DP, et al.: Effect of prior intensive therapy in type 1 diabetes on 10-year progression of retinopathy in the DCCT/EDIC: comparison of adults and adolescents. *Diabetes* 59:1244–1253, 2010

Whittemore R, Grey M, Lindemann E, Ambrosino J, Jaser S: Development of an internet coping skills training program for teenagers with type 1 diabetes. *Comput Inform Nurs* 28:103–111, 2010

Williams AS, Schnarrenberger PA: A comparison of dosing accuracy: visually impaired and sighted people using insulin pens. *J Diabetes Sci Technol* 4:514–521, 2010

Wood JR, Laffel LMB: Technology and intensive management in youth with type 1 diabetes: state of the art. *Curr Diab Rep* 7:104–113, 2007

Ziegler R, Heidtmann B, Hilgard D, Hofer S, Rosenbauer J, Holl R, et al.: Frequency of SMBG correlates with HbA1c and acute complications in children and adolescents with type 1 diabetes. *Pediatr Diabetes* 12:11–17, 2011

Zrebiec JF: Internet communities: do they improve coping with diabetes? *Diabetes Educ* 31:825–828, 830–832, 834, 836, 2005

Zrebiec JF, Jacobson AM: What attracts patients with diabetes to an Internet support group? A 21-month longitudinal website study. *Diabet Med* 18:154–158, 2001

Lori Laffel, MD, MPH, is Chief of the Pediatric, Adolescent and Young Adult Section and an Investigator in the Section on Genetics and Epidemiology at the Joslin Diabetes Center, and an Associate Professor of Pediatrics at Harvard Medical School, in Boston, MA.

Chapter 12
Bariatric Surgery

Brooke A. Bailer, PhD, Thomas A. Wadden, PhD,
Lucy F. Faulconbridge, PhD, and David B. Sarwer, PhD

Extreme obesity, defined by a BMI >40 kg/m², now affects 5.7% of adults in the U.S. (Flegal 2010). This condition is associated with increased mortality, particularly from cardiovascular disease, type 2 diabetes, and several cancers (Allison 1999, Calle 2003). It is also associated with an increased risk of psychiatric disorders, as well as with marked impairments in quality of life (Black 1992, Sullivan 1993, Onyike 2003, Kinzl 2006, Kalarchian 2007). Surgical intervention is the most effective treatment for extremely obese individuals who have failed to lose weight with behavioral or pharmacological approaches (Buchwald 2004). The Roux-en-Y gastric bypass (RYGB) produces long-term (i.e., 10-year) reductions in initial body weight of ~25%, whereas laparoscopic adjustable banding achieves a loss of 15–20% (Buchwald 2004). Weight loss achieved with these interventions is associated with significant improvements in health, particularly type 2 diabetes (Buchwald 2004, Kral 2007).

Individuals seeking bariatric surgery are required to undergo extensive medical evaluation to determine that they are medically appropriate for surgery. They also typically complete a behavioral-psychosocial assessment, as recommended (in 1991) by a National Institutes of Health (NIH) Consensus Development Conference on Gastrointestinal Surgery for Severe Obesity (NIH conference 1991) and by a more recent expert panel (Mechanick 2009). This chapter describes the behavioral status of obese patients who seek bariatric surgery, as well as changes in mood, eating behavior, and quality of life that can be anticipated following surgery. The chapter combines a review of research findings with observations resulting from long clinical experience working with these individuals.

PREOPERATIVE PSYCHIATRIC STATUS

Psychiatric status varies markedly in applicants for bariatric surgery. At the time of evaluation for surgery, a majority of individuals have essentially normal psychological functioning (Sarwer 2005b). Thus, mental health and other practitioners should be prepared to meet many candidates who have good self-esteem and enjoy their work and personal lives. However, a significant minority of individuals report marked psychological distress. Kalarchian et al. (2007), for example, examined the psychiatric status of 288 consecutive candidates using the Structured Clinical Interview for the DSM-IV (SCID). They found that 37.8% of the sample met criteria for an Axis I disorder at the time of surgical evaluation and 66.3% had a history of an Axis I disorder (Kalarchian 2007). Other investigators have reported similar findings using structured interviews (Kinzl 2006, Rosenberger 2006, Kalarchian 2007, Mauri 2008, Muhlhans 2009).

Affective Disorders

Major depressive disorder (MDD) and dysthymic disorder are among the most common psychiatric conditions observed in surgery candidates (Black 1992, Sarwer 2004, Kinzl 2006, Rosenberger 2006, Kalarchian 2007, Mauri 2008, Muhlhans 2009). Prevalence rates for lifetime history of MDD range from ~15–50%, whereas those for current MDD are 3–25%. The lifetime prevalence of dysthymic disorder, a less severe form of depression, has been estimated at ~5%, with lower rates for current dysthymia (Black 1992, Rosenberger 2006, Kalarchian 2007, Mauri 2008, Muhlhans 2009). (See Chapter 1 on Depression for diagnostic criteria.)

Several risk factors for depression in obese individuals have been identified, the first of which is higher BMI. Onyike et al. (2003), examining data from the National Health and Nutrition Examination Survey, found that individuals with a BMI ≥40 kg/m² had 4.6 times the risk of experiencing major depression in the past month as compared with people of average weight. By contrast, the risk was increased by only 1.9 times in people with a BMI of 35–39.9 kg/m² (Onyike 2003). Higher BMI is associated with impaired physical function and bodily pain which, in turn, are associated with depression (Kalarchian 2007). People with higher BMIs also may experience greater weight-related stigma, as well as greater body image dissatisfaction, each of which is related to greater symptoms of depression (Myers 1999, Sarwer 2005b). Younger surgery candidates also appear to be at greater risk of mood disorders, as are women (Dixon 2003).

Anxiety Disorders

Anxiety disorders also are frequently observed in bariatric surgery candidates, particularly specific phobia, social phobia, panic disorder, and post-traumatic stress disorder (Rosenberger 2006, Kalarchian 2007, Mauri 2008, Muhlhans 2009). Studies that used semistructured clinical interviews have reported a lifetime history of anxiety disorders in ~15–40% of surgery patients (Rosenberger 2006, Kalarchian 2007, Mauri 2008, Muhlhans 2009). The presence of a current anxiety disorder, identified at the time of the assessment, has been observed in 12–24% of candidates (Rosenberger 2006, Kalarchian 2007, Mauri 2008, Muhlhans 2009).

Substance Use

The lifetime prevalence of substance use, including alcohol and drug use, in surgery candidates has been estimated at ~1–35%, with most estimates below 15% (Rosenberger 2006, Kalarchian 2007, Mauri 2008, Muhlhans 2009). Prevalence rates for current substance use have been much lower, ranging from 1–2% (Rosenberger 2006, Kalarchian 2007, Muhlhans 2009). Kalarchian et al. (2007) hypothesized that the discrepancy in lifetime and current prevalence rates may be due to candidates' attempts to present themselves in a positive light during the psychosocial interview, so as to not disqualify themselves from surgery. Alternatively, some patients report having stopped using alcohol and other substances, and replacing their use with overeating.

Personality Disorders

Based on SCID interviews, ~20–30% of surgery candidates have been estimated to meet criteria for an Axis II disorder (Kalarchian 2007, Mauri 2008). These disorders involve a set of personality traits that are associated with chronic social dysfunction. The most common personality disorders among surgery candidates include obsessive-compulsive, avoidant, paranoid, and borderline disorders (Kalarchian 2007, Mauri 2008). In many cases, individuals with personality disorders are not troubled by their conditions. Instead, their often self-centered or manipulative patterns of interpersonal behavior cause difficulties for their friends, family members, or coworkers (Millon 1996).

Methodological Variability in Assessment

For all of the diagnostic categories described so far, differences in method of assessment appear to have contributed to the range of prevalence estimates obtained (Mitchell 2010). Diagnostic procedures have ranged from structured clinical interviews—the ideal method of assessment for research purposes—to unstructured practitioner-based assessment, to the use of self-report measures, which tend to overestimate the prevalence of psychopathology (Dymek-Valentine 2004, Allison 2006). A recent study that examined the frequency of agreement between unstructured practitioner-based evaluations and SCID assessments for current and lifetime psychiatric diagnoses found poor agreement in current and some lifetime Axis I disorders (Mitchell 2010). Retrospective recall of psychiatric symptoms, another methodological variation, also compromises the accuracy of diagnoses (Niego 2007).

Clinical Significance and Treatment of Preoperative Psychiatric Disorders

Investigators originally expected that preoperative psychopathology would be associated with suboptimal weight loss following surgery. However, findings in this area have been inconsistent (Bloomston 1997, Powers 1997, Ma 2006). A recent study, for example, found that individuals with a lifetime history of mood or anxiety disorders lost less weight after surgery compared with those without such a history, whereas current Axis I and Axis II disorders did not predict impaired weight loss (Kalarchian 2008). Another investigation found that weight loss was suboptimal in patients with greater psychopathology (i.e., more than one psychiatric diagnosis) compared with those with less psychopathology (i.e., one or no psychiatric diagnoses) (Kinzl 2006). Several studies, however, have reported greater weight loss in patients with depression or a history of psychiatric treatment (Averbukh 2003, Clark 2003, Herpertz 2004, van Hout 2005). In summarizing the literature, Herpertz et al. (2004) concluded that negative affect that is related to patients' distress about their obesity may facilitate weight loss following surgery. By contrast, major depression or other psychopathology that occurs independent of body weight may be associated with suboptimal outcomes, including medical complications (Herpertz 2004). This is an interesting hypothesis that merits further study.

The finding that preoperative psychiatric status does not consistently predict weight loss has led some to question the need for a psychosocial evaluation (Buchwald 2005). Given the frequent occurrence of clinically significant depression and other disorders, which can be treated with behavioral or pharmacologic interventions to relieve patients' suffering, thorough preoperative care should include the treatment of significant psychiatric disorders, as it does the management of severe hypertension, sleep apnea, and other medical conditions. Not surprisingly, a significant minority of bariatric surgery candidates report a history of psychiatric care. Approximately 15–40% of patients report having received psychotherapy, and roughly 40% indicated that they were taking psychotropic medications at the time of their presurgical behavioral assessment (Dixon 2003, Sarwer 2004, Friedman 2007, Crémieux 2010). The most commonly used psychotropic medications have been antidepressants, followed by antianxiety medications, with a small number of candidates reporting the use of antipsychotic medications (Sarwer 2004). Sarwer et al. (2004) found that, in a sample of 90 bariatric surgery candidates, only 3% were taking antipsychotic medications, compared with 30% taking antidepressant medications.

PREOPERATIVE EATING BEHAVIOR

Patients with extreme obesity have higher energy requirements (as determined by indirect calorimetry) than people of average weight (James 1978). Thus, extremely obese individuals consume more calories than their average-weight peers, although this amount may be equal to only a few hundred extra calories per day, the amount needed to maintain the excess adiposity (James 1978). Thus, practitioners may be surprised to find that many bariatric surgery patients do not report consuming excessively large amounts of food. However, a subset of surgery candidates suffer from binge eating and other eating disorders.

Prevalence of Binge Eating Disorder

Binge eating disorder (BED) is characterized by the consumption of an objectively large amount of food in a short period of time (i.e., 2 hours), in combination with a feeling of loss of control while eating (Spitzer 1992). It is also associated with an increased risk of other psychopathology, including depression and anxiety (Sarwer 2005b, Kalarchian 2007, Jones-Corneille 2010). BED is distinguished from bulimia nervosa by a lack of compensatory behaviors following the binge episode, such as vomiting, laxative use, or excessive exercise. Overall prevalence estimates of BED in surgery candidates have ranged from 2–50% (Hsu 1997, Powers 1999, Saunders 1999, Glinski 2001, Guisado 2001, de Zwaan 2003, Dymek-Valentine 2004, Allison 2006, Zimmerman 2007).

Self-report measures tend to overestimate the prevalence of BED, as compared with the use of structured or semistructured clinical interviews conducted by experienced assessors (Allison 2006). Paradoxically, overweight and obese patients tend to underestimate the amount of food that must be eaten to qualify as an objectively large amount—a value that has been defined as approximately twice the amount most people would eat under comparable circumstances (Wadden 2004). Prevalence estimates also vary according to whether a binge frequency requirement of at least twice per week (for the last 6 months) is used, as stipulated in the DSM-IV (American Psychiatric Association 2000), as compared with only once a week, as proposed for DSM-V (American Psychiatric Association 2000). Structured clinical interviews, using strict DSM-IV criteria, have yielded prevalence rates for BED of ~4–25% (Glinski 2001, Guisado 2001, Dymek-Valentine 2004, Allison 2006, Zimmerman 2007).

The effect of preoperative BED on weight loss following surgery has been a topic of debate (Wadden 2011). Several early reports suggested that BED was associated with suboptimal weight loss following surgery (Pekkarinen 1994, de Zwaan 2002, Sallet 2007), leading some investigators to recommend that patients receive (preoperative) cognitive behavioral treatment for their binge eating (Ashton 2009). Many of these early studies, however, had significant methodological limitations (Wadden 2011). More recent investigations have found little or no difference in weight loss 1 to 2 years after surgery in patients who did and did not have preoperative BED (Burgmer 2005, White 2006, Fujioka 2008, Alger-Mayer 2009, Wadden 2011). Wadden et al. (2011), for example, found that patients with BED lost 22.1% of initial weight at 1 year, compared with 24.1% for those who, prior to surgery, were free of a current eating disorder ($P > 0.30$). Patients' experience of postoperative loss of control over their eating—whether present or not before surgery—appears to be associated with suboptimal weight loss (Burgmer 2005, White 2010). Evaluation of subjective feelings of loss of control should be monitored before surgery and at milestone visits following surgery. Referral for cognitive behavioral treatment should be made as needed (White 2010, Wadden 2011).

Night Eating Syndrome

Prevalence rates of night eating syndrome (NES) in surgery candidates have ranged from ~2–55% (Rand 1997, Powers 1999, Allison 2006, Colles 2006). NES is characterized by an abnormally increased food intake in the evening and nighttime (O'Reardon 2004, Allison 2005). Patients with NES ingest at least 25% of daily food intake after the evening meal, and they experience nocturnal awakenings (at least 2 times per week) that are associated with eating (Allison 2010). To qualify for this diagnosis, patients must have an awareness of their nocturnal eating episodes, which distinguishes NES from sleep-related eating disorder (SRED). The patient's eating behavior must be associated with distress or impairment in functioning in order for an individual to meet criteria for NES (Allison 2010).

Allison et al. (2006), using a combination of self-report measure and semistructured clinical interview, found that ~5% of surgery patients met criteria for NES at the time of the presurgical interview. The conflicting prevalence rates for NES appear to be attributable to the use of different criteria for diagnosing the disorder and to the use of different methods of assessment. Little information is available concerning the effect of preoperative NES on weight loss following surgery.

PREOPERATIVE QUALITY OF LIFE

As noted previously, at the time of evaluation for surgery, a majority of candidates have essentially normal psychiatric status. Nonetheless, these individuals may experience impaired quality of life as a result of their excess weight.

Health-Related Quality of Life

The strain of carrying excess weight can impede even the most basic physical functions and personal care tasks (Larsson 2001a, Larsson 2001b). Numerous investigations have found that extremely obese individuals report significant impairment in performing activities such as walking, climbing stairs, bathing, and dressing (Larsson 2001a, Larsson 2001b) and that such difficulties are among the most distressing aspects of their obesity (Duval 2006). Health-related quality of life (HRQoL) is a broad term that describes an individual's functional status across a variety of domains, such as physical, mental, and social performance (Kral 1992, Wadden 2002). The domains that appear to be the most impaired in bariatric surgery candidates as a result of their excess weight are physical functioning and pain (Dixon 2001, Fabricatore 2005). Obesity-related conditions, including sleep apnea, type 2 diabetes, and osteoarthritis, appear to further exacerbate impairments in quality of life (White 2004).

A recent meta-analysis of 54 studies, conducted between 1980 and 2006, examined HRQoL in three groups: *1)* bariatric surgery candidates, *2)* obese individuals seeking nonsurgical treatment, and *3)* non–treatment-seeking overweight and obese participants (van Nunen 2007). The analysis found that individuals who sought surgical treatment reported significantly more impairment in HRQoL across several domains, including physical functioning and physical role limitations, than did obese individuals in the other two groups. Additional studies of non–treatment-seeking individuals have shown that the highest BMI levels are associated with the greatest impairments in quality of life (Jia 2005).

Several studies have examined the relations among BMI, HRQoL, and mood. Kalarchian et al. (2007) found that bariatric surgery patients with significant bodily pain and numerous role limitations were at increased risk for having a current Axis I diagnosis—typically mood (e.g., major depression) or anxiety disorders (e.g., panic)—compared with surgery patients without these physical conditions. Fabricatore et al. (2005) also examined the relationship between BMI, HRQoL, and symptoms of depression in 306 bariatric surgery candidates. Patients were classified as having impaired or unimpaired quality of life and were divided into three BMI categories (40–49.9 kg/m^2, 50–59.9 kg/m^2, and >60 kg/m^2) (Fabricatore 2005). Depression scores on the Beck Depression Inventory (BDI) generally varied by HRQoL impairment but not by BMI class. For example, individuals with class II and III obesity who did not report impaired physical functioning, bodily pain, or physical role limitations had lower depression scores than individuals in the same BMI category who reported these conditions, as shown in Figures 12.1 and 12.2. Moreover, BDI scores did not increase with higher BMI categories for individuals who were free of impairments in HRQoL. (Not all differences for HRQoL, within each BMI category, were statistically significant because of the small sample sizes, but all results were in the same direction.) These findings suggest that HRQoL may act as a mediator between BMI level and depression (Fabricatore 2005).

Body Image and Sexual Functioning

Body image. A significant minority of obese individuals experience marked body image dissatisfaction (Sarwer 2005b). As early as 1967, Stunkard and Mendelson (1967) described a group of obese patients with body image "disparagement" who believed their bodies were "ugly and despicable" and that others viewed them with "hostility and contempt." Their body image disparagement took the form of an overwhelming preoccupation with their obesity, often to the exclusion of any other personal characteristics. More recently, Sarwer et al. (1998) appeared to

Figure 12.1. Mean symptoms of depression among surgery candidates across BMI group and whether the individual indicated significant or nonsignificant levels of physical functioning impairment on the SF-36. Bars with different letters differ significantly from each other as determined by Tukey's honestly significant difference comparison ($p < 0.05$). The horizontal line indicates the level at which depressive symptoms become clinically significant. Reprinted from Fabricatore (2005) with permission from the publisher.

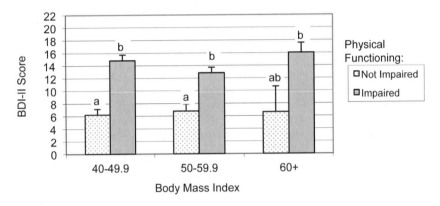

Figure 12.2. Mean symptoms of depression among surgery candidates across BMI group and whether the individual indicated significant or nonsignificant levels of impairment in bodily pain on the SF-36. Bars with different letters differ significantly from each other as determined by Tukey's honestly significant difference comparison ($p < 0.05$). The horizontal line indicates the level at which depressive symptoms become clinically significant. Reprinted from Fabricatore (2005) with permission from the publisher.

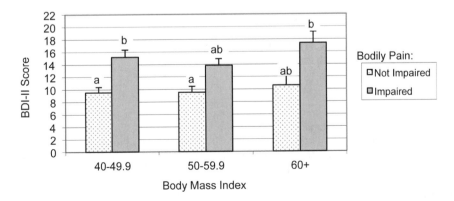

observe a similar phenomenon in 8% of the obese individuals who enrolled in a clinical trial. This subset of individuals met criteria for body dysmorphic disorder, defined as a preoccupation with an imagined or slight defect in appearance that causes clinically significant distress or impairment in social, occupational, or other areas of functioning (Sarwer 2005a). Patients with this disorder scored an average of 13.2 on the BDI (indicative of mild depression), compared with normal scores (i.e., mean of 7.2) for patients who reported body image dissatisfaction but did not meet criteria for body dysmorphic disorder (Sarwer 1998). Neither Stunkard (1967) nor Sarwer's (1998) patients were candidates for bariatric surgery, and only a minority of surgery candidates present with body image disparagement of this degree.

Adami et al. (1999) examined body image dissatisfaction in 30 bariatric surgery candidates compared with 30 never-obese control subjects. Bariatric surgery candidates reported significantly greater body image concerns than the never-obese control subjects, particularly in the areas of general body dissatisfaction, feeling fat, and perceptions of lower body fatness, as measured by the Eating Disorders Inventory body dissatisfaction subscale, the Body Shape Questionnaire, and the Body Attitude Questionnaire (Adami 1999). Grilo et al. (2005) found that low self-esteem and BED predicted greater body image dissatisfaction in surgery candidates, results that also have been reported in non–surgery-seeking obese individuals (Barry 2003, Grilo 2005). In a study of 131 female surgery candidates, Rosenberger et al. (2006) found significant body image dissatisfaction that was predicted by the presence of depressed mood, low self-esteem, and high levels of perfectionism.

Sexual function. Problems with sexual functioning are common among people seeking bariatric surgery (Assimakopoulos 2006, Kolotkin 2006, Dallal 2008, Kolotkin 2008). Bond et al. (2009) reported that ~60% of female surgery candidates met criteria for female sexual dysfunction (FSD); older age and menopause predicted FSD in this sample. These individuals reported greater levels of sexual dysfunction across all domains assessed (i.e., desire, arousal, lubrication, orgasm, satisfaction, and pain), when compared with a healthy control group (Bond 2009). Male surgery candidates also have been found to report greater impairments in sexual functioning, as compared with the general population (Dallal 2008). Impairment has been observed across all domains, including sexual drive, erectile function, ejaculatory function, and sexual satisfaction (Dallal 2008).

CHANGES IN PSYCHIATRIC STATUS FOLLOWING BARIATRIC SURGERY

Affective Disorders

Numerous studies have concluded that extremely obese patients experience improvements in psychosocial status following weight loss with bariatric surgery (Powers 1997, Mamplekou 2005, Rosik 2005, Assimakopoulos 2010, Kruseman 2010). The Swedish Obese Subjects (SOS) study provides perhaps the best assessment of changes in mood and anxiety following surgery (Karlsson 1998). This trial included a carefully matched control group that received traditional diet and exercise counseling. Self-reported depression scores fell significantly more at 1 year in surgically treated than control patients (40 vs. 10% reductions, respectively). Similar improvements were observed in anxiety. At 2 years, mean weight loss, which was induced primarily by vertical banded gastroplasty, was ~23% of initial weight. At both this time and at a 4-year follow-up evaluation, mood and anxiety levels tended to increase from their nadir at 1 year (Karlsson 1998, Sullivan 2001). Larger weight losses, however, at both times were associated with greater improvements in both depression and anxiety. At a 10-year follow-up conducted in a subset of patients, improvements in depression remained significantly greater in surgically treated than control participants, but groups did not differ significantly in changes in anxiety (Karlsson 2007).

In an uncontrolled study, Dixon et al. (2003) reported favorable improvements in depression following a 20% reduction in initial weight achieved with laparoscopic adjustable gastric banding. The mean presurgical score of 17.7 on the BDI indicated symptoms of mild depression. One year after surgery, this value fell to 7.8 and remained at 9.0 at year 4 in the subset of patients evaluated. These latter values indicate minimal symptoms of depression (Dixon 2003).

Additional long-term studies are needed to identify factors that may be associated with the rebound in symptoms of depression and anxiety that often occur 1 to 2 years postsurgery in many patients (Karlsson 2007, Kruseman 2010). These conditions may return toward baseline levels as patients stop losing weight or begin to regain a small amount of weight, the latter being common 18 to 24 months postsurgery (Sjostrom 2007). Moreover, people who, prior to surgery, have a history of mood or anxiety disorders may continue to have these problems after bariatric surgery despite large weight losses (Herpertz 2004).

Risk of Suicide after Surgery

Several cohort studies have noted higher than expected rates of suicide among individuals who have undergone bariatric surgery. Higa et al. (2000) reported 1 completed suicide out of 1,040 surgeries in their examination of all-cause mortality in postbariatric surgery patients. Hsu et al. (1998), in reviewing the literature, reported 8 completed suicides out of 1,785 bariatric surgery patients during a follow-up period of 14 years. Waters et al. (1991) reported 3 deaths from suicide over a 3-year period in a cohort of 157 postbariatric surgery patients. Omalu et al. (2005) described 3 cases of suicide in obese individuals following bariatric surgery (without describing their sample size). The prevalence of suicide in the U.S. population is ~11 deaths/year per every 100,000 people (www.cdc.gov/ncipc/wisqars).

A large case-control study of extremely obese patients who had bariatric surgery also suggested a higher than expected rate of suicide (Adams 2007). Adams et al. (2007) examined ~10,000 surgically treated patients and 9,600 obese non–treatment-seeking individuals from the same geographic area who were identified from driver's license applications. Subjects were matched for age, sex, and BMI and assessed for differences in cause-specific (e.g., cardiovascular, cancer) and all-cause mortality. During a mean follow-up period of 7 years, almost 50% more surgery patients (n = 43) committed suicide than did control participants (n = 24). The difference was not statistically significant but suggests a trend that warrants further study (Adams 2007).

If there is a higher than expected rate of suicide in bariatric surgery patients, what factors may explain it? The limited data suggest that patients who are at the greatest risk of suicidal behavior following bariatric surgery are likely to be those with preoperative depression and other psychopathology. Of the three completed suicides described by Waters et al. (1991), all three individuals had preoperative mood disorders (i.e., anxiety and depression). Psychiatric complications improved in the first 6–12 months after bariatric surgery but returned over time. A similar picture emerged in the case report by Omalu et al. (2005) All three individuals who committed suicide following surgery had a preoperative history of recurrent major depression. These latter individuals took their lives an average of 21.6 months after surgery, while maintaining weight losses of 25 to 41% of initial weight (Omalu 2005).

Adams et al. (2007) found a higher rate of suicide in their bariatric surgery patients compared with weight-matched control subjects, but their study did not include information about preoperative psychopathology in either the surgically treated or control participants. Thus, it is possible that individuals who sought surgery had higher rates of depression and suicidal ideation than did people in the control group and were at increased risk of self-inflicted death, regardless of whether they underwent surgery.

POSTOPERATIVE CHANGES IN EATING BEHAVIOR

Binge Eating Disorder

Several studies have reported marked improvements in BED following bariatric surgery (Kalarchian 1999, Powers 1999, Kalarchian 2002, Herpertz 2004). Kalarchian et al. (2002), for example, examined patients 4 months after surgery and observed a total cessation of binge episodes. Wadden et al. (2011) similarly observed the complete absence of binge eating episodes at 6 months postsurgery in patients who, before surgery, reported binge eating on an average of 9.5 of the prior 28 days. These findings are probably attributable to the dramatic reduction in the size of the stomach, which limits the volume of food that patients can consume.

Although binge eating declines sharply in the short term after bariatric surgery, a significant minority of patients continue to report experiencing a sense of loss of control over their eating (Hsu 1996, Hsu 1997, White 2006). Several studies have reported that this experience predicts suboptimal weight loss 2 or more years postsurgery (Pekkarinen 1994, Kalarchian 2002, White 2006, Sallet 2007, Colles 2008, Fujioka 2008, Alger-Mayer 2009, White 2010). Other investigators have reported that actual binge episodes (in which patients consume an objectively large amount of food) often return over long-term follow-up (Kruseman 2010). A recent study of patients 8.5 years after surgery found that 51% reported "irregular" episodes of binge eating in the previous month (Kruseman 2010).

Prevalence of Night Eating Syndrome in Bariatric Surgery Patients

The few studies that have examined the effects of bariatric surgery on NES have obtained inconsistent results. Rand et al. (1997) concluded that the prevalence of NES decreased slightly from 31 to 27% at 32 months postoperatively (Rand 1997). Another study reported that the prevalence of NES was unchanged following surgery (Adami 1999). Both studies suffered from methodological weaknesses (i.e., retrospective design, small sample) that limited the integrity of the results. More recently, Colles et al. (2008) assessed the prevalence of NES prospectively in 129 surgical patients, using both a self-report questionnaire and a semistructured interview (conducted over the phone). The prevalence of NES declined significantly from 17.1% before surgery to 7.8% 12 months following surgery. Notably, more than half of the participants who met criteria for NES 1 year postsurgery did not have the diagnosis preoperatively (Colles 2008). More research is clearly warranted to clarify the effect of bariatric surgery on symptoms of NES. Further, it is possible that patients who do not want to bring attention to behavior that impacts their weight-loss trajectory postsurgery may present a biased self-report of their eating habits.

Dietary Adherence

Suboptimal weight loss is observed in up to 20% of patients in the first postoperative year and is usually associated with poor adherence to dietary and behavioral recommendations, including eating a low-calorie diet (Pories 1987, Brolin 1989, Hsu 1998). Sarwer et al. (2008) examined predictors of postoperative weight loss and found that (in addition to male sex and increased cognitive restraint) patients who reported the highest dietary adherence (on a 9-point Likert scale) lost 28% more weight than those who reported the lowest adherence. Kruseman et al. (2010) followed patients for 8 years and found that adherence to the postsurgical, low-calorie diet decreased significantly after the first year. The authors divided patients into two groups, according to the amount of excess weight they lost. The group with impaired weight loss reported eating ~300 kcal/day more than the successful group (which lost >50% of excess weight) (Kruseman 2010).

Vomiting and plugging. Vomiting has been reported by approximately one-third of surgery patients (Brolin 1994, Pekkarinen 1994, Wyss 1995, Saunders 1999, Mitchell 2001, Kinzl 2002). It occurs most frequently in the first few months following surgery and then decreases over time (Stunkard 1985). However, some individuals report vomiting for years after surgery (Adami 1995, Wyss 1995, Powers 1997, Balsiger 2000, Mitchell 2001). Postsurgical vomiting does not appear to be a form of purging behavior, even when it is self-induced. Instead, it appears to be a reflexive response to overeating or a reaction to intolerable foods. Vomiting may also occur when foods become stuck in the surgical pouch or upper digestive track. This latter occurrence is referred to as plugging or frothing. This typically occurs in response to eating foods such as breads or pastas, as well as meats that are tough and dry (Wyss 1995, Powers 1997, Mitchell 2001).

Gastric dumping. Gastric dumping, a complication observed in RYGB patients, is characterized by nausea, severe diarrhea, heart palpitations, faintness, and fatigue (Sugarman 1987, Sugarman 1989, Mitchell 2001). It typically occurs following consumption of sugary foods and is observed in 50–70% of gastric bypass patients (Sugarman 1987, Pories 1995). The frequency of dumping declines over time. The unpleasant symptoms of gastric dumping reinforce patients to avoid the consumption of sugary foods (Wadden 2007).

POSTOPERATIVE QUALITY OF LIFE

Health-Related Quality of Life

The large weight losses achieved with bariatric surgery dramatically improve (if not normalize) physical function and other aspects of quality of life, including walking, climbing stairs, bathing, and dressing (Wyss 1995, Karlsson 1998, van Gemert 1998, Choban 1999, Hörchner 1999, Weiner 1999, Hell 2000, Schok 2000, Carmichael 2001, Dymek 2001, Kolotkin 2001, Larsen 2003, Müller 2008, Sears 2008, Batsis 2009, Kolotkin 2009, Sarwer 2010). Nguyen et al. (2009), for example, studied patients with a mean presurgical BMI of 48 kg/m² and found, at both 3- and 6-month postoperative assessments, that their physical function had improved to that of the general population. O'Brien et al. (2006) studied less obese patients (mean BMI = 33.7 kg/m²) who underwent laparoscopic adjustable gastric banding. Patients' scores on all SF-36® Health Survey scales fell in the significantly impaired range at baseline but rose to meet or exceed normative levels 2 years after surgery, following a 22% reduction in initial weight. Physical functioning scores improved significantly more in surgically treated patients than in participants in this study who were randomly assigned to lifestyle modification plus pharmacotherapy (O'Brien 2006).

Weight loss and improvements in physical function also may be associated with significant reductions in weight-related pain, as well as correction (or improvement) of weight-related postural abnormalities that limit mobility. The SOS study found that "work-restricting" pain in the neck, back, hips, knees, and ankles, as well as effort-related calf pain, was significantly more common among obese people than those in the general population (Peltonen 2003, Karason 2005). Patients who underwent bariatric surgery reported significantly greater improvement (or resolution) in these types of pain over 2 years than did similarly obese control subjects who received nonsurgical weight reduction. Surgically treated patients also were significantly less likely to develop such pains. The reduction in pain in weight-bearing joints, such as the knees and ankles, appears to be more durable than the relief that patients initially report in their lower backs and non–weight-bearing body areas. Improvement in the former areas can be observed at least 6 years after bariatric surgery (Peltonen 2003).

Improvements in HRQoL are closely correlated with weight loss. A recent study that examined the 10-year trends in HRQoL in the SOS study found that improvements in HRQoL peaked at 6 months to 1 year postsurgery. Thereafter, HRQoL declined from years 1–6, during which time patients regained some of their lost weight. The authors reported a stabilization of weight regain *and* of HRQoL from years 6–10, suggesting that changes in HRQoL mirror those in body weight (Karlsson 2007). This trend has been replicated in other studies (van Hout 2008, Batsis 2009, Kolotkin 2009, Sarwer 2010).

Body Image and Sexual Functioning

Body image. Weight loss achieved with bariatric surgery is also associated with improvements in body image (Solow 1974, Gentry 1984, Camps 1996, Adami 1998). In a recent study of 200 patients, Sarwer et al. (2010) observed a 30% improvement in scores on the Body Shape Questionnaire at 20, 40, and 92 weeks postsurgery. Participants also reported improvements in body image–related quality of life (BIQoL), a construct that assesses the impact that positive or negative body image has on several aspects of quality of life. BIQoL continued to improve through week 40 and was stable between weeks 40 and 92. These positive long-term findings are important in light of clinical reports that body image dissatisfaction may increase over time, as surgery patients begin to notice loose, sagging skin on their breasts, abdomen, thighs, and arms (Sarwer 2010).

Sexual function. Numerous studies have reported that sexual functioning improves after surgery (Larsen 1990, Camps 1996, Kinzl 2001, Kolotkin 2006, Sanchez-Santos 2006, Kolotkin 2008, Assimakopoulos 2010, Bond 2011). Bond et al. (2011), for example, found significant improvements in FSD in 54 female surgery patients when assessed 6 months postoperatively. Almost two-thirds of the patients reported that their FSD had resolved (Bond 2011). Similar improvements have been reported in men (Dallal 2008). Dallal et al. (2008) examined sexual functioning in 97 men 19 months postoperatively and observed improvements in all domains assessed (i.e., sexual drive, erectile function, ejaculatory function, and sexual satisfaction). Weight loss predicted the extent of the improvement in sexual function in the sample, with higher weight losses associated with greater improvements in sexual functioning (Dallal 2008).

Summary

As noted previously, psychosocial evaluation of weight loss surgery candidates was first recommended by the NIH Consensus Development Conference on Gastrointestinal Surgery for Severe Obesity in 1991, as well as an expert panel in 2008, and is currently practiced by virtually all weight-loss surgery programs (NIH conference 1991, Devlin 2004, Kalarchian 2007, Kral 2007). The most recent recommendations for presurgical evaluation and postsurgical care represent a consensus of clinical opinion reached by an expert panel of providers from the American Association of Clinical Endocrinologists (AACE), The Obesity Society (TOS), and the American Society for Metabolic & Bariatric Surgery (ASMBS). Clinical opinion has been guided by findings from the correlational and observational studies described previously in this chapter. However, there have been few, if any, randomized controlled trials that have addressed issues such as the benefits of conducting an initial behavioral evaluation of candidates or of the efficacy of providing behavioral counseling 12 to 24 months postsurgery to improve eating and activity behaviors in patients who showed suboptimal weight loss. Controlled trials of such issues are needed but their present absence should not prevent patients from receiving appropriate clinical interventions that would appear to address their needs.

The content and structure of the behavioral evaluations has been described by several investigators (Wadden 2006a, Greenberg 2009). Currently there is not uniformity of approach, although the purpose of all evaluations is to identify behavioral and psychosocial factors that are considered contraindications to surgery (e.g., substance abuse and bulimia nervosa) or could result in suboptimal weight loss, as well as to identify potential obstacles that might impede long-term weight management (Mechanick 2009). Three recent studies reported that ~3% of surgery candidates were deemed inappropriate for surgery, and 8–32% were recommended for psychiatric care or nutritional counseling prior to surgery (Sarwer 2004, Pawlow 2005, Friedman 2007). Postponing surgery for psychiatric or nutritional counseling is rare, and the benefit of doing so has not been sufficiently studied.

RECOMMENDATIONS FOR CLINICAL CARE

1. Uncontrolled psychiatric complications, such as major depression, should be treated prior to surgery to alleviate patients' suffering (Mechanick 2009). Weight loss induced by surgery clearly does not appear to be a sufficient treatment for chronic psychiatric conditions, as suggested by the limited evidence on depression and suicide following surgery (Waters 1991, Omalu 2005, Adams 2007). Patients with preoperative psychopathology also should be assessed at regular intervals following surgery to ensure that they achieve optimal control over psychiatric conditions (Greenberg 2009). All patients who undergo bariatric surgery should be provided access to mental health professionals to assist them, when needed, in adjusting to changes in physical and psychosocial functioning following surgery. Such changes are very positive in the vast majority of surgically treated individuals.
2. Candidates for bariatric surgery should be assessed by a mental health professional who also has expertise in obesity and is a member of the perioperative team (Fabricatore 2006). Practitioners can screen for depression using an interview, as described elsewhere (Wadden 2006a, Wadden 2006b, Wadden 2006c), supplemented by a paper-and-pencil questionnaire, such as the nine-item depression scale of the Patient Health Questionnaire (PHQ-9) (Spitzer 1999). Although weight loss generally improves mood, it is not a primary treatment for major depression or other psychiatric conditions (Herpertz 2004, Wadden 2006a). Thus, psychiatric care should not be delayed in expectation that weight loss will resolve significant mental health problems (Herpertz 2004).
3. HRQoL should be an essential component of the psychosocial presurgical evaluation, as well as being monitored postprocedure. This evaluation component may identify issues associated with depressed mood and weight-loss outcomes.
4. As with other domains of psychological distress, pre- and postsurgical monitoring of clinically significant body image issues, including sexual function, should be assessed and monitored.
5. Given findings from Omalu et al. (2005) that substantial weight loss alone was not sufficient to alleviate depression and suicidal behavior, the increased risk of suicidal behavior in bariatric surgery patients underscores the need for candidates to undergo a thorough preoperative behavioral evaluation and be provided appropriate psychiatric care for depression and other disorders, and for such care to continue postsurgery.
6. History of eating patterns and disordered eating behaviors (also see Chapter 2) should be evaluated and monitored pre- and postsurgically at regularly scheduled medical management visits.
7. As with other disordered eating patterns, NES should be assessed presurgery and monitored postsurgically.

8. Patients with impaired weight loss may benefit from postsurgical counseling to improve adherence to dietary recommendations.

BIBLIOGRAPHY

Adami GF, Meneghelli A, Bressani A, Scopinaro N: Body image in obese patients before and after stable weight reduction following bariatric surgery. *J Psychosomatic Res* 46:275–281, 1999

Adami GF, Gandolfo P, Campostano A, Meneghelli A, Ravera G, Scopinaro N: Body image and body weight in obese patients. *Int J Eat Disord* 24:299–306, 1998

Adami GF, Gandolfo BB, Scopinaro N: Binge eating in massively obese patients undergoing bariatric surgery. *Int J Eat Disord* 17:45–50, 1995

Adams TD, Gress RE, Smith SC, Halverson RC, et al.: Long-term mortality after gastric bypass surgery. *N Engl J Med* 357:753–761, 2007

Alger-Mayer S, Rosati C, Polimeni JM, Malone M: Preoperative binge eating status and gastric bypass surgery: a long-term outcome study. *Obes Surg* 19:139–145, 2009

Allison DB, Fontaine KR, Manson JE, Stevens J, VanItallie TB: Annual deaths attributable to obesity in the United States. *JAMA* 282:1530–1538, 1999

Allison KC, Lundgren JD, O'Reardon JP, Galiebter A, et al.: Proposed diagnostic criteria for night eating syndrome. *Int J Eat Disord* 43:241–247, 2010

Allison KC, Wadden TA, Sarwer DB, Fabricatore AN, et al.: Night eating syndrome and binge eating disorder among persons seeking bariatric surgery: prevalence and related features. *Obesity (Silver Spring)* 14 (Suppl. 2):S77–S82, 2006

Allison KC, Stunkard AJ: Obesity and eating disorders. *Psychiatr Clin North Am* 28:55–67, 2005

American Psychiatric Association: *Diagnostic and Statistical Manual of Mental Disorders (DSM-IV-TR)*. 4th ed. Washington, DC, American Psychiatric Association, 2000

Ashton K, Drerup M, Windover A, Heinberg L: Brief, four-session group CBT reduces binge eating behaviors among bariatric surgery candidates. *Surg Obes Relat Dis* 5:257–262, 2009

Assimakopoulos K, Karaivazoglou K, Panayiotopoulos S, Hyphantis T, Iconomou G, Kalfarentzos F: Bariatric surgery is associated with reduced depressive symptoms and better sexual function in obese female patients: a one-year follow-up study. *Obes Surg* 21:362–366, 2010

Assimakopoulos K, Panayiotopoulos S, Iconomou G, Karaivazoglou K, et al.: Assessing sexual function in obese women preparing for bariatric surgery. *Obes Surg* 16:1087–1091, 2006

Averbukh Y, Heshka S, El-Shoreya H, Flancbaum L, et al.: Depression score predicts weight loss following Roux-en-Y gastric bypass. *Obes Surg* 13:833–836, 2003

Balsiger BM, Poggio JL, Mai J, Kelly KA, Sam MG: Ten and more years after vertical banded gastroplasty as primary operation for morbid obesity. *J Gastrointest Surg* 4:598–605, 2000

Barry DT, Grilo CM, Masheb RM: Comparison of patients with bulimia nervosa, obese patients with binge eating disorder, and nonobese patients with binge eating disorder. *J Nerv Ment Dis* 191:589–594, 2003

Batsis JA, Lopez-Jimenez F, Collazo-Clavell ML, Clark MM, Somers VK, Sarr MG: Quality of life after bariatric surgery: a population-based cohort study. *Am J Med* 122:1055.e1–1055.e10, 2009

Black DW, Goldstein RB, Mason EE: Prevalence of mental disorder in 88 morbidly obese bariatric clinic patients. *Am J Psychiatry* 149:227–234, 1992

Bloomston M, Zervos EE, Camps MA, Goode SE, Rosemurgy AS: Outcome following bariatric surgery in super versus morbidly obese patients: does weight matter? *Obes Surg* 7:414–419, 1997

Bond DS, Wing RR, Vithiananthan S, Sax HC, et al.: Significant resolution of female sexual dysfunction after bariatric surgery. *Surg Obes Relat Dis* 7:1–7, 2011

Bond DS, Vithiananthan S, Leahey TM, Thomas JG, et al.: Prevalence and degree of sexual dysfunction in a sample of women seeking bariatric surgery. *Surg Obes Relat Dis* 5:698–704, 2009

Brolin RE, Robertson LB, Kenler HA, Cody RP: Weight loss and dietary intake after vertical banded gastroplasty and Roux-en-Y gastric bypass. *Ann Surg* 220:782–790, 1994

Brolin RE: Gastric restrictive surgery. *JAMA* 262:1188, 1989

Buchwald H, Consensus Conference Panel: Consensus conference statement bariatric surgery for morbid obesity: health implications for patients, health professionals, and third-party payers. *Surg Obes Relat Dis* 1:371–381, 2005

Buchwald H, Avidor Y, Braunwald E, Jensen MD, et al.: Bariatric surgery: a systematic review and meta-analysis. *JAMA* 292:1724–1737, 2004

Burgmer R, Grigutsch K, Zipfel S, Wolf AM, et al.: The influence of eating behavior and eating pathology on weight loss after gastric restriction operations. *Obes Surg* 15:684–691, 2005

Calle EE, Rodriguez C, Walker-Thurmond K, Thun MJ: Overweight, obesity, and mortality from cancer in a prospectively studied cohort of U.S. adults. *N Engl J Med* 348:1625–1638, 2003

Camps MA, Zervos E, Goode S, Rosemurgy AS: Impact of bariatric surgery on body image perception and sexuality in morbidly obese patients and their partners. *Obes Surg* 6:356–360, 1996

Carmichael AR, Sue-Ling HM, Johnston D: Quality of life after the Magenstrasse and Mill procedure for morbid obesity. *Obes Surg* 11:708–715, 2001

Centers for Disease Control and Prevention, National Center for Injury Prevention and Control: Web-based Injury Statistics Query and Reporting System (WISQARS™). Available at www.cdc.gov/ncipc/wisqars. Accessed 25 June 2012

Choban PS, Onyejekwe J, Burge JC, Flancbaum L: A health status assessment of the impact of weight loss following Roux-en-Y gastric bypass for clinically severe obesity. *J Am Coll Surg* 188:491–497, 1999

Clark MM, Balsiger BM, Sletten CD, Dahlman KL, et al.: Psychosocial factors and 2-year outcome following bariatric surgery for weight loss. *Obes Surg* 13:739–745, 2003

Colles SL, Dixon JB, O'Brien PE: Grazing and loss of control related to eating: two high-risk factors following bariatric surgery. *Obesity (Silver Spring)* 16:615–622, 2008

Colles SL, Dixon JB: Night eating syndrome: impact on bariatric surgery. *Obes Surg* 16:811–820, 2006

Crémieux PY, Ledoux S, Clerici C, Crémieux F, Buessing M: The impact of bariatric surgery on comorbidities and medication use among obese patients. *Obes Surg* 20:861–870, 2010

Dallal RM, Chernoff A, O'Leary MP, Smith JA, Braverman JD, Quebbermann BB: Sexual dysfunction is common in the morbidly obese male and improves after gastric bypass surgery. *J Am Coll Surg* 207:859–864, 2008

de Zwaan M, Mitchell JE, Howell LM, Monson N, et al.: Characteristics of morbidly obese patients before gastric bypass surgery. *Compr Psychiatry* 44:428–434, 2003

de Zwaan M, Lancaster KL, Mitchell JE, Howell LM, et al.: Health-related quality of life in morbidly obese patients: effect of gastric bypass surgery. *Obes Surg* 12:773–780, 2002

Devlin MJ, Goldfein JA, Flancbaum L, Bessler M, Eisenstadt R: Surgical management of obese patients with eating disorders: a survey of current practice. *Obes Surg* 14:1252–1257, 2004

Dixon JB, Dixon ME, O'Brien PE: Depression in association with severe obesity: changes with weight loss. *Arch Intern Med* 163:2058–2065, 2003

Dixon JB, Dixon ME, O'Brien PE: Quality of life after lap-band placement: influence of time, weight loss, and comorbidities. *Obes Res* 9:713–721, 2001

Duval K, Marceau P, Lescelleur O, Hould FS, et al.: Health-related quality of life in morbid obesity. *Obes Surg* 16:574–579, 2006

Dymek MP, le Grange D, Neven K, Alverdy J: Quality of life and psychosocial adjustment in patients after Roux-en-Y gastric bypass: a brief report. *Obes Surg* 11:32–39, 2001

Dymek-Valentine M, Rienecke-Hoste R, Alverdy J: Assessment of binge eating disorder in morbidly obese patients evaluated for gastric bypass: SCID versus QEWP-R. *Eat Weight Disord* 9:211–216, 2004

Fabricatore AN, Crerand CE, Wadden TA, Sarwer DB, Krasucki JL: How do mental health professionals evaluate candidates for bariatric surgery? Survey results. *Obes Surg* 16:567–573, 2006

Fabricatore AN, Wadden TA, Sarwer DB, Faith M: Health-related quality of life and symptoms of depression in extremely obese persons seeking bariatric surgery. *Obes Surg* 15:304–309, 2005

Flegal KM, Carroll MD, Ogden CL, Curtin LR: Prevalence and trends in obesity among US adults, 1999–2008. *JAMA* 303:235–241, 2010

Friedman KE, Applegate KL, Grant J: Who is adherent with preoperative psychological treatment recommendations among weight loss surgery candidates? *Surg Obes Relat Dis* 3:376–382, 2007

Fujioka K, Yan E, Wang HJ, Li Z: Evaluating preoperative weight loss, binge eating disorder, and sexual abuse history on Roux-en-Y gastric bypass outcome. *Surg Obes Relat Dis* 4:137–143, 2008

Gentry K, Halverson JD, Heisler S: Psychologic assessment of morbidly obese patients undergoing gastric bypass: a comparison of preoperative and postoperative adjustment. *Surgery* 95:215–220, 1984

Glinski J, Wetzler S, Goodman E: The psychology of gastric bypass surgery. *Obes Surg* 11:581–588, 2001

Greenberg I, Sogg S, M Perna F: Behavioral and psychological care in weight loss surgery: best practice update. *Obesity (Silver Spring)* 17:880–884, 2009

Grilo CM, Masheb RM, Brody M, Burke-Martindale CH, Rothschild BS: Binge eating and self-esteem predict body image dissatisfaction among obese men and women seeking bariatric surgery. *Int J Eat Disord* 37:347–351, 2005

Guisado JA, Vaz FJ, Lopez-Ibor JJ, Rubio MA: Eating behavior in morbidly obese patients undergoing gastric surgery: differences between obese people with and without psychiatric disorders. *Obes Surg* 11:576–580, 2001

Hell E, Miller KA, Moorehead MK, Samuels N: Evaluation of health status and quality of life after bariatric surgery: comparison of standard Roux-en-Y gastric bypass, vertical banded gastroplasty and laparoscopic adjustable silicone gastric banding. *Obes Surg* 10:214–219, 2000

Herpertz S, Kielmann R, Wolf AM, Hebebrand J, Senf W: Do psychosocial variables predict weight loss or mental health after obesity surgery? A systematic review. *Obes Res* 12:1554–1569, 2004

Higa KD, Boone KB, Ho T: Complications of the laparoscopic Roux-en-Y gastric bypass: 1040 patients—what have we learned? *Obes Surg* 10:509–513, 2000

Hörchner R, Tuinebreijer W: Improvement of physical functioning of morbidly obese patients who have undergone a lap-band operation: one-year study. *Obes Surg* 9:399–402, 1999

Hsu LK, Benotti PN, Dwyer J, Roberts SB, et al.: Nonsurgical factors that influence the outcome of bariatric surgery: a review. *Psychosom Med* 60:338–346, 1998

Hsu LK, Sullivan SP, Benotti PN: Eating disturbances and outcome of gastric bypass surgery: a pilot study. *Int J Eat Disord* 21:385–390, 1997

Hsu LK, Betancourt S, Sullivan SP: Eating disturbances before and after vertical banded gastroplasty: a pilot study. *Int J Eat Disord* 19:23–34, 1996

James WP, Davies HL, Bailes J, Dauncey MJ: Elevated metabolic rates in obesity. *Lancet* 1:1122–1125, 1978

Jia H, Lubetkin E: The impact of obesity on health-related quality-of-life in the general adult US population. *J Pub Health* 27:156–164, 2005

Jones-Corneille LR, Wadden TA, Sarwer DB, Faulconbridge LF, et al.: Axis I psychopathology in bariatric surgery candidates with and without binge eating disorder: results of structured clinical interviews. *Obesity Surg* 22:389–397, 2010

Kalarchian MA, Marcus MD, Levine MD: Relationship of psychiatric disorders to 6-month outcomes after gastric bypass. *Surg Obes Relat Dis* 4:544–549, 2008

Kalarchian MA, Marcus MD, Levine MD, Courcoulas AP, et al.: Psychiatric disorders among bariatric surgery candidates: relationship to obesity and functional health status. *Am J Psychiatry* 164:328–334, 2007

Kalarchian MA, Marcus MD, Wilson GT, Labouvie EW, Brolin RE, LaMarca LB: Binge eating among gastric bypass patients at long-term follow-up. *Obes Surg* 12:270–275, 2002

Kalarchian MA, Wilson GT, Brolin RE, Bradley L: The effects of bariatric surgery on binge eating and related psychopathology. *Eat Weight Disord* 4:1–5, 1999

Karason K, Peltonen M, Lindroos AK, Sjostrom L, Lonn L, Torgerson JS: Effort-related calf pain in the obese and long-term changes after surgical obesity treatment. *Obes Res* 13:137–145, 2005

Karlsson J, Taft C, Rydén A, Sjostrom L, Sullivan M: Ten-year trends in health-related quality of life after surgical and conventional treatment for severe obesity: the SOS intervention study. *Int J Obes* 31:1248–1261, 2007

Karlsson J, Sjostrom L, Sullivan M: Swedish Obese Subjects (SOS): an intervention study of obesity: two-year follow-up of health-related quality of life (HRQL) and eating behavior after gastric surgery for severe obesity. *Int J Obes* 22:112–126, 1998

Kinzl JF, Schrattenecker M, Traweger C, Mattesich M, Fiala M, Biebl W: Psychosocial predictors of weight loss after bariatric surgery. *Obesity Surgery* 16:1609–1614, 2006

Kinzl JF, Trefalt E, Fiala M, Biebl W: Psychotherapeutic treatment of morbidly obese patients after gastric banding. *Obes Surg* 12:292–294, 2002

Kinzl JF, Trefalt E, Fiala M, Hotter A, Biebl W, Aiger F: Partnership, sexuality, and sexual disorders in morbidly obese women: consequences of weight loss after gastric banding. *Obes Surg* 11:455–458, 2001

Kolotkin RL, Crosby RD, Gress RE, Hunt SC, Adams TD: Two-year changes in health-related quality of life in gastric bypass patients compared with severely obese controls. *Surg Obes Relat Dis* 5:250–256, 2009

Kolotkin RL, Binks M, Crosby RD, Ostbye T, Mitchell JE, Hartley G: Improvements in sexual quality of life after moderate weight loss. *Int J Impot Res* 20:487–492, 2008

Kolotkin RL, Binks M, Crosby RD, Ostbye T, Gress RE, Adams TD: Obesity and sexual quality of life. *Obesity (Silver Spring)* 14:472–479, 2006

Kolotkin RL, Crosby RD, Williams GR, Hartley GG, Nicol S: The relationship between health-related quality of life and weight loss. *Obes Res* 9:564–571, 2001

Kral JG, Naslund E: Surgical treatment of obesity. *Nature Clin Practice Endocrinology & Metabolismn* 3:574–583, 2007

Kral JG, Sjöström LV, Sullivan MB: Assessment of quality of life before and after surgery for severe obesity. *Am J Clin Nutr* 55 (2 Suppl.):S611–S614, 1992

Kruseman M, Leimgruber A, Zumbach F, Golay A: Dietary, weight, and psychological changes among patients with obesity, 8 years after gastric bypass. *J Am Diet Assoc* 110:527–534, 2010

Larsen F: Psychosocial function before and after gastric banding surgery for morbid obesity: a prospective psychiatric study. *Acta Psychiatr Scan Suppl* 359:1–57, 1990

Larsen JK, Geenen R, van Ramshorst B, Brand N, et al.: Psychosocial functioning before and after laparoscopic adjustable gastric banding: a cross-sectional study. *Obes Surg* 13:629–636, 2003

Larsson UE, Mattsson E: Functional limitations linked to high body mass index, age and current pain in obese women. *Int J Obes Relat Metab Disord* 25:893–899, 2001a

Larsson UE, Mattsson E: Perceived disability and observed functional limitation in obese women. *Int J Obes Relat Metab Disord* 25:1705–1712, 2001b

Ma Y, Pagoto SL, Olendzki BC, Hafner AR, et al.: Predictors of weight status following laparoscopic gastric bypass. *Obes Surg* 16:1227–1231, 2006

Mamplekou E, Komesidou V, Bissias C, Papakonstantinou A, Melissas J: Psychological condition and quality of life in patients with morbid obesity before and after surgical weight loss. *Obes Surg* 15:1177–1184, 2005

Mauri M, Rucci P, Calderone A, Santini F, et al.: Axis I and II disorders and quality of life in bariatric surgery candidates. *J Clin Psychiatry* 69:295–301, 2008

Mechanick JI, Kushner RF, Sugerman HJ, Gonzalez-Campoy JM, et al.: American Association of Clinical Endocrinologists, The Obesity Society, and American Society for Metabolic & Bariatric Surgery medical guidelines for clinical practice for the perioperative nutritional, metabolic, and nonsurgical support of the bariatric surgery patient. *Obesity (Silver Spring)* 17 (Suppl. 1):S1–S70, v, 2009

Millon T, Davis RD: *Disorders of Personality: DSM-IV and Beyond*. New York, John Wiley & Sons, 1996

Mitchell JE, Steffen KJ, de Zwaan M, Ertelt TW, Marino JM, Mueller A: Congruence between clinical and research-based psychiatric assessment in bariatric surgical candidates. *Surg Obes Relat Dis* 6:628–634, 2010

Mitchell JE, Lancaster KL, Burgard MA, Howell LM, et al.: Long-term follow-up of patients' status after gastric bypass. *Obes Surg* 11:464–468, 2001

Muhlhans B, Horbach T, de Zwaan M: Psychiatric disorders in bariatric surgery candidates: a review of the literature and results of a German prebariatric surgery sample. *General Hospital Psychiatry* 31:414–421, 2009

Müller MK, Wenger C, Schiesser M, Clavien PA, Weber M: Quality of life after bariatric surgery: a comparative study of laparoscopic banding vs. bypass. *Obes Surg* 18:1551–1557, 2008

Myers A, Rosen J: Obesity stigmatization and coping: relation to mental health symptoms, body image, and self-esteem. *Int J Obes Relat Metab Disord* 23:221–230, 1999

Nguyen NT, Slone JA, Nguyen XM, Hartman JS, Hoyt DB: A prospective randomized trial of laparoscopic gastric bypass versus laparoscopic adjustable gastric banding for the treatment of morbid obesity: outcomes, quality of life, and costs. *Ann Surg* 250:631–641, 2009

Niego SH, Kofman MD, Weiss JJ, Geliebter A: Binge eating in the bariatric surgery population: a review of the literature. *Int J Eat Disord* 40:349–359, 2007

NIH conference: Gastrointestinal surgery for severe obesity: Consensus Development Conference Panel. *Ann Intern Med* 115:956–961, 1991

O'Brien PE, Dixon JB, Laurie C, Skinner S, et al.: Treatment of mild to moderate obesity with laparoscopic adjustable gastric banding or an intensive medical program. *Ann Intern Med* 144:625–633, 2006

Omalu B, Cho P, Shakir A, Agumadu UH, et al.: Suicides following bariatric surgery for the treatment of obesity. *Surg Obes Relat Dis* 1:447–449, 2005

Onyike CU, Crum RM, Lee HB, Lyketsos CG, Eaton WW: Is obesity associated with major depression? Results from the Third National Health and Nutrition Examination Survey. *Am J Epidemiol* 158:1139–1147, 2003

O'Reardon JP, Ringel BL, Dinges DF, Allison KC, et al.: Circadian eating and sleeping patterns in the night eating syndrome. *Obes Res* 12:1789–1796, 2004

Pawlow LA, O'Neil PM, White MA, Byrne TK: Findings and outcomes of psychological evaluations of gastric bypass applicants. *Surg Obes Relat Dis* 1:523–527, discussion 528–529, 2005

Pekkarinen T, Koskela K, Huikuri K, Mustajoki: Long-term results of gastroplasty for morbid obesity: binge-eating as a predictor of poor outcome. *Obes Surg* 4:248–255, 1994

Peltonen M, Lindroos AK, Torgerson JS: Musculoskeletal pain in the obese: a comparison with a general population and long-term changes after conventional and surgical obesity treatment. *Pain* 104:549–557, 2003

Pories WJ, Swanson MS, MacDonald KG, Long SB, et al.: Who would have thought it? An operation proves to be the most effective therapy for adult-onset diabetes mellitus. *Ann Surg* 222:339–350, discussion 350–352, 1995

Pories WJ, Caro JF, Flickinger EG, Meelheim HD, Swanson MS: The control of diabetes mellitus (NIDDM) in the morbidly obese with the Greenville Gastric Bypass. *Ann Surg* 206:316–323, 1987

Powers PS, Perez A, Boyd F, Rosemurgy A: Eating pathology before and after bariatric surgery: a prospective study. *Int J Eat Disord* 25:293–300, 1999

Powers PS, Rosemurgy A, Boyd F, Perez A: Outcome of gastric restriction procedures: weight, psychiatric diagnoses, and satisfaction. *Obes Surg* 7:471–477, 1997

Rand CSW, Macgregor AMC, Stunkard AJ: The night eating syndrome in the general population and among postoperative obesity surgery patients. *Int J Eat Disord* 22:65–69, 1997

Rosenberger PH, Henderson KE, Grilo CM: Psychiatric disorder comorbidity and association with eating disorders in bariatric surgery patients: a cross-sectional study using structured interview-based diagnosis. *J Clin Psychiatry* 67:1080–1085, 2006

Rosik CH: Psychiatric symptoms among prospective bariatric surgery patients: rates of prevalence and their relation to social desirability, pursuit of surgery, and follow-up attendance. *Obes Surg* 15:677–683, 2005

Sallet PC, Sallet JA, Dixon JB, Collis E, et al.: Eating behavior as a prognostic factor for weight loss after gastric bypass. *Obes Surg* 17:445–451, 2007

Sanchez-Santos R, Del Barrio MJ, Gonzalez C, Madico C, et al.: Long-term health-related quality of life following gastric bypass: influence of depression. *Obes Surg* 16:580–585, 2006

Sarwer DB, Wadden TA, Moore RH, Eisenberg MH, et al.: Changes in quality of life and body image after gastric bypass surgery. *Surg Obes Relat Dis* 6:608–614, 2010

Sarwer DB, Wadden TA, Moore RH, Baker AW, et al.: Preoperative eating behavior, postoperative dietary adherence, and weight loss after gastric bypass surgery. *Surg Obes Relat Dis* 4:640–646, 2008

Sarwer DB, Thompson JK, Cash TF: Body image and obesity in adulthood. *Psychiatr Clin North Am* 28:69–87, 2005a

Sarwer DB, Wadden TA, Fabricatore AN: Psychosocial and behavioral aspects of bariatric surgery. *Obes Res* 13:639–648, 2005b

Sarwer DB, Cohn NI, Gibbons LM, Magee L, et al.: Psychiatric diagnoses and psychiatric treatment among bariatric surgery candidates. *Obes Surg* 14:1148–1156, 2004

Sarwer DB, Wadden TA, Foster GD: Assessment of body image dissatisfaction in obese women: specificity, severity, and clinical significance. *J Consult Clin Psychol* 66:651–654, 1998

Saunders R: Binge eating in gastric bypass patients before surgery. *Obes Surg* 9:72–76, 1999

Schok M, Geenen R, de Wit P, Brand N, van Antwerpen T, van Ramshorst B: Quality of life after laparoscopic adjustable gastric banding for severe obesity: postoperative and retrospective preoperative evaluations. *Obes Surg* 10:502–508, 2000

Sears D, Fillmore G, Bui M, Rodriquez J: Evaluation of gastric bypass patients 1 year after surgery: changes in quality of life and obesity-related conditions. *Obes Surg* 18:1522–1525, 2008

Sjostrom L, Narbro K, Sjostrom D, Karason K, et al.: Effects of bariatric surgery on mortality in Swedish obese subjects. *N Engl J Med* 357:741–752, 2007

Solow C, Silberfarb PM, Swift K: Psychosocial effects of intestinal bypass surgery for severe obesity. *N Engl J Med* 290:300–304, 1974

Spitzer RL, Kroenke K, Williams JB: Validation and utility of a self-report version of PRIME-MD: the PHQ primary care study. *JAMA* 282:1737–1744, 1999

Spitzer RL, Devlin M, Walsh TB, Hasin D, et al.: Binge eating disorder: a multisite field trial of the diagnostic criteria. *Int J Eat Disord* 11:191–203, 1992

Stunkard A, Foster GD, Glassman J, Rosato E: Retrospective exaggeration of symptoms: vomiting after gastric surgery for obesity. *Psychosom Med* 47:150–155, 1985

Stunkard A, Mendelson M: Obesity and body image: characteristics of disturbances in the body image of some obese persons. *Am J Psychiatry* 123:1296–1300, 1967

Sugarman HJ, Londrey GL, Kellum JM: Weight loss with vertical banded gastro-plasty and Roux-Y gastric bypass for morbid obesity with selective vs. random assignment. *Am J Surg* 157:93–102, 1989

Sugarman HJ, Starkey JV, Birkenhauer R: A randomized prospective trial of gas-tric bypass versus vertical banded gastroplasty for morbid obesity and their effects on sweets versus non-sweets eaters. *Ann Surg* 205:613–624, 1987

Sullivan M, Karlsson J, Sjostrom L, et al.: Why quality of life measures should be used in the treatment of patients with obesity. In *International Textbook of Obe-sity.* Bjorntrop P, Ed. London, John Wiley and Sons, 2001

Sullivan M, Karlsson J, Sjostrom L, Backman L, et al.: Swedish Obese Subjects (SOS): an intervention study of obesity: baseline evaluation of health and psy-chosocial functioning in the first 1743 subjects examined. *Int J Obes Relat Metab Disord* 17:503–512, 1993

van Gemert WG, Adang EM, Greve JW, Soeters PB: Quality of life assessment of morbidly obese patients: effect of weight-reducing surgery. *Am J Clin Nutr* 67:197–201, 1998

van Hout GC, Fortuin FA, Pelle AJ, van Heck GL: Psychosocial functioning, per-sonality, and body image following vertical banded gastroplasty. *Obes Surg* 18:115–120, 2008

van Hout G, Verschure SK, van Heck G: Psychosocial predictors of success fol-lowing bariatric surgery. *Obes Surg* 15:553–560, 2005

van Nunen A, Wouters E, Vingerhoets A, Hox JJ, Geenen R: The health-related quality of life of obese persons seeking or not seeking surgical or non-surgical treatment: a meta-analysis. *Obes Surg* 17:1357–1366, 2007

Wadden TA, Faulconbridge LF, Jones-Corneille LR, Sarwer DB, et al.: Binge eat-ing disorder and the outcome of bariatric surgery at one year: a prospective, observational study. *Obesity (Silver Spring)* 19:1220–1228, 2011

Wadden TA, Sarwer DB, Fabricatore AN, Jones L, Stack R, Williams NS: Psycho-social and behavioral status of patients undergoing bariatric surgery: what to expect before and after surgery. *Med Clin North Am* 9:451–469, 2007

Wadden TA, Butryn ML, Sarwer DB, Fabricatore AN, et al.: Comparison of psy-chosocial status in treatment-seeking women with class III vs. class I-II obe-sity. *Obesity (Silver Spring)* 14 (Suppl. 2):S90–S98, 2006a

Wadden TA, Foster GD: Weight and Lifestyle Inventory (WALI). *Obesity (Silver Spring)* 14 (Suppl. 2):S99–S118, 2006b

Wadden TA, Sarwer DB: Behavioral assessment of candidates for bariatric sur-gery: a patient-oriented approach. *Obesity (Silver Spring)* 14 (Suppl 2):S53–S62, 2006c

Wadden TA, Foster GD, Sarwer BD, Anderson DA, et al.: Dieting and the devel-opment of eating disorders in obese women: results of a randomized con-trolled trial. *Am J Clin Nutr* 80:560–568, 2004

Wadden, TA, Phelan S: Assessment of quality of life in obese individuals. *Obesity Research* 10 (Suppl. 1):S50–S7, 2002

Waters GS, Pories WJ, Swanson MS, Meelheim HD, Flickinger EG, May HJ: Long-term studies of mental health after the Greenville gastric bypass operation for morbid obesity. *Am J Surg* 161:154–158, 1991

Weiner R, Datz M, Wagner D, Bockhorn H: Quality-of-life outcome after laparoscopic adjustable gastric banding for morbid obesity. *Obes Surg* 9:539–545, 1999

White MA, Kalarchian MA, Masheb RM, Marcus MD, Grilo CM: Loss of control over eating predicts outcomes in bariatric surgery patients: a prospective, 24-month follow-up study. *J Clin Psychiatry* 71:175–184, 2010

White MA, Masheb RM, Rothschild BS, Burke-Martindale CH, Grilo CM: The prognostic significance of regular binge eating in extremely obese gastric bypass patients: 12-month postoperative outcomes. *J Clin Psychiatry* 67:1928–1935, 2006

White MA, O'Neil PM, Kolotkin RL, Byrne TK: Gender, race, and obesity-related quality of life at extreme levels of obesity. *Obes Res* 12:949–955, 2004

Wyss C, Laurent-Jaccard A, Burckhardt P, Jayet A, Gazzola L: Long-term results on quality of life of surgical treatment of obesity with vertical banded gastroplasty. *Obes Surg* 5:387–392, 1995

Zimmerman M, Francione-Witt C, Chelminski I, Young D, et al.: Presurgical psychiatric evaluations of candidates for bariatric surgery, part 1: reliability and reasons for and frequency of exclusion. *J Clin Psychiatry* 68:1557–1562, 2007

Brooke A. Bailer, PhD, is a Postdoctoral Fellow at the Center for Weight and Eating Disorders in the Department of Psychiatry at the Perelman School of Medicine of the University of Pennsylvania in Philadelphia, PA.

Thomas A. Wadden, PhD, is the Director of the Center for Weight and Eating Disorders in the Department of Psychiatry at the Perelman School of Medicine of the University of Pennsylvania in Philadelphia, PA.

Lucy F. Faulconbridge, PhD, is the Director of Research at the Center for Weight and Eating Disorders in the Department of Psychiatry at the Perelman School of Medicine of the University of Pennsylvania in Philadelphia, PA.

David B. Sarwer, PhD, is the Director of Clinical Services at the Center for Weight and Eating Disorders in the Department of Psychiatry at the Perelman School of Medicine of the University of Pennsylvania in Philadelphia, PA.

Chapter 13
Psychosocial Adjustment to Diabetes and Critical Periods of Psychological Risk

RICHARD R. RUBIN, PhD, AND MARK PEYROT, PhD

Hamburg and Inoff (1983) were among the first to recognize the existence of predictable periods of diabetes-related psychosocial stress, including: *1)* diagnosis of diabetes, *2)* onset of complications, and *3)* treatment regimen transitions. In this section we discuss what is known about psychosocial outcomes during each of these periods along with interventions designed to improve these outcomes. Recommendations for screening and focused interventions are provided for the benefit of clinicians.

DIAGNOSIS

Children and Parents

Several studies suggest that children who develop type 1 diabetes (T1D) experience psychological problems associated with diabetes diagnosis (Wysocki 1989, Kovacs 1995, Northam 1996, Kovacs 1997a, Kovacs 1997b), but others found little or no change in psychological status during the year after diagnosis (Grey 1997, Jacobson 1997). Even studies that found psychological problems associated with diagnosis (primarily adjustment disorder and depression) reported that episodes of these problems were time-limited and that essentially all children recovered from these problems by the end of the first year after diagnosis (Kovacs 1995, Northam 1996). On the other hand, Kovacs (1995) reported that among children with an adjustment disorder in response to diabetes diagnosis, the 5-year cumulative probability of a new psychiatric disorder was 0.48, compared with 0.16 among other children in the study.

Kovacs (1985b) found that mothers (who generally bear the majority of responsibility for care of a child with diabetes) had a pattern of adjustment to diabetes diagnosis similar to children, whereas fathers appeared to experience little distress at any time.

Risk factors for diagnosis-associated psychological problems in children diagnosed with T1D include female gender, family stress, and nonintact family structure (Amer 1999) as well as avoidant coping behaviors (Grey 1997). The psychological adjustment to a diagnosis of type 2 diabetes (T2D) in children is understudied because until recently, T2D in children had not been considered sufficiently common to warrant systematic investigation.

Grey et al. (1995) studied 8- to 14-year-old children newly diagnosed with diabetes and a nondiabetic peer comparison group. Children's adjustment problems at diagnosis disappeared at 1 year postdiagnosis but reappeared at 2 years postdiagnosis, a pattern similar to that found by Kovacs and colleagues (1985a, 1985b, 1990a, 1990b). Grey et al. (1995) argued that, although adjustment immediately after diagnosis is crucial, their data suggest that a second "critical period" of adjustment occurs in the second year after diagnosis and that intervention is important during the critical second year of life with diabetes for prevention of psychosocial deterioration. A recent study comparing the adjustment experiences of parents of youngsters with T1D with parents of children diagnosed with cancer reported that the timing of interventions is important early in the disease course as well as later when the school-aged child confronts new developmental challenges at adolescence (Boman 2004).

Adults

There have been few formal studies of psychological adjustment to diagnosis, especially of adjustment-related psychiatric disorders and the impact of diagnosis on spouses and other members of the patient's social network. One large international study asked patients (about two-thirds of whom had T2D) to recall their reactions to being diagnosed with diabetes (Skovlund 2005). Eighty-five percent of patients reported strong negative emotions (including shock, anger, anxiety, depression, and helplessness) at this time. Another study suggests these reactions may be more intense among those with T1D (Lo 2001). Emotional reactions to diagnosis in adults may also be influenced by social support, personal resources, and coping style (Willoughby 2000, Lo 2001).

Experiencing strong negative emotions at diagnosis may predict later problems, including poorer self-reported regimen adherence, diabetes control, and quality of life, and higher levels of diabetes-related psychological distress (Skovlund 2005), especially when combined with ineffective coping (Pibernik-Okanovic 1996). On the other hand, although the diagnosis of diabetes may be experienced as an assault on personal identity, many patients grapple with these identity issues and integrate the new identity as a person with diabetes into their lives (Goldman 1998).

Interventions

Studies of psychosocial interventions at diabetes diagnosis are rare and restricted to children. Laron (1979) described a special psychosocial crisis intervention clinic for newly diagnosed children, and Galatzer (1982) reported positive outcomes for this intervention over a period of 3–15 years, including improved regimen adherence and psychosocial adjustment and a two-thirds reduction in the need for psychological intervention compared with children who had not received the special intervention at diagnosis. Another study reported null findings at two years postdiagnosis for a randomized clinical trial of conventional care versus psychosocial group counseling (Sundelin 1996).

Summary

Psychological problems at diagnosis of diabetes are common in adults and children and in the parents of diagnosed children. In addition, these problems, though they often resolve quickly, are predictive of negative long-term clinical and psychological outcomes. Finally, risk factors for acute and long-term psychological problems, including female gender, lack of support, family stress, and avoidant coping styles, have been identified.

DIABETES COMPLICATIONS

The presence of diabetes complications (particularly the presence of two or more complications) and the severity of complications appear to be associated with psychological distress, including clinically meaningful symptoms of depression or anxiety and lower scores on quality of life measures (Jacobson 1994, Keinanen-Kiukaanniemi 1996, Anderson 1997, Peyrot 1997, Trief 1998). Polonsky et al. (1995) found that diabetes-related distress also was higher among people with short-term and long-term diabetes complications.

Others, studying specific diabetes complications, have found that the presence of neuropathy, cardiovascular disease, or end-stage renal disease (ESRD) was associated with decreased health-related quality of life (Ahroni 1994, Klein 1998); the presence of ESRD was associated with markedly increased functional impairment (Rodin 1990); and the presence of nephropathy was associated with greater health worries and reduced perceived health in patients with T1D (Parkerson 1993). Another study found lower health-related quality of life in patients with gastroparesis (a neuropathic complication of diabetes) (Farup 1998).

Several researchers have found increased depression and negative life experiences during the 2 years after diagnosis with proliferative diabetic retinopathy (Wuslin 1987, Wuslin 1989). These psychosocial disruptions existed regardless of the severity of the visual impairment and were maintained even after lost vision was regained. These psychosocial consequences of visual impairment may not be unique to individuals with diabetes (Robertson 2006). Interestingly, one study found that a history of psychiatric illness was a risk factor for development of diabetic retinopathy, an association possibly due to elevated glycohemoglobin levels in this group (Cohen 1997).

Diabetic neuropathy also seems to be associated with psychological distress (Carrington 1996, Vileikyte 2005, Watson-Miller 2006). One study found that the association between neuropathy symptoms and depression symptom scores was partially mediated by two sets of psychosocial variables: *1)* perception of diabetic neuropathy symptom unpredictability and lack of treatment control, and *2)* restrictions in activities of daily living and changes in social self-perception (Vileikyte 2005). Another study found that the psychological status of mobile amputees was better than that of patients with diabetic foot ulcers but not as good as that of patients who had neither amputations nor foot ulcers (Watson-Miller 2006).

Both men and women with diabetes appear to be at increased risk for sexual dysfunction (Enzlin 2002, Enzlin 2003). It has been estimated that 50% of diabetic men with impotence problems have a significant emotional overlay attributable to depression or anxiety that contributes to erectile dysfunction (Whitehead 1983). Other researchers have found a significant association between sexual problems and depression among diabetic men (Cavan 1987, Lustman 1990) and women (Leedom 1986). These psychological factors may both exacerbate and be exacerbated by organic pathology in the development and maintenance of sexual dysfunction (Schiavi 1979).

Summary

Psychological problems are common in patients who suffer from diabetes complications. The possibility that these problems could be a risk factor for developing additional complications or exacerbating existing complications (via less active self-care and higher blood glucose levels) points to a benefit of effective treatment for psychological distress.

TREATMENT REGIMEN TRANSITIONS

Treatment regimen transitions (i.e., addition of new categories of medication) for patients with T2D may be associated with psychological distress. A number of studies found that patients treating their diabetes without medication had higher scores on diabetes quality-of-life scales (Jacobson 1994) than those using oral hypoglycemic agents, and better overall quality of life (Keinanen-Kiukaanniemi 1996) than those taking any hypoglycemic agent. Similarly, those taking oral hypoglycemic agents reported better health-related and diabetes-related quality of life (Jacobson 1994, Glasgow 1997) than those taking insulin, and those switching to insulin reported reduced well-being (Van der Does 1998). In contrast, some studies found no significant association between type of therapy (no medication, oral agents, insulin) and quality of life in patients with T2D (Mayou 1990) and no differences in depression or anxiety between patients treated with insulin and those not using insulin (Peyrot 1997).

Intensification of insulin therapy in patients with T1D, as in the Diabetes Control and Complications Trial Research Group (1996) intensive treatment arm, does not appear to be associated with reduced well-being. In fact, other studies found improvements in global life satisfaction, anxiety, and depression in patients intensifying their insulin therapy (Langewitz 1997) and improved treatment satisfaction and diabetes burden in patients who increased the number of injections they took each day or switched from injections to continuous subcutaneous insulin infusion (CSII) (Chantelau 1997). Still other studies indicate that switching from syringes to pens or CSII as a means of insulin delivery is associated with improved health-related quality of life (Hornquist 1995, Chantelau 1997) and that psychosocial outcomes are better in patients using pens or CSII than in those using syringes to deliver insulin (DeVries 2002, Linkeschova 2002).

Summary

Treatment regimen transitions associated with deterioration of beta cell function in patients with T2D may be associated with psychological distress.

RECOMMENDATIONS FOR CLINICAL CARE

Diagnosis

1. Resolving distress at diagnosis is a worthy goal in its own right; it may also improve health status directly by reducing the negative neuroendocrine and physiologic effects of stress and indirectly by reestablishing an emotional state that facilitates learning positive patterns of diabetes self-care (Hamburg 1983, Brown 1985, Holmes 1986). At diagnosis of diabetes, clinicians should identify patients who are depressed and those where family adaptation is poor, and provide appropriate psychological support, especially in individuals at high risk.

2. Diabetes-specific distress may not be identified using general measures of mood or psychiatric symptoms. Thus it is also recommended that diabetes-specific measures such as the Problem Areas in Diabetes (PAID-Revised) be incorporated in all evaluation processes.

Diabetes Complications

1. Clinicians should conduct routine psychosocial assessments when complications occur. Content area should include mood, quality of well-being (general and diabetes-specific), medical, social, and financial resources.
2. Since symptom unpredictability and changes in self-perception can be pathways through which complications affect depression symptoms, clinicians should use interventions designed to help patients understand the likely course of their complication(s) and the interventions designed to foster and maintain a positive sense of self, since these interventions could have a positive impact on psychological well-being.
3. Sexual problems are frequent in patients with diabetes; since these problems affect psychological health, clinicians should routinely ask about sexual functioning and well-being and discuss psychological and medical options for improving sexual functioning.

Treatment Regimen Transitions

1. Clinicians should help patients understand the progressive nature of T2D (i.e., the natural decline in insulin secretion) to mitigate feelings of guilt and consequent distress associated with the need to begin taking oral medications or insulin.
2. Clinicians are advised against using the threat of taking oral medication or insulin in an effort to encourage more active self-care, as this may cause distress and increase resistance to initiating appropriate therapies.
3. To reduce treatment burden and enhance treatment satisfaction and quality of life, clinicians should identify and prescribe treatment regimens and medication delivery systems (e.g., pens and pumps for insulin delivery) that are the easiest for patients to use.

ACKNOWLEDGEMENTS

The authors would like to thank Tim Wysocki and Barbara Anderson for their input. The authors are responsible for the use of their contributions.

BIBLIOGRAPHY

Ahroni JH, Boyko EJ, Davignon DR, Pecaro RE: The health and functional status of veterans with diabetes. *Diabetes Care* 17:318–321, 1994

Amer KS: Children's adaptation to insulin-dependent diabetes mellitus: a critical review of the literature. *Pediatr Nurs* 25:627–631, 1999

Anderson RM, Fitzgerald JT, Wisdom K, Davis WK, Hiss RG: A comparison of global versus disease-specific quality-of-life measures in patients with NIDDM. *Diabetes Care* 20:299–305, 1997

Boman KK, Viksten J, Kogner P, Samuelsson U: Serious illness in childhood: the different threats of cancer and diabetes from a parent perspective. *J Pediatr* 145:373–379, 2004

Brown SA: Diabetes and grief. *Diabetes Educ* 6:409–416, 1985

Carrington AL, Mawdsley SK, Morley M, Kincey J, Boulton AJ: Psychological status of diabetic people with and without lower limb disability. *Diabetes Res Clin Pract* 32:19–25, 1996

Cavan DA, Barnett AH, Leatherdale BA: Diabetic impotence: risk factors in a clinic population. *Diab Res* 5:145–148, 1987

Chantelau E, Schiffers T, Schutze J, Hansen B: Effect of patient-selected intensive insulin therapy on quality of life. *Patient Educ Couns* 30:167–173, 1997

Cohen ST, Welch G, Jacobson AM, de Groot M, Samson J: The association of lifetime psychiatric illness and increased retinopathy in patients with type 1 diabetes mellitus. *Psychosomatics* 38:98–108, 1997

DeVries JH, Snoek FJ, Kostense PJ, Masurel N, Heine RJ: A randomized trial of continuous subcutaneous insulin infusion and intensive injection therapy in type 1 diabetes for patients with long-standing poor glycemic control. *Diabetes Care* 25:2074–2080, 2002

Diabetes Control and Complications Trial Research Group: Influence of intensive diabetes treatment on quality-of-life outcomes in the Diabetes Control and Complications Trial. *Diabetes Care* 19:195–203, 1996

Enzlin P, Mathieu C, Van den Bruel A, Vanderschueren D, Demyttenaere K: Prevalence and predictors of sexual dysfunction in patients with type 1 diabetes. *Diabetes Care* 26:409–414, 2003

Enzlin P, Mathieu C, Van den Bruel A, Bosteels J, Vanderschueren D, Demyttenaere K: Sexual dysfunction in women with type 1 diabetes: a controlled study. *Diabetes Care* 25:672–677, 2002

Farup CE, Leidy NK, Murray M, Williams GR, Helbers L, Quigley EM: Effect of domperidone on the health-related quality of life of patients with symptoms of diabetic gastroparesis. *Diabetes Care* 21:1699–1706, 1998

Galatzer A, Amir S, Gil R, Karp M, Laron Z: Crisis intervention program in newly diagnosed diabetic children. *Diabetes Care* 5:414–419, 1982

Glasgow RE, Ruggiero L, Eakin EG, Dryfoos J, Chobanian L: Quality of life and associated characteristics in a large national sample of adults with diabetes. *Diabetes Care* 20:562–567, 1997

Goldman JB, MacLean HM: The significance of identity in the adjustment to diabetes among insulin users. *Diabetes Educ* 24:741–748, 1998

Grey M, Lipman T, Cameron ME, Thurber FW: Coping behaviors at diagnosis and in adjustment one year later in children with diabetes. *Nurs Res* 46:312–317, 1997

Grey M, Cameron ME, Lipman TH, Thurber FW: Psychosocial status of children with diabetes in the first 2 years after diagnosis. *Diabetes Care* 18:1330–1336, 1995

Hamburg BA, Inoff GE: Coping with predictable crises of diabetes. *Diabetes Care* 6:409–416, 1983

Holmes DM: The person and diabetes in psychosocial context. *Diabetes Care* 9:194–206, 1986

Hornquist JO, Wikby A, Stenstrom U, Andersson PO: Change in quality of life among type 1 diabetes. *Diab Res Clin Pract* 28:63–72, 1995

Jacobson AM, Hauser ST, Willett JB, Wolfsdorf JI, Dvorak R, Herman L, de Groot M: Psychological adjustment to IDDM: 10-year follow-up of an onset cohort of child and adolescent patients. *Diabetes Care* 20:811–818, 1997

Jacobson AM, de Groot M, Samson JA: The evaluation of two measures of quality of life in patients with type I and type II diabetes. *Diabetes Care* 17:267–274, 1994

Keinanen-Kiukaanniemi S, Ohinmaa A, Pajunpaa H, Koivukangas P: Health related quality of life in diabetic patients measured by the Nottingham Health Profile. *Diabet Med* 13:382–388, 1996

Klein BE, Klein R, Moss SE: Self-rated health and diabetes of long duration. The Wisconsin Epidemiologic Study of Diabetic Retinopathy. *Diabetes Care* 21:236–240, 1998

Kovacs M, Goldston D, Obrosky DS, Bonar LK: Psychiatric disorders in youths with IDDM: rates and risk factors. *Diabetes Care* 20:36–44, 1997a

Kovacs M, Obrosky DS, Goldston D, Drash A: Major depressive disorder in youths with IDDM: a controlled prospective study of course and outcome. *Diabetes Care* 20:45–51, 1997b

Kovacs M, Ho V, Pollock MH: Criterion and predictive validity of the diagnosis of adjustment disorder: a prospective study of youths with new-onset insulin-dependent diabetes mellitus. *Am J Psychiatry* 152:523–528, 1995

Kovacs M, Iyengar S, Goldston D, Obrosky DS, Marsh J: Psychological functioning among mothers of children with insulin-dependent diabetes mellitus: a longitudinal study. *J Consult Clin Psychol* 58:189–195, 1990a

Kovacs M, Iyengar S, Goldston D, Stewart J, Obrosky DS, Marsh J: Psychological functioning of children with insulin-dependent diabetes mellitus: a longitudinal study. *J Pediatr Psychol* 15: 619–632, 1990b

Kovacs M, Feinberg TL, Paulauskas S, Finkelstein R, Pollock M, Crouse-Novak M: Initial coping responses and psychosocial characteristics of children with insulin-dependent diabetes mellitus. *J Pediatr* 106:827–834, 1985a

Kovacs M, Finkelstein R, Feinberg TL, Crouse-Novak M, Paulauskas S, Pollock M: Initial psychologic responses of parents to the diagnosis of insulin-dependent diabetes mellitus in their children. *Diabetes Care* 8:568–575, 1985b

Langewitz W, Wossmer B, Iseli J, Berger W: Psychological and metabolic improvement after an outpatient teaching program for functional intensified insulin therapy (FIT). *Diab Res Clin Pract* 37:157–164, 1997

Laron Z, Galatzer A, Amir S, Gil R, Karp M, Minouni M: A multidisciplinary, comprehensive, ambulatory treatment scheme for diabetes mellitus in children. *Diabetes Care* 2:342–348, 1979

Leedom LJ, Procci WP, Don D, Meehan WP: Sexual dysfunction and depression in diabetic women (Abstract). *Diabetes* 35 (Suppl. 1):23A, 1986

Linkeschova R, Raoul M, Bott U, Berger M, Spraul M: Less severe hypoglycemia, better metabolic control, and improved quality of life in type 1 diabetes mellitus with continuous subcutaneous insulin infusion (CSII) therapy: an observational study of 100 consecutive patients followed for a mean of 2 years. *Diabet Med* 19:746–751, 2002

Lo R, MacLean D: The dynamics of coping and adapting to the impact when diagnosed with diabetes. *Aust J Adv Nurs* 19:26–32, 2001

Lustman PJ, Clouse RE: Relationship of psychiatric illness to impotence in men with diabetes. *Diabetes Care* 13:893–95, 1990

Mayou R, Bryant B, Turner R: Quality of life in non-insulin-dependent diabetes and a comparison with insulin-dependent diabetes. *Journal of Psychosomatic Research* 34:1–11, 1990

Northam E, Anderson P, Adler R, Werther G, Warne G: Psychosocial and family functioning in children with insulin-dependent diabetes at diagnosis and one year later. *J Pediatr Psychol* 21:699–717, 1996

Parkerson GR, Connis RT, Broadhead WE, Patrick DL, Taylor TR, Chiu-Kit JT: Disease-specific versus generic measurement of health-related quality of life in insulin-dependent diabetic patients. *Medical Care* 31:629–639, 1993

Peyrot M, Rubin RR: Levels and risks of depression and anxiety symptomatology among diabetic adults. *Diabetes Care* 20:585–590, 1997

Pibernik-Okanovic M, Roglic G, Prasek M, Metelko Z: Emotional adjustment and metabolic control in newly diagnosed diabetic persons. *Diab Res Clin Pract* 34:99–105, 1996

Polonsky WH, Anderson BJ, Lohrer, PA, Welch G, Jacobson AM, Aponte JE, Schwartz CE: Assessment of diabetes-related distress. *Diabetes Care* 18:754–760, 1995

Robertson N, Burden ML, Burden AC: Psychological morbidity and problems of daily living in people with visual loss and diabetes: do they differ from people without diabetes? *Diabet Med* 23:1110–1116, 2006

Rodin G: Quality of life in adults with insulin-dependent diabetes mellitus. *Psychotherapy Psychosomatics* 54:132–139, 1990

Schiavi PC, Hogan B: Sexual problems in diabetes mellitus: psychological aspects. *Diabetes Care* 2:9–17,1979

Skovlund SE, Peyrot M: The Diabetes Attitudes, Wishes, and Needs (DAWN) Program: a new approach to improving outcomes of diabetes care. *Diabetes Spectrum* 18:136–142, 2005

Sundelin J, Forsandfer G, Mattson SE: Family-oriented support at the outset of diabetes mellitus: a comparison of two group conditions during 2 years following diagnosis. *Acta Paediatr* 85:49–55, 1996

Trief PM, Grant W, Elbert K, Weinstock RS: Family environment, glycemic control, and the psychosocial adaptation of adults with diabetes. *Diabetes Care* 21:241–245, 1998

Van der Does FE, De Neeling JN, Snoek FJ, Kostense PJ, Grootenhuis PA, Bouter LM, Heine RJ: Randomized study of two different levels of glycemic control within the acceptable range in type 2 diabetes. *Diabetes Care* 21:2085–2093, 1998

Vileikyte L, Leventhal H, Gonzalez JS, Peyrot M, Rubin RR, Ulbrecht JS, Garrow A, Waterman C, Cavanagh PR, Boulton AJ: Diabetic peripheral neuropathy and depressive symptoms: the association revisited. *Diabetes Care* 28:2378–2383, 2005

Watson-Miller S: Living with a diabetic foot ulcer: a phenomenological study. *J Clin Nurs* 15:1336–1337, 2006

Whitehead ED, Klyde BJ, Zussman S, Wayne N, Shinbach K, Davis D: Male sexual dysfunction and diabetes mellitus. *New York State J Med* 83:1174–1179, 1983

Willoughby DF, Kee C, Demi A: Women's psychosocial adjustment to diabetes. *J Adv Nurs* 32:1422–1430, 2000

Wuslin LR, Jacobson AM: Visual and psychological function in PDR (Abstract). *Diabetes* 38 (Suppl. 1):242A, 1989

Wuslin LR, Jacobson AM, Rand LI: Psychosocial aspects of diabetic retinopathy. *Diabetes Care* 10:367–373, 1987

Wysocki T, Huxtable K, Linscheid TR, Wayne W: Adjustment to diabetes mellitus in preschoolers and their mothers. *Diabetes Care* 12:524–529, 1989

Richard R. Rubin, PhD, is Professor in the Departments of Medicine and Pediatrics at The Johns Hopkins University School of Medicine in Baltimore, MD.

Mark Peyrot, PhD, is Professor in the Department of Sociology, Loyola University Maryland in Baltimore, MD.

Chapter 14
Special Issues in Children and Adolescents

TIM WYSOCKI, PHD

BARBARA J. ANDERSON, PHD

The complex daily diabetes regimen affects child development and family life throughout the pediatric age range (Anderson 1980, Silverstein 1994, Wolfsdorf 1994). This section reviews normal development and research on diabetes among: *1)* infants (0–2 years of age), *2)* toddlers and preschoolers (2–5 years), *3)* school-age children (6–11 years), and *4)* adolescents (12–18 years). Despite the global increase in new diagnoses of type 1 diabetes (T1D) in infants, toddlers, and preschoolers (Gardner 1997, Soltesz 2006, Vehik 2011), there have yet been no large multicenter clinical trials studying children with diabetes under 6 years of age and their families. Thus, the level of evidence for research discussed in the first two sections (infants and toddlers/preschoolers) is relatively weak.

DIABETES IN INFANCY

For the first two years of life, the central psychological task is establishing a mutually strong and trusting emotional attachment between the infant and the primary caregivers (Erikson 1950). Although there have been no large studies or clinical trials of diabetes in infancy, there are several small clinical studies that illustrate the impact of diabetes on infant–parent attachment. In one qualitative study (Hatton 1995), mothers of infants with diabetes reported a diminished bond with their children and a loss of the ideal mother–child relationship. In another small, descriptive study (Sullivan-Bolyai 2003), mothers reported feeling "constant vigilance" because their children were so dependent on them to manage the disease and to recognize dangerous glycemic fluctuations. Due to the complex demands of daily diabetes management, many parents report that finding caregivers who are competent and comfortable caring for a young child with diabetes is often extremely difficult (Kushion 1991, Wolfsdorf 1994, Sullivan-Bolyai 2003). One study (Sullivan-Bolyai 2003) indicated that this chronic stress and lack of social support puts mothers at risk for physical and emotional problems. This highlights the importance of helping parents of infants identify support systems to reduce the stresses on families created by a diagnosis of T1D (Daneman 1999).

DIABETES IN TODDLERS AND PRESCHOOLERS

Toddlers have two central developmental tasks: 1) to separate from the parent or primary caregiver and establish him/herself as a separate person, by developing a sense of autonomy, and 2) to develop a sense of mastery over the environment and the confidence that he/she can act upon and affect the physical and social environment (Erikson 1950). Preschoolers build upon this newly established autonomy to explore and begin to master the world outside the home.

There is not a large empirical research base on this age period, but a few studies document that diabetes during the toddler and preschool years continues to affect the parent-child relationship profoundly. Parents of toddlers with diabetes in a study by Powers et al. (2002) reported more behavioral and feeding problems at mealtimes than did parents of healthy control subjects. Subsequent observational research carried out by this group revealed that despite increased parental concerns, preschoolers with T1D did not have more challenging mealtime behaviors than age-matched healthy control subjects (Patton 2004). Finally, in a larger controlled study of family mealtime interactions, parents of preschoolers with T1D spoke more commands and worked harder at controlling mealtimes, while children ate less (Patton 2008). Clearly, the normal task of feeding a toddler or preschooler becomes more challenging for parents of young children with T1D.

Wysocki et al. (1989) investigated maternal reports of the psychological adjustment of a sample of 20 children with diabetes between 2 and 6 years of age. Compared to a normative sample, children showed significantly more "internalizing" behavior problems on the Child Behavior Checklist (CBCL) (Achenbach 1983), such as depression, anxiety, sleep problems, somatic complaints, or withdrawal. In contrast, Northam et al. (1996) found no significant deviations from normative scores on any scale of the CBCL at diagnosis or 1 year later in a sample of 18 children under 4 years of age. Neither study assessed children's behavior independent of maternal report. Wysocki et al. (1989b) also noted that mothers of very young children with diabetes reported more parenting stress when contrasted with a nondiabetic standardization sample. Powers et al. (2002) also found higher stress levels in parents of children with diabetes compared with parents of nondiabetic children. Both Eiser (1990) and Garrison and McQuiston (1989) have suggested that behavioral changes in the young child and changes in parental experiences are to be expected when *any* chronic illness is present in the preschool-aged child. Therefore, it is important not to conclude from these findings that it is diabetes per se that causes the behavioral adjustment problems or that all mothers of preschoolers with diabetes see their families as severely stressed.

Compared with findings from a sample of older children and adolescents with diabetes, mothers of very young children report more concerns about identifying hypoglycemia (Banion 1983, Wysocki 1989a). And there is a growing body of evidence documenting the negative consequences, or mild cognitive deficits, in young children, possibly resulting from hypoglycemia. A series of studies by Ryan and colleagues (1984, 1985a, 1985b), using a battery of neurobehavioral tests, identified significant differences between youth with diabetes compared with control subjects. Additionally, children diagnosed with diabetes under 5 years of age manifested significant cognitive deficits when evaluated during the adolescent years, possibly resulting from symptomatic or asymptomatic hypoglycemia occurring earlier in life before final maturation of the central nervous system. In another study by Rovet et al. (1987), children diagnosed under 4 years of age scored lower than other children with diabetes diagnosed later in childhood and lower than nondiabetic sibling control subjects on tests of visual-spatial orientation but not on verbal ability. Hypoglycemic seizures were found to occur with greater frequency in the group of children diagnosed under 4 years of age compared with those diagnosed at older ages, suggesting that severe hypoglycemia may impair later cognitive functioning (Eiser 1990). Golden et al. (1989) collected longitudinal data on the frequency of hypoglycemia from the time of diagnosis in a sample of 23 children with diabetes onset prior to the age of 5 years. These investigators documented that it was the frequency of asymptomatic and mildly symptomatic hypoglycemia that was significantly correlated with lower scores on the abstract/visual reasoning scale, indicating that even mild or asymptomatic episodes of hypoglycemia may have a negative cumulative effect on cognitive functioning.

In the previously described studies, no measurements of neurocognitive functioning were made near the time of diagnosis to rule out the possibility that the metabolic decompensation of diabetes onset affected such functioning. Two studies have followed children with diabetes prospectively from diagnosis using neuropsychological assessments. The preliminary findings of Rovet et al. (1990) indicated no evidence of neurocognitive impairment in these children at diagnosis or 1 year later, but the authors reported that they may not have followed subjects long enough to observe any impairment. Northam et al. (1998) compared the performance of children with T1D on standardized measures of general intelligence, attention, speed of processing, memory, learning, and executive skills with the performance of control subjects. At 3 months postdiagnosis, there were no differences between groups, but at 2 years postdiagnosis, children with diabetes demonstrated smaller gains, particularly in the areas of information-processing speed, acquisition of new knowledge, and conceptual reasoning skills. The subset of the diabetes sample that performed the worst were those children with early onset of diabetes, which further suggests an early onset effect (Ryan 1984). However, there has also been evidence in the other direction, from a prospective, longitudinal study of new-onset children in Switzerland with T1D, which concluded that the metabolic condition at diagnosis and long-term metabolic control, rather than frequency of severe hypoglycemia, are risk factors for impaired intellectual development (Schoenle 2002).

In light of findings regarding cognitive deficits associated with severe hypoglycemia, prevention of severe and recurrent hypoglycemia is critically important for toddlers and preschoolers (Ryan 1985a, Ryan 1985b, Rovet 1987, Golden 1989). Thus the now more commonly accepted regimen of intensive insulin therapy, as advocated for individuals over the age of 13 years by the Diabetes Control and Complications Trial (DCCT) (Golden 1985, Drash 1993, DCCT Research Group 1994, Brink 1997, Ryan 1999) must be applied very carefully to these very young and vulnerable patients (Golden 1985, Drash 1993, DCCT Research Group 1994, Brink 1997, Ryan 1999). Achieving optimal glycemic control in this age range is further complicated by the finicky eating habits, erratic physical activity, and rapid growth that are all characteristic of this developmental period. Treatment goals, therefore, must be individualized to provide safe and effective medical treatment yet also permit the young child to master the normal developmental tasks of early childhood.

Continuous subcutaneous insulin infusion (CSII) therapy, or pump therapy, has increasingly been used in young children. Several studies have shown that insulin pump therapy is a safe alternative to multiple daily insulin injections that may reduce the rate of severe hypoglycemic reactions and improve quality of life for families of young children with diabetes (Tubiana-Rufi 1996, Litton 2002, Saha 2002, DiMeglio 2004, Shehadeh 2004). Based on these studies, it appears that CSII therapy is an effective and safe alternative for very young children, given that their families have the educational and support resources to use this complex technology. As with all management issues, the decision to start pump therapy must be individualized to each family's lifestyle and abilities.

If multiple daily injections are used, glargine, a recently introduced long-acting insulin analog with no appreciable peak action, has been shown to significantly reduce hypoglycemia, especially nocturnal hypoglycemia, in children (Hathout 2003, Tan 2004). By decreasing hypoglycemia, and thus reducing stress for families of young children with diabetes, these new management tools have the potential to improve quality of life for these families.

DIABETES IN SCHOOL-AGED CHILDREN

The primary developmental tasks of the school-aged child include making a smooth adjustment from the home to the school setting; forming close friendships with children of the same sex; developing new intellectual, athletic, and artistic skills; and forming a positive sense of self (Erikson 1950, Erikson 1968).

Studies of school-aged children with diabetes have linked low self-esteem and poor social-emotional adjustment to poorly controlled diabetes (Johnson 1980, Ryden 1994). Dumont et al. (1995) found that recurrent diabetic ketoacidosis (DKA) over 8 years postdiagnosis was associated with significantly higher ratings of behavior problems and lower levels of social competence. Liss et al. (1998) found that children who had been hospitalized with DKA in the preceding year reported lower levels of self-esteem and social competence than children who had no DKA in that period. Significantly more youths in the DKA group met the diagnostic criteria for at least one psychiatric disorder (88 vs. 28%).

Participation or attendance in school is disrupted if the child has chronically poor glycemic control (Balik 1986), which may result in educational setbacks and interfere with peer relationships and self-esteem (Pond 1995). Minimizing the occurrence of hypoglycemia at school is crucial in light of studies (Puczynski 1990) indicating that memory and concentration may continue to be impaired even after the physical symptoms of hypoglycemia have subsided.

In contrast to the lack of large studies with younger children, there has been more research on how family environment variables relate to glycemic control among school-aged children. Waller et al. (1986) conducted one of the first empirical descriptive studies of families with children with diabetes under the age of 12 years. Among school-aged patients, more diabetes-related family guidance and control were associated with better metabolic outcomes, and diabetes-related parental warmth and caring were important for optimal outcomes. Liss et al. (1998) also found that children hospitalized with DKA reported less diabetes-related parental warmth and caring. Non–diabetes-specific family factors, such as conflict, stress, and family cohesion, have also been linked to glycemic control and adherence (Marteau 1987, Hauser 1990, Auslander 1993, Jacobson 1994, Miller-Johnson 1994, Goldston 1995, Viner 1996). For example, high levels of family stress were correlated with poorer glycemic control in children under 12 years of age (Viner 1996). In contrast, Kovacs et al. (1989) have not found relationships between general family factors and metabolic control or treatment adherence in a longitudinal study of school-aged children. However, a second longitudinal study of school-aged children with newly diagnosed diabetes by Jacobson and colleagues (1990, 1994) revealed that the child's perception of family conflict measured at diagnosis was the strongest predictor of poor adherence to insulin administration, meal planning, exercise, and blood glucose monitoring tasks over a 4-year follow-up period.

The connection between conflict, adherence, and glycemic control was also examined by Miller-Johnson et al. (1994). Parent–child conflict was a significant correlate of both adherence and glycemic control. The authors suggested that conflict may interfere with glycemic control by disrupting treatment adherence. In a study of parenting styles, regimen adherence, and glycemic control in 4- to 10-year-olds with T1D and their parents, "authoritative parenting" characterized by parental support and affection was related to better regimen adherence and glycemic control (Davis 2001). "Authoritative parenting," in which conflict is minimized as parents set consistent, realistic limits on children's behavior while displaying warmth and sensitivity to their child's needs and feelings, has been linked to improved behavioral outcomes in general child development as well as in diabetes-specific adjustment of school-aged children (Anderson 2004). Finally, family environments that are more structured and rule-governed are associated with better glycemic control in school-aged children with T1D (Cohen 2004).

Empirical studies support the conclusion that older school-aged children who are given greater responsibility for their diabetes management make more mistakes in their self-care, are less adherent, and are in poorer metabolic control than those whose parents are more involved (Burns 1986, Anderson 1990, Weissberg-Benchell 1995, Wysocki 1996b, Anderson 1997). From these studies, it has become increasingly clear that parental involvement in diabetes management is required throughout the school-age developmental period.

DIABETES IN ADOLESCENTS

A central developmental task of adolescence is becoming an individual and separating from one's parents psychologically as manifested in the development of goals, values, preferences, and opinions that are influenced by, yet distinct from, those of one's parents (Lerner 2004, Adams 2005, Arnett 2010). Negotiating these crucial challenges of adolescence certainly becomes more complex in the context of family management of childhood diabetes (Bobrow 1985, Hanson 1990, Wysocki 1993, Ryden 1994, Viner 1996, Wysocki 2002). Although many families do well with this delicate balancing act, some struggle at times and still others suffer serious, chronic problems in coping with diabetes and its management. This section summarizes the extensive current knowledge about psychological variables that influence the effectiveness of family management of diabetes during adolescence and evaluates controlled trials of psychological interventions targeting adaptation to diabetes among adolescents and their families.

Achieving and maintaining tight glycemic control is more difficult in adolescence due to diminished insulin sensitivity (Amiel 1986). Compounding the metabolic effects of this normal physiological phenomenon, many behavioral and psychological characteristics of adolescents may also influence diabetes outcomes, such as rebelliousness, risk-taking, peer influences, and decreased parental monitoring. Although adolescents demonstrate steady increases in diabetes knowledge (Johnson 1982, Eastman 1983, Johnson 1984) and skills (Delamater 1988, Delamater 1989) and assume increasing responsibility for diabetes care (La Greca 1990, Wysocki 1992a, Wysocki 1996b), treatment adherence tends to decline from late childhood throughout adolescence (Johnson 1986, Viner 1996, Harris 2000, Schilling 2002, Iannotti 2006, Schilling 2009, Lewin 2010). Coupled with this, family communication and problem-solving skills become increasingly important determinants of the effectiveness of family management of diabetes (Balik 1986, Wysocki 1993, Miller-Johnson 1994). Adolescents who experience more parental involvement, monitoring, and collaborative teamwork in diabetes management tend to achieve and maintain better diabetes outcomes (Anderson 1997, Palmer 2004, Weibe 2005, Ellis 2007, Ellis 2008, Helgeson 2008, Wysocki 2008b, Helgeson 2009b, Wysocki 2009). Social support from peers and siblings is also an important influence on adolescents' adaptation to diabetes (La Greca 1995, Burroughs 1997, Greco 2001, Bearman 2002, La Greca 2002, Pendley 2002, Wysocki 2006a, Helgeson 2009a). Adolescents who exhibit concomitant psychopathology, particularly anxiety (Kovacs 1996, Kovacs 1997a, Herzer 2010), depression (Kovacs 1996, Kovacs 1997a, Kovacs 1997b, Hood 2006, McGrady 2009), and eating disorders (Steel 1987, Colas 1991, Bryden 1999, Jones 2000, Colton 2004, Grylli 2005, Peveler 2005, Colton 2007, Young-Hyman 2010), face greater risks of poor diabetes outcomes and excessive health care utilization. As discussed earlier, numerous studies have shown that diabetes raises the risk of cognitive and learning disorders, particularly among children diagnosed with diabetes as preschoolers (Achenbach 1983, Banion 1983, Ryan 1984, Garrison 1989, Wysocki 1989b, Eiser 1990, Rovet 1993, Northam 1996, Ryan 1997, Holmes 1999, Northam 2001, Ferguson 2005, Hershey 2010), but the extent to which such disorders may affect adaptation to diabetes has not been studied. Both severe hypoglycemia and chronic hyperglycemia have been implicated in the etiology of cognitive and neuroanatomical changes associated with T1D (Ryan 1997, Ferguson 2005, Hershey 2010). Finally, there is evidence that a negative developmental trajectory around diabetes management during adolescence may persist into early adulthood, accelerating the risk of long-term medical and psychological complications of diabetes (Wysocki 1992a, Bryden 2001, Bryden 2003), underscoring the importance of the empirical validation of psychological interventions that can prepare families to cope more effectively with diabetes during this challenging developmental period.

Numerous interventions targeting adolescent and family management of diabetes have been evaluated (Delamater 2001, Hampson 2001, Rubin 2001). These have included evaluations reporting beneficial effects of various psycho-educational strategies including behavior modification techniques (Lowe 1979, Epstein 1981, Schafer 1982, Carney 1983, Gross 1983, Gross 1985, Wysocki 1989a), group or individual training in diabetes-specific social skills (Kaplan 1985, Satin 1989, Grey 1998, Grey 1999, Grey 2000), coping skills (Grey 1998, Grey 1999, Grey 2000, Hains 2001, Silverman 2003), problem solving (Anderson 1989, Cook 2002), and stress management techniques (Fowler 1976, Rose 1983, Delamater 1990, Boardway 1993, McNabb 1994, Mendez 1997). Motivational interviewing has shown promise in several initial clinical trials (Channon 2005, Channon 2007). Applications of telemedicine approaches to diabetes self-management behaviors have also demonstrated promise (Farmer 2005, Mulvaney 2010). Trials of various family therapy modalities have yielded beneficial effects on diabetes outcomes (Delamater 2001, Hampson 2001, Rubin 2001), particularly evaluations of behaviorally oriented family interventions such as behavioral family systems therapy (Wysocki 2006b, Wysocki 2007, Wysocki 2008a) and multisystemic therapy (Ellis 2004, Ellis 2005). Several studies have also affirmed the benefits of preventive strategies, including an 8-week self-management training program for families of newly diagnosed youths (Delamater 1990) and a clinic-based intervention designed to promote parent–child teamwork in family diabetes management (Anderson 1999, Anderson 2001, Laffel 2003).

Overall, the results of these behavioral and psychological intervention studies conducted with adolescents with T1D suggest that clinically significant treatment effects on behavioral and psychological outcomes are commonly obtained, whereas comparable effects on glycemic outcomes have been more elusive (Delamater 2001, Hampson 2001, Rubin 2001). None of these trials has involved large, multicenter samples, and few have met all of the optimal criteria for randomized controlled trials (Chambless 2001, Stinson 2003). Also, a wide variety of intervention approaches have been studied, with few replications reported by other research groups. More research is needed to verify the effectiveness of these methods with larger, diverse samples, to explore the moderators and mediators of intervention effectiveness, and to analyze the cost-effectiveness and feasibility of translation of these methods into routine clinical practice.

The increased prevalence of type 2 diabetes (T2D) in the pediatric age-group (Rosenbloom 1999, American Diabetes Association 2000, Rosenbloom 2003) and of "hybrid" forms of diabetes (e.g., maturity-onset diabetes of youth; "type 1.5 diabetes") (Rosenbloom 2003) create new clinical and scientific challenges. There are many parallels to the management of T1D during adolescence, but T2D carries with it special psychological considerations that may impede generalization of research findings across these conditions. Compared with T1D, T2D is more likely to have later onset, to occur disproportionately among racial and ethnic minorities and those with lower socioeconomic status, to correlate with a positive family history among first-degree relatives, and to be associated with obesity and inactivity (Rosenbloom 1999, Young-Hyman 2001, Rosenbloom 2003, Young-Hyman 2003, Sperling 2005). Unfortunately, compared to T1D, T2D, particularly in children and adolescents, has received very little research attention from behavioral scientists (Rosenbloom 1999, Young-Hyman 2001, Rosenbloom 2003, Young-Hyman 2003, Sperling 2005, Wysocki 2005).

There is an extensive body of literature demonstrating that behavioral interventions can be effective in promoting long-term weight control (Brownell 1983, Epstein 1994, Jelalian 1999, Jeffrey 2000, Dubbert 2004) and increased physical activity (Sallis 1999, Dubbert 2004) among youths, but much of this research has been done with self-selected samples of participants. Controlled trials of such interventions with youths who have been diagnosed with T2D, or who are at high risk for this diagnosis, are needed to determine the extent to which these earlier promising results may generalize to these populations and to identify variables that predict treatment outcomes.

The Studies to Treat Or Prevent Pediatric Type 2 Diabetes (STOPP-T2D) trials of the National Institutes of Health were two of the first large studies of these cohorts of youth with or at risk for T2D. First, the HEALTHY Study was a school-based multicomponent intervention focused on diabetes risk reduction in youth attending minority, lower socioeconomic status (SES) middle schools (HEALTHY Study Group 2010). Forty-two schools across the country were randomized to either the comprehensive school-based intervention or to an assessment-only control group, and youth were studied from 6th through 8th grade. Results indicated that the prevalence of overweight and obese students decreased in both the intervention and control schools, with no significant differences between the school groups. However the youth in the school-based intervention did show significantly greater reduction in indices of adiposity such as BMI z-scores, waist circumference, and fasting insulin levels. The study investigators suggest that these changes in adiposity markers may reduce the risk of childhood-onset T2D; however, this hypothesis awaits further study.

A second STOPP-T2D study, the recently completed TODAY study (Treatment Options for Type 2 Diabetes in Adolescents and Youth) compared three treatments—a metformin-only arm, a metformin-plus–intensive lifestyle intervention arm, and a metformin-plus-rosiglitazone arm in youth 10–17 years of age with recently diagnosed T2D who had a BMI score ≥ the 85th percentile at baseline (TODAY Study Group 2012). The majority of the study youth were from minority racial/ethic and lower-SES backgrounds, and 90% had a parent or grandparent with T2D, often with diabetes complications. Results of this randomized controlled trial with this high-risk cohort indicated that over the average 3.8 years of study duration, 51% of youth in the metformin-alone arm had treatment failure. The addition of rosiglitazone, but not the intensive lifestyle intervention, was superior to metformin alone, yet 39% of youth in the two-drug arm had treatment failure; and 47% of youth had treatment failure in the metformin-plus–lifestyle intervention arm. These drug failure rates are discouraging and suggest that pediatric T2D is very difficult to treat and that most youth with T2D will require multiple oral agents and/or insulin within a few years after diagnosis. These two major studies provide the first rigorous information to guide further clinical treatment and research investigations of the high-risk cohort of youth with and at risk for T2D.

RECOMMENDATIONS FOR CLINICAL CARE

Based upon the extensive research literature reviewed, the following recommendations for clinical management of diabetes in children and adolescents are suggested:

1. **Promote family teamwork, communication, and conflict resolution skills:** Clinicians should encourage healthy family communication about diabetes and help family members to develop effective problem-solving and conflict resolution skills to maintain productive parent–child teamwork for successful diabetes management.
2. **Detect adjustment problems early**: Early detection of depression, anxiety disorders, eating disorders, and learning disabilities enhances the range

and effectiveness of treatment options and may minimize adverse effects on diabetes management.

3. **Refer for appropriate services and encourage adequate use of those services**: Ideally, refer patients and families to specialized psychological or psychiatric services that are connected to the diabetes team. If that is not available, seek to cultivate a referral relationship with qualified and interested pediatric mental health professionals.

4. **Advocate for health promotion on a community level**: The development of school and community-based programs that encourage healthy eating, regular physical activity, and weight control could promote prevention of T2D as well as more effective management of T1D.

5. **Counsel patients and families regarding advances in medical care**: Programmable insulin pumps, continuous glucose sensors, carbohydrate counting, flexible insulin regimens, and other such advances are likely to become increasingly available (Chapter 11). Careful selection and preparation of candidates for these advances may enhance their chances of enjoying improved glycemic control and quality of life as a consequence.

6. **Seek continuing education regarding psychological aspects of diabetes**: There is an extensive and growing body of empirical research on the psychological and behavioral aspects of diabetes. Clinicians who achieve and maintain familiarity with that research will be better equipped to implement these recommendations.

BIBLIOGRAPHY

Achenbach TM, Edelbrock CS: *Manual for the Child Behavior Checklist and Revised Child Behavior Profile.* Burlington, VT, University of Vermont Press, 1983

Adams GR, Berzonsky MD: *The Blackwell Handbook of Adolescence.* New York, Blackwell Publishing, 2005

American Diabetes Association: Type 2 diabetes in children and adolescents. *Pediatrics* 105:671–680, 2000

Amiel SA, Sherwin RS, Simonson DC, Lauritano AA, Tamborlane WV: Impaired insulin action in puberty: a contributing factor to poor glycemic control in adolescents with diabetes. *N Engl J Med* 315:215–219, 1986

Anderson B, Ho J, Brackett J, Finkelstein D, Laffel L: Parental involvement in diabetes management tasks: relationships to blood glucose monitoring adherence and metabolic control in young adolescents with insulin-dependent diabetes mellitus. *J Pediatr* 130:257–265, 1997

Anderson BJ: Family conflict and diabetes management in youth: clinical lessons from child development and diabetes research. *Diabetes Spectrum* 17:22–26, 2004

Anderson BJ, Loughlin C, Goldberg E, Laffel L: Comprehensive, family-focused outpatient care for very young children living with chronic disease: lessons from a program in pediatric diabetes. *Child Serv Soc Policy Res Pract* 4:235–250, 2001

Anderson BJ, Brackett J, Ho J, Laffel LM: An office-based intervention to maintain parent-adolescent teamwork in diabetes management. *Diabetes Care* 22:713–721, 1999

Anderson BJ, Auslander WF, Jung KC, Miller JP, Santiago JV: Assessing family sharing of diabetes responsibilities. *J Pediatr Psychol* 15:477–492, 1990

Anderson BJ, Wolf FM, Burkhart MT, Cornell RG, Bacon GE: Effects of a peer group intervention on metabolic control of adolescents with IDDM: randomized outpatient study. *Diabetes Care* 12:184–188, 1989

Anderson BJ, Auslander WF: Research on diabetes management and the family: a critique. *Diabetes Care* 3:696–702, 1980

Arnett J: *Adolescence and Emerging Adulthood: A Multicultural Approach*. 4th ed. Boston, Prentice Hall, 2010

Auslander WF, Bubb J, Rogge M, Santiago JV: Family stress and resources: potential areas of intervention in children recently diagnosed with diabetes. *Health Soc Work* 18:101–113, 1993

Balik B, Haig B, Moynihan PM: Diabetes and the school-aged child. *MCN Am J Matern Child Nurs* 11:324–330, 1986

Banion CR, Miles MS, Carter MC: Problems of mothers in management of children with diabetes. *Diabetes Care* 6:548–551, 1983

Bearman KJ, La Greca AM: Assessing friend support of adolescents' diabetes care: the diabetes social support questionnaire—friends version. *J Pediatr Psychol* 27:417–428, 2002

Boardway RH, Delamater AM, Tomakowsky J, Gutai JP: Stress management training for adolescents with diabetes. *J Pediatr Psychol* 18:29–45, 1993

Bobrow ES, AvRuskin TW, Siller J: Mother-daughter interactions and adherence to diabetes regimens. *Diabetes Care* 8:146–151, 1985

Brink SJ, Moltz K: The message of the DCCT for children and adolescents. *Diabetes Spectrum* 10:259–267, 1997

Brownell KD, Kelman JH, Stunkard AJ: Treatment of obese children with and without their mothers: changes in weight and blood pressure. *Pediatr* 71:515–523, 1983

Bryden KS, Dunger DB, Mayou RA, Peveler RC, Neil HA: Poor prognosis of young adults with type 1 diabetes: a longitudinal study. *Diabetes Care* 26:1052–1057, 2003

Bryden KS, Peveler RC, Stein A, Neil A, Mayou RA, Dunger DB: Clinical and psychological course of diabetes from adolescence to young adulthood. *Diabetes Care* 24:1536–1540, 2001

Bryden KS, Neil A, Mayou RA, Peveler RC, Fairburn CG, Dunger DB: Eating habits, body weight, and insulin misuse. *Diabetes Care* 22:1956–1960, 1999

Burns KL, Green P, Chase HP: Psychosocial correlates of glycemic control as a function of age in youth with IDDM. *J Adoles Health Care* 7:311–319, 1986

Burroughs TE, Harris MA, Pontious SL, Santiago JV: Research on social support in adolescents with IDDM: a critical review. *Diabetes Educ* 23:438–448, 1997

Carney RM, Schechter K, Davis T: Improving adherence to blood glucose monitoring in insulin-dependent diabetic children. *Behav Ther* 14:247–254, 1983

Chambless DL, Ollendick TH: Empirically supported psychological interventions: controversies and evidence. *Ann Rev Psychol* 52:685–716, 2001

Channon SJ, Huws-Thomas M, Rollnick S, Hood K, Cannings-John R, Rogers C, Gregory JW: A multicenter randomized controlled trial of motivational interviewing in teenagers with diabetes. *Diabetes Care* 30:1390–1395, 2007

Channon S, Huws-Thomas MV, Gregory JW, Rollnick S: Motivational interviewing with teenagers with diabetes. *Clin Child Psychol Psychiatr* 10:43–51, 2005

Cohen DM, Lumley MA, Naar-King S, Partridge T, Cakan N: Child behavior problems and family functioning as predictors of adherence and glycemic control in economically disadvantaged children with type 1 diabetes: a prospective study. *J Pediatr Psychol* 29:171–184, 2004

Colas C, Mathieu P, Techobroutsky G: Eating disorders and retinal lesions in type 1 (insulin-dependent) diabetic women. *Diabetologia* 34:288, 1991

Colton P, Olmsted M, Daneman D, Rydall A, Rodin G: Disturbed eating behavior and eating disorders in preteen and early teenage girls with type 1 diabetes. *Diabetes Care* 27:1654–1659, 2004

Colton PA, Olmsted MP, Daneman D, Rydall AC, Rodin G: Five-year prevalence and persistence of disturbed eating behavior and eating disorders in girls with type 1 diabetes. *Diabetes Care* 30:2861–2862, 2007

Cook S, Herold K, Edidin DV, Briars R: Increasing problem solving in adolescents with type 1 diabetes: the choices diabetes program. *Diabetes Educ* 28:115–123, 2002

Daneman D, Frank M, Perlman K, Wittenberg J: The infant and toddler with diabetes: challenges of diagnosis and management. *Paediatr Child Health* 4:57–63, 1999

Davis CL, Delamater AM, Shaw KH, LaGreca AM, Eidson MS, Perez-Rodriguez JE: Parenting styles, regimen adherence, and glycemic control in 4-10-year-old children with diabetes. *J Pediatr Psychol* 26:123–129, 2001

Delamater AM, Jacobson AM, Anderson B, Cox D, Fisher L, Lustman P, Rubin R, Wysocki T: Psychosocial therapies in diabetes: report of the psychosocial therapies working group. *Diabetes Care* 24:1286–1292, 2001

Delamater AM, Bubb J, Davis SG, Smith JA, Schmidt L, White NH: Randomized prospective study of self-management training with newly diagnosed diabetic children. *Diabetes Care* 13:492–498, 1990

Delamater AM, Davis S, Bubb J, Smith J, White NH, Santiago JV: Self-monitoring of blood glucose by adolescents with diabetes: technical skills and utilization of data. *Diabetes Educ* 15:56–61, 1989

Delamater AM, Smith JA, Kurtz SM, White NH: Dietary skills and adherence in children with type 1 diabetes mellitus. *Diabetes Educ* 14:33–36, 1988

Diabetes Control and Complications Trial Research Group: Effect of intensive diabetes treatment on the development and progression of long-term complications in adolescents with insulin-dependent diabetes mellitus: Diabetes Control and Complications Trial. *J Pediatr* 125:177–188, 1994

DiMeglio LA, Pottorff TM, Boyd SR, France L, Fineberg N, Eugster EA: A randomized, controlled study of insulin pump therapy in diabetic preschoolers. *J Pediatr* 145:380–384, 2004

Drash AL: The child, the adolescent, and the Diabetes Control and Complications Trial. *Diabetes Care* 16:1515–1516, 1993

Dubbert PM, King AC, Marcus BH, Sallis JF: Promotion of physical activity through the life span. In *Handbook of Clinical Health Psychology. Volume 2: Disorders of Behavior and Health*. Boll TJ, Raczynski JM, Leviton LC, Eds. Washington, DC, American Psychological Association, 2004, p. 147–181

Dumont RH, Jacobson AM, Cole C, Hauser ST, Wolfsdorf JI, Willett JB, Milley JE, Wertlieb D: Psychosocial predictors of acute complications of diabetes in youth. *Diabet Med* 12:612–618, 1995

Eastman BG, Johnson SB, Silverstein J, Spillar R, McCallum M: Understanding of hypo- and hyperglycemia by youngsters with diabetes and their parents. *J Pediatr Psychol* 8:229–243, 1983

Eiser C: *Chronic Childhood Disease: An Introduction to Psychological Theory and Research*. New York, Cambridge University Press, 1990

Ellis DA, Templin T, Podolski C, Frey M, Naar-King S, Moltz K: The Parental Monitoring of Diabetes Care scale: development, reliability and validity of a scale to evaluate parental supervision of adolescent illness management. *J Adol Health* 42:146–153, 2008

Ellis DA, Podolski CL, Frey M, Naar-King S, Wang B, Moltz K: The role of parental monitoring in adolescent health outcomes: impact on regimen adherence in youth with type 1 diabetes. *J Pediatr Psychol* 32:907–917, 2007

Ellis DA, Frey M, Naar-King S, Templin T, Cunningham P, Cakan N: Use of multi-systemic therapy to improve regimen adherence among adolescents with type 1 diabetes in chronic poor metabolic control: a randomized controlled trial. *Diabetes Care* 28:1604–1610, 2005

Ellis DA, Naar-King S, Frey M, Templin T, Rowland M, Greger N: Use of multisystemic therapy to improve regimen adherence among adolescents with type 1 diabetes in poor metabolic control: a pilot investigation. *J Clin Psychol Med Settings* 11:315–324, 2004

Epstein LH, Valoski A, Wing RR, McCurley J: Ten-year outcomes of behavioral family-based treatment for childhood obesity. *Health Psychol* 13:373–383, 1994

Epstein LH, Beck S, Figueroa J, Farkas G, Kazdin AE, Daneman D, Becker DJ: The effects of targeting improvement in urine glucose on metabolic control in children with insulin-dependent diabetes mellitus. *J App Behav Anal* 14:365–375, 1981

Erikson EH: *Identity: Youth and Crisis*. New York, W. W. Norton, 1968

Erikson EH: *Childhood and Society*. New York, W. W. Norton, 1950

Farmer AJ, Gibson OJ, Dudley C, Bryden KS, Hayton PM, Tarasenko L, Neil A: A randomized controlled trial of the effect of real-time telemedicine support on glycemic control in young adults with type 1 diabetes (ISRCTN 46889446). *Diabetes Care* 28:2697–2702, 2005

Ferguson SC, Blane A, Wardlaw J, Frier BM, Perros P, McCrimmon RJ, Deary IJ: Influence of early onset age of type 1 diabetes on cerebral structure and cognitive function. *Diabetes Care* 28:1431–1437, 2005

Fowler J, Budzynski T, Vandebergh R: Effects of an EMG biofeedback relaxation program on control of diabetes: a case study. *Biofeedback Self Regul* 1:105–112, 1976

Gardner SG, Bingley PJ, Sawtell PA, Weeks S, Gale EA: Rising incidence of insulin-dependent diabetes in children aged under 5 years in the Oxford region: time trend analysis. The Bart's Oxford Study Group. *BMJ* 315:712–717, 1997

Garrison WT, McQuiston S: *Chronic Illness during Childhood and Adolescence*. Newbury Park, CA, Sage Publications, 1989

Golden MP, Ingersoll GM, Brack CJ, Russell BA, Wright JC, Huberty TJ: Longitudinal relationship of asymptomatic hypoglycemia to cognitive function in IDDM. *Diabetes Care* 12:89–93, 1989

Golden MP, Russell BP, Ingersoll GM, Gray DL, Hummer KM: Management of diabetes in children younger than 5 years of age. *Am J Dis Child* 139:448–452, 1985

Goldston DB, Kovacs M, Obrosky S, Iyengar S: A longitudinal study of life events and metabolic control among youths with insulin-dependent diabetes mellitus. *Health Psychol* 14:409–414, 1995

Greco P, Pendley JS, McDonell K, Reeves G: A peer group intervention for adolescents with type 1 diabetes and their best friends. *J Pediatr Psychol* 26:485–490, 2001

Grey M, Boland E, Davidson M, Li J, Tamborlane W: Coping skills training for youth on intensive therapy has long-lasting effects on metabolic control and quality of life. *J Pediatr* 137:107–113, 2000

Grey M, Boland E, Davidson M, Yu C, Tamborlane W: Coping skills training for youth with diabetes on intensive therapy. *Appl Nurs Res* 12:3–12, 1999

Grey M, Boland E, Davidson M, Yu C, Sullivan-Bolyai S, Tamborlane WV: Short-term effects of coping skills training as adjunct to intensive therapy in adolescents. *Diabetes Care* 21:902–908, 1998

Gross AM, Magalnick LJ, Richardson P: Self management training with families of insulin-dependent diabetic children: a long term controlled investigation. *Child Fam Behav Ther* 3:141–153, 1985

Gross AM, Heimann L, Shapiro R, Schultz RM: Children with diabetes: social skills training and HbA1c levels. *Behav Modif* 7:151–163, 1983

Grylli V, Hafferl-Gattermayer A, Wagner G, Schober E, Karwautz A: Eating disorders and eating problems among adolescents with type 1 diabetes: exploring relationships with temperament and character. *J Pediatr Psychol* 30:197–206, 2005

Hains AA, Davies WH, Parton E, Silverman AH: Brief report: a cognitive behavioral intervention for distressed adolescents with type 1 diabetes. *J Pediatr Psychol* 26:61–66, 2001

Hampson SE, Skinner TC, Hart J, Storey L, Gage H, Foxcroft D, Kimber A, Shaw K, Walker J: Effects of educational and psychosocial interventions for adolescents with diabetes mellitus: a systematic review. *Health Technol Assess* 5:1–79, 2001

Hanson CL, Rodrigue J, Henggeler SW, Harris MA, Klesges R, Carle D: The perceived self-competence of adolescents with insulin-dependent diabetes mellitus: deficit or strength? *J Pediatr Psychol* 15:605–618, 1990

Harris MA, Wysocki T, Sadler M, Wilkinson K, Harvey LM, Buckloh LM, Mauras N, White NH: Validation of a structured interview for the assessment of diabetes self management. *Diabetes Care* 23:1301–1304, 2000

Hathout EH, Fujishige L, Geach J, Ischandar M, Mauro S, Mace JW: Effect of therapy with insulin glargine (Lantus) on glycemic control in toddlers, children, and adolescents with diabetes. *Diabetes Technol Ther* 5:801–806, 2003

Hatton DL, Canam C, Thorne S, Hughes AM: Parents' perceptions of caring for an infant or toddler with diabetes. *J Adv Nurs* 22:569–577, 1995

Hauser ST, Jacobson AM, Lavori P, Wolfsdorf JI, Herskowitz RD, Milley JE, Bliss R, Gelfand E, Wertlieb D, Stein J: Adherence among children and adolescents with insulin-dependent diabetes mellitus over four-year longitudinal follow-up: II. Immediate and long-term linkages with the family milieu. *J Pediatr Psychol* 15:527–542, 1990

HEALTHY Study Group, Foster GD, Linder B, Baranowski T, Cooper DM, Goldberg L, et al.: A school-based intervention for diabetes risk reduction. *N Engl J Med* 363:443–453, 2010

Helgeson VS, Lopez LC, Kamarck T: Peer relationship and diabetes: retrospective and ecological momentary assessment approaches. *Health Psychol* 28:273–282, 2009a

Helgeson VS, Siminerio L, Escobar O, Becker D: Predictors of metabolic control among adolescents with diabetes: a 4-year longitudinal study. *J Pediatr Psychol* 34:254–270, 2009b

Helgeson VS, Reynolds K, Siminerio L, Escobar O, Becker D: Parent and adolescent distribution of responsibility for self-care: links to health outcome. *J Pediatr Psychol* 33:497–508, 2008

Hershey T, Perantie DC, Wu J, Weaver PM, Black KJ, White NH: Hippocampal volumes in youth with type 1 diabetes. *Diabetes* 59:236–241, 2010

Herzer M, Hood KK: Anxiety symptoms in adolescents with type 1 diabetes: association with blood glucose monitoring and glycemic control. *J Pediatr Psychol* 35:415–425, 2010

Holmes CS, Cant M, Fox MA, Lampert NL, Greer T: Disease and demographic risk factors for disrupted cognitive functioning in children with insulin-dependent diabetes mellitus (IDDM). *Sch Psychol Rev* 28:215–227, 1999

Hood KK, Huestis S, Maher A, Butler D, Volkening LA, Laffel LM: Depressive symptoms in children and adolescents with type 1 diabetes: association with diabetes-specific characteristics. *Diabetes Care* 29:1389–1391, 2006

Iannotti RJ, Nansel TR, Schneider S, Haynie DL, Simons-Morton B, Sobel DO, Zeitzoff L, Plotnick LP, Clark L: Assessing regimen adherence of adolescents with type 1 diabetes. *Diabetes Care* 29:2263–2267, 2006

Jacobson AM, Hauser ST, Lavori P, Willett JB, Cole CF, Wolfsdorf JI, Dumont RH, Wertlieb D: Family environment and glycemic control: a four-year prospective study of children and adolescents with insulin-dependent diabetes mellitus. *Psychosom Med* 56:401–409, 1994

Jacobson AM, Hauser ST, Lavori P, Wolfsdorf JI, Herskowitz RD, Milley JE, Bliss R, Gelfand E, Wertlieb D, Stein J: Adherence among children and adolescents with insulin-dependent diabetes mellitus over four-year longitudinal follow-up: I. The influence of patient coping and adjustment. *J Pediatr Psychol* 15:511–526, 1990

Jeffrey RW, Epstein LH, Wilson GT, Drewnowski A, Stunkard AJ, Wing RR: Long-term maintenance of weight loss: current status. *Health Psychol* 19:5–16, 2000

Jelalian E, Saelens B: Empirically supported treatments in pediatric psychology: pediatric obesity. *J Pediatr Psychol* 24:223–248, 1999

Johnson SB, Silverstein J, Rosenbloom A, Carter R, Cunningham W: Assessing daily management of childhood diabetes. *Health Psychol* 5:545–564, 1986

Johnson SB: Knowledge, attitudes and behavior: correlates of health in childhood diabetes. *Clinical Psychology Review* 5:545–564, 1984

Johnson SB, Pollak R, Silverstein J, Rosenbloom A, Spillar R, McCallum M, Harkavy J: Cognitive and behavioral knowledge about insulin-dependent diabetes among children and parents. *Pediatr* 69:708–713, 1982

Johnson SB: Psychological factors in juvenile diabetes: a review. *J Behav Med* 3:95–102, 1980

Jones JM, Lawson ML, Daneman D, Olmsted MP, Rodin G: Eating disorders in adolescent females with and without type 1 diabetes: cross sectional study. *BMJ* 320:1563–1566, 2000

Kaplan RM, Chadwick MW, Schimmel LE: Social learning intervention to promote metabolic control in type 1 diabetes mellitus: pilot experiment results. *Diabetes Care* 8:152–155, 1985

Kovacs M, Goldston D, Obrosky DS, Bonar LK: Psychiatric disorders in youths with IDDM: rates and risk factors. *Diabetes Care* 20:36–44, 1997a

Kovacs M, Goldston D, Obrosky DS, Drash A: Major depressive disorder in youths with IDDM. *Diabetes Care* 20:45–51, 1997b

Kovacs M, Mukerji P, Iyengar S, Drash A: Psychiatric disorder and metabolic control among youths with IDDM. A longitudinal study. *Diabetes Care* 19:318–323, 1996

Kovacs M, Kass RE, Schnell TM, Goldston D, Marsh J: Family functioning and metabolic control of school-aged children with IDDM. *Diabetes Care* 12:409–414, 1989

Kushion W, Salisbury PJ, Seitz KW, Wilson BE: Issues in the care of infants and toddlers with insulin dependent diabetes mellitus. *Diabetes Educ* 17:107–110, 1991

La Greca AM, Bearman KJ: The diabetes social support questionnaire-family version: evaluating adolescents' diabetes-specific support from family members. *J Pediatr Psychol* 27:665–676, 2002

La Greca AM, Auslander WF, Greco P, Spetter D, Fisher EB, Santiago JV: I get by with a little help from my family and friends: adolescents' support for diabetes care. *J Pediatr Psychol* 26:279–282, 1995

La Greca AM, Follansbee DM, Skyler JS: Developmental and behavioral aspects of diabetes management in youngsters. *Children's Health Care* 19:132–139, 1990

Laffel LM, Vangsness L, Connell A, Goebel-Fabri A, Butler D, Anderson BJ: Impact of ambulatory, family-focused teamwork intervention on glycemic control in youth with type 1 diabetes. *J Pediatr* 142:409–416, 2003

Lerner RM, Steinberg L: *Handbook of Adolescent Psychology.* 2nd ed. New York: Wiley, 2004

Lewin AB, Storch E, Wiliams LB, Duke DC, Silverstein J, Geffken GR: Brief report: normative data on a structured interview for diabetes adherence in childhood. *J Pediatr Psychol* 35:177–182, 2010

Liss DS, Waller DA, Kennard BD, McIntire D, Capra P, Stephens J: Psychiatric illness and family support in children and adolescents with diabetic ketoacidosis: a controlled study. *J Am Acad Child Adolesc Psychiatry* 37:536–544, 1998

Litton J, Rice A, Friedman N, Oden J, Lee MM, Freemark M: Insulin pump therapy in toddlers and preschool children with type 1 diabetes mellitus. *J Pediatr* 141:490–495, 2002

Lowe K, Lutzker J: Increasing compliance to a medical regimen with a juvenile diabetic. *Behav Ther* 10:57–64, 1979

Marteau TM, Bloch S, Baum JD: Family life and diabetic control. *J Child Psychol Psychiat* 28:823–833, 1987

McGrady ME, Laffel L, Drotar D, Repaske D, Hood KK: Depressive symptoms and glycemic control in adolescents with type 1 diabetes: mediational role of blood glucose monitoring. *Diabetes Care* 32:804–806, 2009

McNabb W, Quinn M, Murphy D, Thorp F, Cook S: Increasing children's responsibility for self-care: the in-control study. *Diabetes Educ* 20:121–124, 1994

Mendez FJ, Belendez M: Effects of a behavioral intervention on treatment adherence and stress management in adolescents with IDDM. *Diabetes Care* 20:1370–1375, 1997

Miller-Johnson S, Emery RE, Marvin RS, Clarke W, Lovinger R, Martin M: Parent-child relationships and the management of diabetes mellitus. *J Consult Clin Psychol* 62:603–610, 1994

Mulvaney S, Rothman RL, Wallston KA, Lybarger C, Dietrich MS: An Internet-based program to improve self-management in adolescents with type 1 diabetes. *Diabetes Care* 33:602–604, 2010

Northam EA, Anderson PJ, Jacobs R, Hughes M, Warne GL, Werther GA: Neuropsychological profiles of children with type 1 diabetes 6 years after disease onset. *Diabetes Care* 24:1541–1546, 2001

Northam EA, Anderson PJ, Werther GA, Warne GL, Adler RG, Andrewes D: Neuropsychological complications of IDDM in children 2 years after disease onset. *Diabetes Care* 21:379–384, 1998

Northam E, Anderson P, Adler R, Werther G, Warne G: Psychosocial and family functioning in children with insulin-dependent diabetes at diagnosis and one year later. *J Pediatr Psychol* 21:699–717, 1996

Palmer D, Berg CA, Wiebe DJ, Beveridge R, Korbel CD, Upchurch R, Swinyard M, Lindsay R, Donaldson D: The role of autonomy and pubertal status in understanding age differences in maternal involvement in diabetes responsibility across adolescence. *J Pediatr Psychol* 29:35–46, 2004

Patton SR, Dolan LM, Powers SW: Differences in family mealtime interactions between young children with type 1 diabetes and controls: implications for behavioral intervention. *J Pediatr Psychol* 33:885–893, 2008

Patton SR, Dolan LM, Mitchell MJ, Byars KC, Standiford D, Powers SW: Mealtime interactions in families of pre-schoolers with type 1 diabetes. *Pediatr Diabetes* 5:190–198, 2004

Pendley JS, Kasmen LJ, Miller DL, Donze J, Swenson C, Reeves G: Peer and family support in children and adolescents with type 1 diabetes. *J Pediatr Psychol* 27:429–438, 2002

Peveler RC, Bryden KS, Neil HA, Fairburn CG, Mayou RA, Dunger DB, Turner HM: The relationship of disordered eating habits and attitudes to clinical outcomes in young adult females with type 1 diabetes. *Diabetes Care* 28:84–88, 2005

Pond JS, Peters ML, Pannell DL, Rogers CS: Psychosocial challenges for children with insulin-dependent diabetes mellitus. *Diabetes Educ* 21:297–299, 1995

Powers SW, Byars KC, Mitchell MJ, Patton SR, Standiford DA, Dolan LM: Parent report of mealtime behavior and parenting stress in young children with type 1 diabetes and in healthy control subjects. *Diabetes Care* 25:313–318, 2002

Puczynski MS, Puczynski SS, Reich J, Kaspar JC, Emanuele M: Mental efficiency and hypoglycemia. *J Dev Behav Pediatr* 11:170–174, 1990

Rose MI, Firestone P, Heick HM, Faught AK: The effect of anxiety management training on the control of juvenile diabetes. *J Behav Med* 6:381–395, 1983

Rosenbloom AL, Silverstein JH: *Type 2 Diabetes in Children and Adolescents: A Guide to Diagnosis, Epidemiology, Pathogenesis, Prevention, and Treatment*. Alexandria, VA, American Diabetes Association, 2003

Rosenbloom AL, Joe JR, Winter WE: Emerging epidemic of type 2 diabetes in youth. *Diabetes Care* 22:345–354, 1999

Rovet JF, Ehrlich RM, Czuchta D, Akler M: Psychoeducational characteristics of children and adolescents with insulin-dependent diabetes mellitus. *J Learn Disabil* 26:7–22, 1993

Rovet JF, Ehrlich RM, Czuchta D: Intellectual characteristics of diabetic children at diagnosis and one year later. *J Pediatr Psychol* 15:775–788, 1990

Rovet JF, Ehrlich RM, Hoppe M: Intellectual deficits associated with early onset of insulin-dependent diabetes mellitus in children. *Diabetes Care* 10:510–515, 1987

Rubin RR, Peyrot M: Psychological issues and treatments for people with diabetes. *J Clin Psychol* 57:457–478, 2001

Ryan CM, Becker DJ: Hypoglycemia in children with type 1 diabetes mellitus. Risk factors, cognitive function, and management. *Endocrinol Metab Clin North Am* 28:883–900, 1999

Ryan CM: Effects of diabetes mellitus on neuropsychological function: a lifespan perspective. *Semin Clin Neuropsychiatry* 2:4–14, 1997

Ryan C, Longstreet C, Morrow L: The effects of diabetes mellitus on the school attendance and school achievement of adolescents. *Child: Care, Health, & Development* 11:229–240, 1985a

Ryan C, Vega A, Drash A: Cognitive deficits in adolescents who developed diabetes early in life. *Pediatr* 75:921–927, 1985b

Ryan C, Vega A, Longstreet C, Drash A: Neuropsychological changes in adolescents with insulin-independent diabetes. *J Consult Clin Psychol* 52:335–342, 1984

Ryden O, Nevander L, Johnsson P, Hansson K, Kronvall P, Sjoblad S, Westbom L: Family therapy in poorly controlled juvenile IDDM: effects on diabetes control, self-evaluation, and behavioral symptoms. *Acta Paediatr* 83:285–291, 1994

Saha ME, Huuppone T, Mikael K, Juuti M, Komulainen J: Continuous subcutaneous insulin infusion in the treatment of children and adolescents with type 1 diabetes mellitus. *J Pediatr Endocrinol Metab* 15:1005–1010, 2002

Sallis JF: Influences on physical activity of children, adolescents, and adults. In *Toward a Better Understanding of Physical Fitness and Activity*. Corbin CB, Pangrazi RP, Eds. Scottsdale, AZ, Holcomb Hathaway, 1999, p. 27–32

Satin W, La Greca AM, Zigo S, Skyler JS: Diabetes in adolescence: effects of multifamily group intervention and parent simulation of diabetes. *J Pediatr Psychol* 14:259–276, 1989

Schafer LC, Glasgow RE, McCaul KD: Increasing the adherence of diabetic adolescents. *J Behav Med* 5:353–362, 1982

Schilling L, Dixon J, Knafl K, Lynn M, Murphy K, Dumser S, Grey M: A new self-report measure of self-management of type 1 diabetes for adolescents. *Nurs Res* 58:228–236, 2009

Schilling L, Grey M, Knafl K: A review of measures of self management of type 1 diabetes by youth and their parents. *Diabetes Educator* 28:796–808, 2002

Schoenle EJ, Schoenle D, Molinari L, Largo RH: Impaired intellectual development in children with type 1 diabetes: association with HbAlc, age at diagnosis and sex. *Diabetologia* 45:108–114, 2002

Shehadeh N, Battelino T, Galatzer A, Naveh T, Hadash A, de Vries L, Phillip M: Insulin pump therapy for 1-6 year old children with type 1 diabetes. *Isr Med Assoc J* 6:284–286, 2004

Silverman AH, Haines AA, Davies WH, Parton E: A cognitive behavioral adherence intervention for adolescents with type 1 diabetes. *J Clin Psychol Med Settings* 10:119–127, 2003

Silverstein JH, Johnson S: Psychosocial challenge of diabetes and the development of a continuum of care. *Pediatr Ann* 23:300–305, 1994

Snyder J: Behavioral analysis and treatment of poor diabetic self-care and antisocial behavior: a single-subject experimental study. *Behav Ther* 18:251–263, 1987

Soltesz G, Patterson C, Dahlquist G: Global trends in childhood type 1 diabetes. In *Diabetes Atlas*. 3rd ed. Chapter 2.1. Brussels, Belgium, International Diabetes Federation, 2006, p. 153–190

Sperling M, Ize-Ludlow D: The classification of diabetes mellitus: a conceptual framework. *Pediatr Clin N Amer* 52:1533–1552, 2005

Steel JM, Young RJ, Lloyd GG, Clark BF: Clinically apparent eating disorders in young diabetic women: associations with painful neuropathy and other complications. *BMJ* 294:859–862, 1987

Stinson JN, McGrath PJ, Yamada JT: Clinical trials in the Journal of Pediatric Psychology: Applying the CONSORT Statement. *J Pediatr Psychol* 28:59–167, 2003

Sullivan-Bolyai S, Deatrick J, Gruppuso P, Tamborlane W, Grey M: Constant vigilance: mothers' work parenting young children with type 1 diabetes. *J Pediatr Nurs* 18:21–29, 2003

Tan CY, Wilson DM, Buckingham B: Initiation of insulin glargine in children and adolescents with type 1 diabetes. *Pediatr Diabetes* 5:80–86, 2004

Thomas AM, Peterson L, Goldstein D: Problem solving and diabetes regimen adherence by children and adolescents with IDDM in social pressure situations: a reflection of normal development. *J Pediatr Psychol* 22:541–561, 1997

TODAY Study Group, Zeitler P, Hirst K, Pyle L, Linder B, Copeland K, et al.: A clinical trial to maintain glycemic control in youth with type 2 diabetes. *N Engl J Med* 366:2247–2256, 2012

Tubiana-Rufi N, de Lonlay P, Bloch J, Czernichow P: Remission of severe hypoglycemic incidents in young diabetic children treated with subcutaneous infusion. *Arch Pediatr* 3:969–976, 1996

Vehik K, Dabelea D: The changing epidemiology of type 1 diabetes: why is it going through the roof? *Diabetes Metab Res Rev* 27:3–13, 2011

Viner R, McGrath M, Trudinger P: Family stress and metabolic control in diabetes. *Arch Dis Child* 74:418–421, 1996

Waller D, Chipman JJ, Hardy BW, Hightower MS, North AJ, Williams SB, Babick AJ: Measuring diabetes-specific family support and its relation to metabolic control: a preliminary report. *J Am Acad Child Psychol* 25:415–418, 1986

Weibe DJ, Berg CA, Korbel C, Palmer DL, Beveridge RM, Upchurch R, Lindsay R, Swinyard MT, Donaldson DL: Children's appraisals of maternal involvement in coping with diabetes: enhancing our understanding of adherence, metabolic control, and quality of life across adolescence. *J Pediatr Psychol* 30:167–178, 2005

Weissberg-Benchell J, Glasgow AM, Tynan WD, Wirtz P, Turek J, Ward J: Adolescent diabetes management and mismanagement. *Diabetes Care* 18:77–82, 1995

Wolfsdorf JI, Anderson BA, Pasquarello C: Treatment of the child with diabetes. In *Joslin's Diabetes Mellitus.* 13th ed. Kahn CR, Weir G, Eds. Philadelphia, Lea & Febiger, 1994, p. 430–451

Wysocki T, Nansel TR, Holmbeck G, Chen RS, Laffel L, Anderson BJ, Weissberg-Benchell J: Collaborative involvement of primary and secondary caregivers: associations with youths' diabetes outcomes. *J Pediatr Psychol* 34:869–881, 2009

Wysocki T, Harris MA, Buckloh L, Mertlich D, Lochrie A, Taylor A., Sadler M, White NH: Randomized controlled trial of behavioral family systems therapy for diabetes: maintenance and generalization of effects on parent-adolescent communication. *Behav Ther* 39:33–46, 2008a

Wysocki T, Iannotti R, Weissberg-Benchell J, Hood K, Laffel L, Anderson BJ, Chen R: Diabetes problem solving by youths with type 1 diabetes and their caregivers: measurement, validation and longitudinal associations with glycemic control. *J Pediatr Psychol* 33:875–884, 2008b

Wysocki T, Harris MA, Buckloh LM, Mertlich D, Lochrie AS, Mauras N, White NH: Randomized controlled trial of behavioral family systems therapy for diabetes: maintenance of effects on diabetes outcomes in adolescents. *Diabetes Care* 30:555–560, 2007

Wysocki T, Greco P: Social support and diabetes management in childhood and adolescence: influence of parents and friends. *Current Diabetes Reports* 6:117–122, 2006a

Wysocki T, Harris MA, Buckloh LM, Mertlich D, Lochrie AS, Taylor A, Sadler M, Mauras N, White NH: Effects of behavioral family systems therapy for diabetes on adolescents' family relationships, treatment adherence and metabolic control. *J Pediatr Psychol* 31:928–938, 2006b

Wysocki T, Buckloh LM, Lochrie A, Antal H: The psychologic context of pediatric diabetes. *Pediatr Clin N Amer* 52:1755–1778, 2005

Wysocki T: Parents, teens, and diabetes. *Diabetes Spectrum* 15:6–8, 2002

Wysocki T, Meinhold PA, Taylor A, Hough BS, Barnard MU, Clarke WL, Bellando BJ, Bourgeois MJ: Psychometric properties and normative data for the Diabetes Independence Survey - Parent Version. *Diabetes Educ* 22:587–591, 1996a

Wysocki T, Taylor A, Hough BS, Linscheid TR, Yeates KO, Naglieri JA: Deviation for developmentally appropriate self-care autonomy. Association with diabetes outcomes. *Diabetes Care* 19:119–125, 1996b

Wysocki T: Associations among parent-adolescent relationships, metabolic control and adjustment to diabetes in adolescents. *J Pediatr Psychol* 18:443–454, 1993

Wysocki T, Hough BS, Ward KM, Green LB: Diabetes mellitus in the transition to adulthood: adjustment, self-care, and health status. *J Dev Behav Pediatr* 13:194–201, 1992a

Wysocki T, Meinhold P, Abrams K, Barnard M, Clarke WL, Bellando BJ, Bourgeois MJ: Parental and professional estimates of self-care independence of children and adolescents with insulin-dependent diabetes mellitus. *Diabetes Care* 15:43–52, 1992b

Wysocki T, Green LB, Huxtable K: Blood glucose monitoring by diabetic adolescents: compliance and metabolic control. *Health Psychol* 8:267–284, 1989a

Wysocki T, Huxtable K, Linscheid TR, Wayne W: Adjustment to diabetes mellitus in pre-schoolers and their mothers. *Diabetes Care* 2:524–529, 1989b

Young-Hyman D, Davis C: Disordered eating behavior in individuals with diabetes: importance of context, evaluation, and classification. *Diabetes Care* 33:683–689, 2010

Young-Hyman D, Schlundt DG, Herman-Wenderoth L, Bozylinski K: Obesity, appearance, and psychosocial adaptation in young African American children. *J Pediatr Psychol* 28:463–472, 2003

Young-Hyman D, Schlundt DG, Herman L, DeLuca F, Counts D: Evaluation of the insulin resistance syndrome in 5- to 10-year-old overweight/obese African-American children. *Diabetes Care* 24:1359–1364, 2001

Tim Wysocki, PhD, is Principal Research Scientist and Director of the Center for Pediatric Psychology Research in the Department of Biomedical Research at Nemours Children's Clinic in Jacksonville, FL.

Barbara J. Anderson, PhD, is Professor of Pediatrics and Associate Head of the Psychology Section at Baylor College of Medicine in Houston, TX.

Chapter 15
Lifespan Development Issues for Adults

Paula M. Trief, PhD

Developmental theorists propose that there are four main domains of life that define the tasks of early adulthood and midlife. These include: work/employment goals and activities, marriage/partnered relationships, child-bearing/parenthood, and leisure time activities (Wrightsman 1994). Although social and cultural factors may have changed the time trajectories and work/family paths chosen (Mollenkopf 2005, Osgood 2005), evidence that work and personal relationships predict mood, quality of life, and mastery over health (Brim 2003) confirm that the choices made in these domains are critical to the course of adulthood. Diabetes can have an impact on each of these areas of life function, and problems in these domains can have a significant impact on diabetes. All domains but leisure time activities are addressed in this chapter.

TRANSITION TO ADULT CARE

Traditional grouping of developmental categories yields classifications of children, adolescents, adults, or older adults. However, there is recent evidence that another category, that of "young adult" (YA), might be an important one, especially when discussing diabetes patients. Arnett (2004) has argued that the ages between 18 and 25 years define the period of "emerging adulthood," especially for white, middle- or upper-class individuals, who use this time to explore their identities, goals, and choices in the domains of partnering, parenting, and work. Evidence that YAs with type 1 diabetes (T1D) are more likely to be lost to medical follow-up (Whittaker 2004), to be nonadherent to care and have poorer medical outcomes (Bryden 2001, Bryden 2003), to die (often from lack of insulin leading to DKA), and to commit suicide (Health Canada 2003, Roberts 2004) has led to increased attention to this age-group. In fact, recognition of this not infrequent lapse in care and poor medical outcomes has led to the American Diabetes Association developing a position paper regarding the transition from pediatric to young adult care (ADA 2011c).

All of the literature thus far pertains to YAs who have T1D. Although an increasing number of youth are developing type 2 diabetes (T2D), this is a relatively new phenomenon, and the data are just beginning to be gathered and disseminated (TODAY Study Group 2007). Thus, this chapter focuses on YAs with T1D.

Transition refers to the developmental task of moving from adolescence to adulthood. During this time, YAs must assume greater responsibility for their health care and autonomy in making their health care decisions. They are establishing their adult identities, with new goals, relationships, and demands for their overall lives as well as for the diabetes-related aspects of their lives.

Although evidence suggests that YAs with T1D are as psychosocially mature as their peers (Pacaud 2007), it is also accepted that the unique demands of T1D (e.g., intensive self-care, extensive involvement with the health care system) present YAs with challenges with which they may struggle to cope during these transition years (Weissberg-Benchell 2007). Studies have also identified a small but clinically significant subgroup of YA patients with a constellation of medical and psychological morbidities, including poor glycemic control, faster progression to microvascular complications, and mental health disorders (e.g., depression, disordered eating) (Rydall 1997, Bryden 1999, Bryden 2001, Bryden 2003, Peveler 2005), who are in need of continued multidisciplinary support to help them manage their disease and concurrent life transition.

Transition also refers to the transfer of care from the pediatric health care system and providers to the adult health care system and providers. In one study, up to 50% of YAs reported difficulties with this transition (Anderson 2004). When YAs were asked what they needed for a smoother transition, they emphasized continuity of contact with their providers and also providers who have an understanding of their life situations (Dovey-Pearce 2005). When clinicians were asked similar questions, they noted their need for developmentally specific patient education materials and training, especially since T1D is a chronic disease that begins in childhood (McDonagh 2004, McDonagh 2006). Two studies describe transition programs for YAs with T1D. These transition programs were found to be feasible and acceptable (Van Walleghem 2006), and one (uncontrolled) study reported that participation in the program resulted in better clinic attendance and glycemic control as well as lower hospital admission rates for DKA (Holmes-Walker 2007).

WORK/EMPLOYMENT GOALS AND ACTIVITIES

When one moves into adulthood, a key developmental task is to identify work that is meaningful, gratifying, and helpful in achieving one's life goals. Diabetes can have a significant impact on these choices and actions.

Effect of Diabetes on Work

Studies have shown that diabetes can have a significant impact on work-related issues for society and for the individual with diabetes. Large population-based studies have assessed the impact of diabetes (combining patients with T1D and T2D) on work-related domains. Diabetes predicts significant losses in worker productivity, including lost income due to early retirement, sick days and disability, and premature mortality (Mayfield 1999, Vijan 2004, Herquelot 2011). Employers pay more for workers who have diabetes through medical and pharmacy claims and lost productivity (Ramsey 2002), whereas workers experience impaired physical and mental health, work and earn less, and are more likely to be unemployed (Mayfield 1999, Valdmanis 2001, Bastida 2002, Holmes 2003).

Diabetes self-management also has a significant impact on work issues. Patients with T2D who use insulin report that having diabetes may affect their choice of work, including how work might affect their self-care regimen (Trief 1999). For example, the choice may be based on their need to maintain a regular schedule as opposed to changing shifts, on the amount of physical activity involved in the job, on the availability of insurance benefits, or on whether they can structure their time to test their blood glucose or eat frequent meals. Once they are employed, diabetes can affect relationships at work, as a diabetes patient might need greater coworker or supervisor support (Trief 1999, Duke 2004, Munir 2005).

Within the group of workers with diabetes, it has also been shown that those in poor glycemic control (and men with poor lipid control) are more likely to report absenteeism (Tunceli 2007) and those with diabetes-related complications are more likely to be unemployed (Von Korff 2005). In one randomized controlled trial (RCT) that targeted improved glycemic control for patients with T2D using active medication therapy (glipizide GITS), positive work and function outcomes were predicted by improved glycemic control. Improved A1C led to higher rates of retained employment, less absenteeism, and fewer restricted-activity and bed days (Testa 1998). Thus, it is clear that diabetes health plays a significant role in work-related outcomes that are relevant both to employers and employees.

A major fear of employers and coworkers is that a person with diabetes may experience hypoglycemia while at work and thus put him/herself or others at risk for injury, even though severe hypoglycemia in the workplace is uncommon and rarely causes serious problems (Leckie 2005). Hypoglycemia usually occurs in individuals who have T1D or those who have T2D and use insulin, but it is generally associated with warning signs, can be prevented and treated, and only rarely results in major impairment. The concern persists, despite evidence that severe hypoglycemic episodes (defined as those requiring help from another person) rarely occur in the workplace; overall incidence was 0.14 episodes per person per year in a sample of individuals with T1D (Leckie 2005).

This concern, and others relevant to the impact of diabetes at work, may result in employment discrimination. One study reported that people with diabetes were more likely than other workers with medical impairments to report discrimination in terms of job retention (i.e., discipline, suspension, or termination) (McMahon 2005).

To address this concern, the American Diabetes Association (ADA) adopted a formal position on employment in 1984, stating, "Any person with diabetes, whether insulin dependent or non–insulin-dependent, should be eligible for any employment for which he/she is otherwise qualified" (ADA 2011a). Under the provisions of the Americans with Disabilities Act, a person with diabetes may be entitled to a "reasonable accommodation" that would enable him/her to successfully manage the diabetes while working. Examples of such accommodations would be: being able to take frequent short breaks to eat, and access to a refrigerator to store medications. The complications associated with diabetes may also require accommodations (e.g., reading aids for the visually impaired) (www.eeoc. gov/facts/diabetes.html). The ADA has compiled a set of guidelines for evaluating individuals with diabetes for employment and what types of workplace accommodations may be needed for workers with diabetes (ADA 2011a). Although little is known about the frequency with which these accommodations are requested, and whether they are provided or denied, workers with diabetes were less likely than workers with other medical impairments to report discrimination during hiring or reasonable accommodation requests (McMahon 2005).

Effect of Work on Diabetes

Successful employment can affect health directly and indirectly. Individuals who are unemployed often have relatively low incomes. Having a low income increases the likelihood that a person will not receive important diabetes care, such as seeing an endocrinologist, or having a yearly A1C test or biannual eye exam (McCall 2004). Working at low-wage jobs often entails working in an environment (i.e., fast, repetitive, high physical demands) that does not promote good health and may partially explain the higher incidence of illness in low-wage workers (Kaplan 1994). Studies have suggested that "job strain" (high work demands and low job control) and "effort-reward imbalance" (low security, high job demands, limited career opportunities) contribute to cardiovascular disease (Guralnik 1993, Kivimaki 2002, De Bacquer 2005), and although this area has not received attention specific to diabetes patients, the strong link between diabetes and cardiovascular disease points to an area of potential importance.

Bringing Work and Diabetes Together—Worksite Interventions

Worksite nutrition and physical activity interventions have been proposed to help individuals improve their health and reduce long-term costs to employers (Katz 2005). The number of workplace-sponsored programs addressing obesity is growing, with the majority conducted by large, private employers (Heinen 2009). However, few outcomes from worksite programs have been published, and in the few that have, results were modest and short-term and often the methodologies were poor (Benedict 2008, Barham 2011). A recent meta-analysis of the effectiveness of worksite nutrition and physical activity interventions to promote weight loss report modest weight loss (~ 2.8 pounds) but noted that even modest weight loss can benefit overall health (Anderson 2009).

MARRIAGE/PARTNERING

Development of a healthy marriage/partnered relationship is a major task of adulthood. Studies have shown that medical patients who derive social and emotional support from others, especially family and spouses, demonstrate better immune, cardiovascular, and endocrine function, recover from illness and injury more quickly, report better psychological adaptation to their illness, engage in more healthy behaviors, and demonstrate better adherence to medical care regimens (Kulik 1989, Lyons 1995, Helgeson 1996, Kiecolt-Glaser 2001, DiMatteo 2004).

Conversely, relationships may have negative effects on health outcomes. Marital interaction (i.e., how the support is given and received) impacts both marital quality and health functioning. A major review of marital interaction studies concluded that negative marital interaction can lead to negative health habits and depression and thus indirectly influence health (Campbell 2002). For patients with T1D, higher criticality by a family member has been linked to poorer glycemic control (Klausner 1995).

Effect of Family Support/Marital Quality on Diabetes

For patients with diabetes, the impact of relationship variables may be particularly significant, as the diabetes care regimen (e.g., purchase and preparation of food, exercise, administration of medication, management of hypoglycemia) often involves the spouse (Trief 2003). For patients with both T1D and T2D, greater social support has been linked to better illness adaptation, regimen adherence, and glycemic control (Schafer 1986, Cardenas 1987, Eaton 1992, Trief 1998). More specifically, greater marital satisfaction has been shown to relate to lower risk of developing metabolic syndrome, a precursor to weight-related diabetes (Troxel 2005), and better marital quality (intimacy, adjustment) to relate to better quality of life and regimen adherence for patients with T2D (Trief 2001, Trief 2004).

These data have led some to make a strong argument for adoption of a family-systems perspective of diabetes management for adults (Fisher 1998, Fisher 2000), an approach that has long been encouraged for youth with T1D (McBroom 2009, Wysocki 2009). This approach includes family relationships and environment as targets of intervention, since family stress can affect patient physiology (Saarni 1990, Uchino 1996, Kiecolt-Glaser 2001) and family dynamics can affect self-care (Kulik 1993).

However, the few studies of family or marital interaction and health that have suggested models for intervention provide limited, and disappointing, data on the effect of couples-based interventions on health outcomes (Schmaling 2000). A meta-analysis of RCTs that assessed the benefit of interventions that included family members for adults with chronic illnesses found a positive effect on depression when the spouse was included, but no effect on anxiety, physical disability, or relationship satisfaction (Martire 2004). It also found that decreased mortality was an outcome of family interventions, but only when the intervention was not limited to spouses and did not address relationship issues. A more recent cross-disease meta-analysis of 25 randomized trials of interventions that targeted the couple, not the individual patient, found significant improvements in pain, depression, and marital functioning when partners were included, though the effect was small (Martire 2010). A meta-analysis of weight-loss interventions found a significant, but also small and short-lived benefit of including partners (Black 1990). However, smoking cessation interventions that included spouses did not yield better outcomes (Palmer 2000, McBride 2004).

There is some evidence that spouse involvement in diabetes education and obesity programs yields better outcomes. In a diabetes education program (non-randomized trial), elderly patients with T2D who participated with spouses learned more, reported less stress, and had greater improvement in glycemic control (Gilden 1989). In one randomized weight-loss trial, which included those with and without diabetes, obese women, but not men, lost more weight if they participated with their obese spouses than if they participated alone (Wing 1991). A systematic review of randomized trials of weight-control interventions with family involvement concluded that there is limited support for involvement of spouses, and that the key may be to carefully pick the family member and actively involve him/her in goal-setting and behavior change activities (McLean 2003).

Since many studies are plagued by design limitations, the question of whether, and how, to include family members or partners is still unanswered.

The model used in these studies is spouse participation. However, an extensive literature review concluded that this model is overly simplistic and argued that a "dyad level" model is more appropriate (Lewis 2006). This approach emphasizes the interdependence of partners, in that it is the interaction between them that affects both members of the dyad. The collaborative problem-solving approach that is suggested by this model is being tested in two ongoing randomized trials of patients with T2D. Preliminary data is promising (Trief 2011b), but results are not yet available (Keogh 2007, Trief 2011a).

Effect of Diabetes on the Marital Relationship

Spouses may experience a significant burden in coping with a partner's diabetes. This may include changes in responsibilities (e.g., food preparation, injection administration), roles, and affect of partner (especially if the partner with T2D develops complications or becomes functionally limited). The spouse is often the primary support for the patient yet may need support him/herself (Revenson 1994). Studies of partners of patients with other chronic illnesses show they often report high levels of anxiety and depression, stress-related symptoms, and poorer performance at work (Revenson 1991). These problems affect the partner's mental health as well as the ability of the pair to problem-solve about the disease (Lewis 1989, Brummett 1998). The meta-analysis of family intervention studies that were RCTs concluded that there were positive effects on the family member, especially when the intervention targeted only the family member and addressed relationship issues (Martire 2004).

Research on diabetes partner stress is limited, with evidence that partners of patients with T2D experience as much, or more, distress as the diabetic patient, even if the diabetic patient is not distressed (Fisher 2002). And, their distress relates to other life stressors (e.g., finances, family relationships), not only to diabetes (Fisher 2002). Partners struggle to be helpful and provide appropriate type and timing of support (Revenson 1991) without being intrusive or critical (Peyrot 1988, Bailey 1993, Trief 2003).

Does Gender Matter?

Sex and gender roles (i.e., who does what) also affect how effectively couples cope with diabetes. Women still tend to assume the greater responsibility for maintaining family function, disease management, and provision of emotional support, and they may experience more of a burden as a result (Coyne 1992, Fisher 1993, Fisher 2002). In one study of obese couples in which at least one partner had T2D, women had better outcomes when treated with their spouses, whereas men had better outcomes when treated alone (Gilden 1989). There is also evidence that husbands and wives cope with illness differently (Gottlieb 1991) and that it may be most beneficial if there is congruence between their coping styles (Revenson 1994). For example, women were more satisfied in their relationships than men when there was more "relationship talk" (talk about the state of the relationship), especially when there was an ill spouse in the pair (Badr 2005).

CHILDBEARING/PARENTHOOD

The decision to conceive and bear a child is a momentous one for all adults but can carry extra stresses and burdens when the woman has diabetes. With good self-management and prenatal care, women with diabetes can have safe pregnancies and healthy babies (ADA 2004a, ADA 2004b, ADA 2011b). However, there are added risks, both for the mother and the baby. Prepregnancy diabetes-related complications often worsen during pregnancy. Hyperglycemia increases risk of miscarriage and premature delivery and may cause congenital malformations (e.g., neural tube defects), immature lungs, and macrosomia (www.cdc.gov/NCBDDD/pregnancy_gateway/diabetes.html). Although the focus has been on women with T1D, it is now recognized that women with T2D are also at risk and will likely be placed on insulin during their pregnancy. Thus, the same regimen-based stresses may occur.

Patients have their own fears. In one study, YAs with T1D reported significant concerns about the impact of having diabetes on future parenthood and marriage (Lloyd 1993). Their fears included the fear of "passing it on" to their children, the fear that future complications would limit involvement with the child, and the significant fear that their diabetes may result in premature mortality, thus limiting the years they would have with their child (Lloyd 1993).

Women who develop gestational diabetes (GDM) also represent a population with specific medical and emotional concerns. From 3–5% of pregnancies of healthy women will involve GDM, with the added burden that up to half will develop T2D in the 5–10 years following childbirth. GDM often results in very large babies and thus preterm delivery and/or Caesarean section (c-section), both of which have their own risks to mother and baby. Other fetal conditions (e.g., poor feeding, hypoglycemia) are also more likely when the mother develops GDM. Treatment of GDM includes medical nutrition therapy and daily self-monitoring of blood glucose and insulin when needed. In two randomized trials, this intervention resulted in significantly less neonatal morbidity than routine pregnancy care (Crowther 2005, Landon 2009). The intensity of the treatment will vary based on measurements of the growth of the fetus, which should be made regularly. Less intensified management may be sufficient for normal-growth babies, but more-intensive treatment is indicated for those babies who are large for their fetal age. As stated, women with GDM are at significantly increased risk for the development of T2D. The diagnosis of GDM presents a unique opportunity to intervene to prevent it.

Pregnant women with diabetes (T1D, T2D, or GDM) are urged to maintain tight blood glucose control before and during pregnancy (ADA 2011b). However, this can be a daunting task. Consider the data of the patients with T1D in the Diabetes Control and Complications Trial (DCCT) who were in the intensively treated group. These participants received weekly supportive phone contact, monthly health care team contact, and free medical supplies, yet less than 5% were able to establish normal-range A1C readings (DCCT Research Group 1993). Efforts to control glycemia during GDM pregnancy require close monitoring of blood glucose levels, frequent contact with the health care team, multiple tests for mother and fetus, and insulin initiation and adjustments, with the added emotional and financial stresses associated with all of these steps.

Since obese women are at increased risk for GDM, a broader focus looks at the effect of obesity on pregnancy, whether the woman has diabetes or not. The Institute of Medicine (IOM) reviewed the literature relevant to gestational weight gain (GWG) and concluded that obese women are at increased risk of complications during pregnancy and labor, including death, and that their children are at higher risk of congenital defects than normal-weight women (Poston 2011). Although much of the evidence was not strong, as the studies are all observational, the IOM did revise its guidelines for healthy weight gain during pregnancy (Rasmussen 2008). There have been a few small RCTs of behavioral interventions to reduce GWG that report promising results (Kinnunen 2007, Claesson 2008) and one that found a beneficial effect of restricted weight gain on pregnancy-induced changes in glucose metabolism (Wolff 2008), suggesting that the intervention might also benefit women who have diabetes. Lifestyle modification programs to help women manage their pregnancy weight gain and increase their activity should be helpful.

Given the behavioral changes required to manage weight gain and diabetes during pregnancy (i.e., carbohydrate counting, food restrictions, increasing physical activity, administering insulin), the psychosocial factors that may negatively affect the woman's ability to adhere to the self-care regimen should be assessed and addressed. These may include depression, stress, anxiety, and/or eating disorders, all of which have been shown to relate to poor adherence (Polonsky 1994, Lin 2004, Gonzalez 2008, Katon 2009, Jaser 2010) and may similarly interfere with the pregnant woman's adherence.

New technologies can improve outcomes. Both multiple daily injections (MDI) and insulin pumps (continuous subcutaneous insulin infusion, or CSII) lead to excellent glycemic control in pregnant women with T1D (Cyganek 2010). Significantly, women who planned their pregnancy had better control than those who did not, independent of the type of therapy used.

It is generally accepted that preconception counseling (PC) and pregnancy planning should be the standard of care for women with T1D, as they are critical to decrease the risks associated with their pregnancy (Charron-Prochownik 2008, Kitzmiller 2008). Women who receive PC report lower A1C and fewer negative maternal and fetal outcomes (Kitzmiller 1996, Galindo 2006, Temple 2006, Charron-Prochownik 2008). Yet, in one survey of health educators, only 68% strongly agreed that it is important to provide PC, most had received no training in PC, and 30–40% did not provide PC to their adult or adolescent patients (Michel 2006).

Despite the accepted value of PC and pregnancy planning, there is very little research on how diabetes affects the decision to become pregnant or on quality of life during pregnancy. Also, there is no literature on how diabetes affects parenthood or the psychosocial outcomes following the birth of the child, despite the fact that parenthood is a key developmental task of adulthood. Research about diabetes and parenthood must be addressed.

LIFE COURSE EVALUATION

There are two additional issues that must be clarified to understand the context of this review and recommendations. First, the theories and research reported are derived from patients, mostly Caucasian, living in developed Western countries. The conclusions and recommendations may not be applicable to patients from other racial or ethnic groups (Mollenkopf 2005) or individuals living in developing countries (Eyetsemitan 2003).

Second, the term "adulthood" encompasses a wide span of years and phases of life that should be considered when choosing treatments, goals, and interventions. We have cited the literature that proposes that early adulthood be considered as a distinct "young adult" stage, when individuals are typically transitioning into the responsibilities and demands of adulthood. Similarly, developmental theorists define other life stages, often by examining the gains and losses across the life span. Young adulthood is considered to be a period of many gains and few losses, whereas midlife may involve a balance, and later life may include many losses and few gains (Baltes 1987). The years of middle adulthood (ages 35–50 years) are typically defined by the developmental tasks of building one's work and personal life, to establish stability in one's career and partnerships that form the foundation of one's future. Some have further argued that later life should be defined as three distinct stages as well. They describe those in late middle-age (50–64 years), the young-old (65–74 years), and the old-old (≥75 years). Each stage has normal developmental challenges. Late middle-age is often defined by financial stability and can be a time of "peak performance," when individuals feel confident and in control (Lackman 2001). Individuals are often beginning to change roles, moving from biological tasks (e.g., bearing and parenting children) and social demands (e.g., finding a job, finding a partner) to fewer expectations and demands (Baltrusch 1988). Young-old individuals are focused on finding new goals for this next phase of life, and they begin to brush up against their own mortality. Retirement often occurs in this stage and may lead to freedom and self-expression and/or confusion and loneliness (Newman 1999). Finally, the old-old face unique challenges associated with physical and cognitive decline, decreased social contact, and greater dependence (Baltrusch 1988, Baltes 2003).

Recognizing that these are broad generalizations, recent data show that these trajectories are changing and must include the different stresses of modern life (e.g., eldercare when one is young-old) and less typical developmental paths (e.g., parents without careers, working singles) (Osgood 2005). However, this developmental perspective emphasizes the importance of understanding the challenges and stresses for each individual, as well as his/her sources of gratification and support (Harden 2005).

RECOMMENDATIONS FOR CLINICAL CARE

The health care provider should assess the physical, social, and emotional milestones that the patient is facing, guided by those that are typical for his/her life stage. By understanding the context of the diabetes for that unique individual, the provider will be in a better position to develop and implement the most appropriate intervention, one that will encourage growth and successful adaptation to diabetes. Further, life stage of the individual is not an indicator of or contraindication to implementation of self-care regimens or ability to optimize disease outcomes. Rather, the provider, in collaboration with the patient, works to optimize the regimen, taking into account life stage, limitations associated with physical condition, resources, and expectations for disease management and outcomes.

Transition to Adult Care

1. Assessment of YA patients with T1D should include evaluation of mental health and substance-use problems that will likely interfere with self-care adherence and medical contact (Weissberg-Benchell 2007).
2. The unique challenges of the YA phase of life should be monitored by the health care provider, so that he/she can pay attention to all factors in the life circumstances of the YA that could complicate his/her ability to engage with the health care team and practice good self-care (Weissberg-Benchell 2007).
3. New models of transition care should be developed and assessed for their efficacy. These may include: a "navigator" to assist the YAs in appointments, insurance, and access to other needed services (Van Walleghem 2006, Holmes-Walker 2007).

Work/Employment Goals and Activities

1. Interventions to help patients achieve better glycemic control should be instituted in the workplace and assessed for their efficacy. Helping workers improve their glycemic control and lose weight can potentially reduce the negative effects of diabetes on worker absenteeism, productivity, and disability (Testa 1998, Anderson 2009).
2. Risk of hypoglycemia should be assessed and actively addressed for individual patients and specific work environments. It is important to dispel the common misperception that all diabetes patients are at risk for hypoglycemia and that hypoglycemia, if it does occur, cannot be successfully managed. These views can lead to job discrimination. A risk assessment can also enhance worker safety. The patient's physician can provide guidance to employers by describing the patient's risk, how it might affect the individual in a specific work environment, and what reasonable accommodations would decrease the risk. The ADA (2011a) position paper provides a series of recommendations that should be adhered to: four recommendations concerning comprehensive individual assessment and the importance of health care professionals with up-to-date diabetes expertise performing the assessment, four recommendations concerning appropriate and inappropriate safety assessments, and one recommendation concerning reasonable accommodations.
3. Employers should be encouraged to provide emotional and instrumental support to their employees with diabetes. Support of bosses and coworkers can lead to greater disclosure by the diabetes patient and is likely to result in better diabetes self-management in the workplace (Trief 1999, Duke 2004, Munir 2005).
4. Diabetes patients who are struggling to manage their diabetes while at work should be encouraged to consider a request for a reasonable accommodation. Changes to schedules, work tasks, and/or environments can result in a worker being more successful at work and at self-care. Employers must be guided by the Americans with Disabilities Act. Employees who are unable to secure a reasonable accommodation should be referred to the

Equal Employment Opportunity Commission (EEOC) for guidance and legal support (ADA 2011a).

Marriage/Partnering

1. Health care providers should selectively involve appropriate family members in diabetes education and other interventions to improve diabetes outcomes. The partner may be the most appropriate person to include, but other family members may be more supportive and thus better able to serve this role. Providers should identify and support this person (or people), as he/she supports the DM patient. However, providers should also recognize that participation alone may not affect outcomes. Rather, active involvement in goal-setting and behavior change, and efforts to work collaboratively, may be needed. These interventions may also have beneficial effects on the partner (Fisher 2002, McLean 2003, Martire 2004, Lewis 2006, Martire 2010, Trief 2011b).
2. When working with patients and partners, health care providers should pay attention to the relationship. They should identify patients in conflictual relationships for specific attention, especially when the partner is highly critical and marital quality is poor. Couples may require referrals to couples counseling to work on changing their negative interaction patterns (McLean 2003, Trief 2006).
3. Diabetes is a stressful disease for partners, too, and positive support is important to their physical and mental health. Health care providers should refer partners to appropriate support groups to help them address the emotional challenges that they are experiencing as the couple copes with diabetes (Fisher 2002).

Childbearing/parenthood

1. Health care providers should evaluate the mental health status of the pregnant woman with diabetes throughout her pregnancy. This should include assessment of potential depression, anxiety, and other mental health problems that might interfere with her ability to adhere to the complex care regimen required during pregnancy when one has diabetes. When concerns are identified, the provider should provide needed support and make appropriate mental health referrals. These recommendations are based on research regarding people with diabetes rather than pregnant diabetic women specifically (Polonsky 1994, Lin 2004, Gonzalez 2008, Katon 2009, Jaser 2010), but expert opinion suggests that these recommendations should be applied to pregnant women who have diabetes.
2. Health care providers should emphasize and provide pregnancy planning and preconception counseling for all women of childbearing age who have diabetes (Charron-Prochownik 2008, Kitzmiller 2008, ADA 2011b).
3. Obese women, and women who develop GDM, should be counseled to manage their weight gain during pregnancy in an effort to forestall negative outcomes associated with both obesity and GDM, as well as to increase the likelihood that they will not develop T2D later in life (Claesson 2008, Wolff 2008, Rasmussen 2009, Poston 2011).

BIBLIOGRAPHY

American Diabetes Association: Diabetes and employment. *Diabetes Care* 34 (Suppl. 1):S82–S86, 2011a

American Diabetes Association: Standards of Medical Care in Diabetes-2011. *Diabetes Care* 34 (Suppl. 1), S11–S61, 2011b

American Diabetes Association: Recommendations for transition from pediatric to adult diabetes care systems. *Diabetes Care* 34:2477–2485, 2011c

American Diabetes Association: Gestational diabetes mellitus. *Diabetes Care* 27 (Suppl. 1):S88–S90, 2004a

American Diabetes Association: Preconception care of women with diabetes. *Diabetes Care* 27 (Suppl. 1):S76–S78, 2004b

Anderson BJ, Wolpert HA: A developmental perspective on the challenges of diabetes education and care during the young adult period. *Patient Education and Counseling* 53:347–352, 2004

Anderson LM, Quinn TA, Glanz K, Ramirez G, Kahwati LC, Johnson DB, et al.: The effectiveness of worksite nutrition and physical activity interventions for controlling employee overweight and obesity: a systematic review. *American Journal of Preventive Medicine* 37:340–357, 2009

Arnett JJ: *Emerging Adulthood: The Winding Road from the Late Teens through the Twenties.* New York, Oxford University Press, 2004

Badr H, Acitelli LK: Dyadic adjustment in chronic illness: does relationship talk matter? *Journal of Family Psychology* 19:465–469, 2005

Bailey BJ, Kahn A: Apportioning illness management authority: how diabetic individuals evaluate and respond to spousal help. *Qualitative Health Research* 3:55–73, 1993

Baltes PB, Smith J: New frontiers in the future of aging: from successful aging of the young old to the dilemmas of the fourth age. *Gerontology* 49:123–135, 2003

Baltes PB: Theoretical propositions of life-span developmental psychology: on dynamics between growth and decline. *Developmental Psychology* 23:611–626, 1987

Baltrusch HJ, Seidel J, Stangel W, Waltz ME: Psychosocial stress, aging and cancer. *Annals of the New York Academy of Sciences* 521:1–15, 1988

Barham K, West S, Trief P, Morrow C, Wade M, Weinstock RS: Diabetes prevention and control in the workplace: a pilot project for county employees. *J Public Health Management Practice* 17:233–241, 2011

Bastida E, Pagan JA: The impact of diabetes on adult employment and earnings of Mexican Americans: findings from a community based study. *Health Economics* 11:403–413, 2002

Benedict MA, Arterburn D: Worksite-based weight loss programs: a systematic review of recent literature. *American Journal of Health Promotion* 22:408–416, 2008

Black DR, Gleser LJ, Kooyers KJ: A meta-analytic evaluation of couples weight-loss programs. *Health Psychology* 9:330–347, 1990

Brim OG, Ryff CD, Kessler RC, Eds.: *How Healthy Are We? A National Study of Well-Being at Midlife*. Chicago, University of Chicago Press, 2003

Brummett BH, Babyak MA, Barefoot JC, Bosworth HB, Clapp-Channing NE, Siegler IC, et al.: Social support and hostility as predictors of depressive symptoms in cardiac patients one month after hospitalization: a prospective study. *Psychosom Med* 60:707–713, 1998

Bryden KS, Dunger DB, Mayou RA, Peveler RC, Neil HA: Poor prognosis of young adults with type 1 diabetes: a longitudinal study. *Diabetes Care* 26:1052–1057, 2003

Bryden KS, Peveler RC, Stein A, Neil A, Mayou RA, Dunger DB: Clinical and psychological course of diabetes from adolescence to young adulthood: a longitudinal cohort study. *Diabetes Care* 24:1536–1540, 2001

Bryden KS, Neil A, Mayou RA, Peveler RC, Fairburn CG, Dunger DB: Eating habits, body weight, and insulin misuse. A longitudinal study of teenagers and young adults with type 1 diabetes. *Diabetes Care* 22:1956–1960, 1999

Campbell TA: Physical disorder and effectiveness research in marriage and family therapy. In *Effectiveness Research in Marriage and Family Therapy*. Sprenkle D, Ed. Alexandria, VA, American Association for Marriage and Family Therapy, 2002, p. 311–337

Cardenas L, Vallbona C, Baker S, Yusim S: Adult onset DM: glycemic control and family function. *American Journal of the Medical Sciences* 293:28–33, 1987

Centers for Disease Control and Prevention: Pregnancy: diabetes and pregnancy. Available at www.cdc.gov/NCBDDD/pregnancy_gateway/diabetes.html. Accessed 26 July 2010

Charron-Prochownik D, Hannan MF, Fischl AR, Slocum JM: Preconception planning: are we making progress? *Current Diabetes Reports* 8:294–298, 2008

Claesson IM, Sydsjo G, Brynhildsen J, Cedergren M, Jeppsson A, Nystrom F, Sydsjo A, Joseffsson A: Weight gain restriction for obese pregnant women: a case-control intervention study. *BJOG* 115:44–50, 2008

Coyne JC, Fiske V: Couples coping with chronic and catastrophic illness. In *Family Health Psychology*. Nakamatsu TJ, Stephs MAP, Hobfoll SS, Crowther J, Eds. Washington, DC, Hemisphere, 1992, p. 129-149

Crowther CA, Hiller JE, Moss JR, McPhee AJ, Jeffries WS, Robinson JS, et al.: Effect of treatment of gestational diabetes mellitus on pregnancy outcomes. *N Engl J Med* 352:2477–2486, 2005

Cyganek K, Hebda-Szydlo A, Katra B, Skupien J, Klupa T, Janas I, et al.: Glycemic control and selected pregnancy outcomes in type 1 diabetes women on continuous subcutaneous insulin infusion and multiple daily injections: the significance of pregnancy planning. *Diabetes Technology & Therapeutics* 12:41–47, 2010

De Bacquer D, Pelfrene E, Clays E, Mak R, Moreau M, de Smet P, et al.: Perceived job stress and incidence of coronary events: 3-year follow-up of the Belgian Job Stress Project cohort. *American Journal of Epidemiology* 161:434–441, 2005

Diabetes Control and Complications Research Group: The effect of intensive treatment of diabetes on the development and progression of long-term complications in insulin-dependent diabetes mellitus. *N Engl J Med* 329:977–986, 1993

DiMatteo MR: Social support and patient adherence to medical treatment: a meta-analysis. *Health Psychology* 23:207–218, 2004

Dovey-Pearce G, Hurrell R, May C, Walker C, Doherty Y: Young adults' (16-25 years) suggestions for providing developmentally appropriate diabetes services: a qualitative study. *Health & Social Care in the Community* 13:409–419, 2005

Duke DJ: Diabetes in the workplace. *Diabetes Self-Management* 21:62, 64–66, 2004

Eaton WW, Mengel M, Mengel L, Larson D, Campbell R, Montague RB: Psychosocial and psychopathologic influences on management and control of insulin-dependent diabetes. *International Journal of Psychiatry in Medicine* 22:105–117, 1992

Equal Employment Opportunity Commission: Questions and answers about diabetes in the workplace and the Americans with Disabilities Act. Available at www.eeoc.gov/facts/diabetes.html. Accessed 16 July 2010

Eyetsemitan FE, Gire JT: *Aging and Adult Development in the Developing World.* Westport, CT, Praeger, 2003

Fisher L, Chesla CA, Skaff MA, Mullan J, Kanter R: Depression and anxiety among partners of European-American and Latino patients with type 2 diabetes. *Diabetes Care* 25:1564–1570, 2002

Fisher L, Wiehs KL: Can addressing family relationships improve outcomes in chronic disease? Report of the National Working Group on Family-Based Interventions in Chronic Disease. *Journal of Family Practice* 49:561–566, 2000

Fisher L, Chesla CA, Bartz RJ, Gilliss C, Skaff MA, Sabogal F, et al.: The family and type 2 diabetes: a framework for intervention. *Diabetes Educ* 24:599–607, 1998

Fisher L, Ransom DC, Terry HE: The California Family Health Project: VII. Summary and integration of findings. *Family Process* 32:69–86, 1993

Galindo A, Burguillo AG, Azriel S, Fuente Pde L: Outcome of fetuses in women with pregestational diabetes mellitus. *Journal of Perinatal Medicine* 34:323–331, 2006

Gilden JL, Hendryx M, Casia C, Singh SP: The effectiveness of diabetes education programs for older patients and their spouses. *Journal of the American Geriatric Society* 37:1023–1030, 1989

Gonzalez JS, Safren SA, Delahanty LM, Cagliero E, Wexler DJ, Meigs JB, et al.: Symptoms of depression prospectively predict poorer self-care in patients with type 2 diabetes. *Diabet Med* 25:1102–1107, 2008

Gottlieb BH, Wager F: Stress and support processes in close relationships. In *The Social Context of Coping.* Eckenrode J, Ed. New York, Plenum, 1991, p. 165–188

Guralnik JM, Land KC, Blazer D, Fillenbaum GG, Branch LG: Educational status and active life expectancy among older blacks and whites. *N Engl J Med* 329:110–116, 1993

Harden J: Developmental life stage and couples' experiences with prostate cancer: a review of the literature. *Cancer Nursing* 28:85–98, 2005

Health Canada: *Responding to the Challenge of Diabetes in Canada: First Report of the National Diabetes Surveillance System* (Pub H39-4/21-2003E ed.). Ottawa, ON, Ministry of Health, 2003

Heinen L, Darling H: Addressing obesity in the workplace: the role of employers. *Milbank Quarterly* 87:101–122, 2009

Helgeson VS, Cohen S: Social support and adjustment to cancer: reconciling descriptive, correlational, and intervention research. *Health Psychology* 15:135–148, 1996

Herquelot E, Gueguen A, Bonenfant S, Dray-Spira R: Impact of diabetes on work cessation: data from the GAZEL cohort study. *Diabetes Care* 34:1344–1349, 2011

Holmes J, Gear E, Bottomley J, Gillam S, Murphy M, Williams R: Do people with type 2 diabetes and their careers lose income? (T2ARDIS-4). *Health Policy* 64:291–296, 2003

Holmes-Walker DJ, Llewellyn AC, Farrell K: A transition care programme which improves diabetes control and reduces hospital admission rates in young adults with type 1 diabetes aged 15-25 years. *Diabet Med* 24:764–769, 2007

Jaser SS: Psychological problems in adolescents with diabetes. *Adolescent Medicine: State of the Art Reviews* 21:138–151, x–xi, 2010

Kaplan G: *Reflections on Present and Future Research on Bio-behavioral Risk Factors: New Research Frontiers in Behavioral Medicine, Proceedings of the National Conference.* Washington, DC, NIH, US Government Printing Office, 1994, p. 119–134

Katon W, Russo J, Lin EH, Heckbert SR, Karter AJ, Williams LH, et al.: Diabetes and poor disease control: is comorbid depression associated with poor medication adherence or lack of treatment intensification? *Psychosom Med* 71:965–972, 2009

Katz DL, O'Connell M, Yeh MC, Nawaz H, Njike V, Anderson LM, et al.: Public health strategies for preventing and controlling overweight and obesity in school and worksite settings: a report on recommendations of the Task Force on Community Preventive Services. *MMWR* 54:1–12, 2005

Keogh KM, White P, Smith SM, McGilloway S, O'Dowd T, Gibney J: Changing illness perceptions in patients with poorly controlled type 2 diabetes: a randomized controlled trial of a family-based intervention: protocol and pilot study. *BMC Family Practice* 8:36, 2007

Kiecolt-Glaser JK, Newton TL: Marriage and health: his and hers. *Psychological Bulletin* 127:472–503, 2001

Kinnunen TI, Pasanen M, Aittasalo M, Fogelholm M, Weiderpass E, Luoto R: Reducing postpartum weight retention—a pilot trial in primary health care. *Nutrition Journal* 6:21, 2007

Kitzmiller JL, Block JM, Brown FM, Catalano PM, Conway DL, Coustan DR, et al.: Managing preexisting diabetes for pregnancy: summary of evidence and consensus recommendations for care. *Diabetes Care* 31:1060–1079, 2008

Kitzmiller JL, Buchanan TA, Kjos S, Combs CA, Ratner RE: Pre-conception care of diabetes, congenital malformations, and spontaneous abortions. *Diabetes Care* 19:514–541, 1996

Kivimaki M, Leino-Arjas P, Luukkonen R, Riihimaki H, Vahtera J, Kirjonen J: Work stress and risk of cardiovascular mortality: prospective cohort study of industrial employees. *BMJ* 325:857, 2002

Klausner EJ, Koenigsberg HW, Skolnick N, Chung H, Rosnick P, Pelino D, et al.: Perceived familial criticism and glucose control in IDDM. *International Journal of Mental Health* 24:64–75, 1995

Kulik JA, Mahler A, Heika I: Emotional support as a moderator of adjustment and compliance after coronary artery bypass surgery: a longitudinal study. *Journal of Behavioral Medicine* 16:45–63, 1993

Kulik JA, Mahler HI: Social support and recovery from surgery. *Health Psychology* 8:221–238, 1989

Lackman ME: *Psychology of Adult Development.* Miamisburg, OH, Science Direct, 2001

Landon MB, Spong CY, Thom E, Carpenter MW, Ramin SM, Casey B, Wapner RJ, Varner MW, Rouse DJ, Thorp JM Jr, Sciscione A, Catalano P, Harper M, Saade G, Lain KY, Sorokin Y, Peaceman AM, Tolosa JE, Anderson GB: A multicenter, randomized trial of treatment for mild gestational diabetes. *N Engl J Med* 361:1339–1348, 2009

Leckie AM, Graham MK, Grant JB, Ritchie PJ, Frier BM: Frequency, severity, and morbidity of hypoglycemia occurring in the workplace in people with insulin-treated diabetes. *Diabetes Care* 28:1333–1338, 2005

Lewis FM, Woods NF, Hough EE, Bensley LS: The family's functioning with chronic illness in the mother: the spouse's perspective. *Social Science & Medicine* 29:1261–1269, 1989

Lewis MA, McBride CM, Pollak KI, Puleo E, Butterfield RM, Emmons KM: Understanding health behavior change among couples: an interdependence and communal coping approach. *Social Science & Medicine* 62:1369–1380, 2006

Lin EH, Katon W, Von Korff M, Rutter C, Simon GE, Oliver M, et al.: Relationship of depression and diabetes self-care, medication adherence, and preventive care. *Diabetes Care* 27:2154–2160, 2004

Lloyd CE, Robinson N, Andrews B, Elston MA, Fuller JH: Are the social relationships of young insulin-dependent diabetic patients affected by their condition? *Diabet Med* 10:481–485, 1993

Lyons RF, Sullivan MJL, Rivo PG: *Relationships in Chronic Illness and Disability.* Thousand Oaks, CA, Sage Publications, 1995

Martire LM, Schulz R, Helgeson VS, Small BJ, Saghafi EM: Review and meta-analysis of couple-oriented interventions for chronic illness. *Annals of Behavioral Medicine* 40:325–342, 2010

Martire LM, Lustig AP, Schulz R, Miller GE, Helgeson VS: Is it beneficial to involve a family member? A meta-analysis of psychosocial interventions for chronic illness. *Health Psychology* 23:599–611, 2004

Mayfield JA, Deb P, Whitecotton L: Work disability and diabetes. *Diabetes Care* 22:1105–1109, 1999

McBride CM, Baucom DH, Peterson BL, Pollak KI, Palmer C, Westman E, et al.: Prenatal and postpartum smoking abstinence a partner-assisted approach. *Am J Prev Med* 27:232–238, 2004

McBroom LA, Enriquez M: Review of family-centered interventions to enhance the health outcomes of children with type 1 diabetes. *Diabetes Educ* 35:428–438, 2009

McCall DT, Sauaia A, Hamman RF, Reusch JE, Barton P: Are low-income elderly patients at risk for poor diabetes care? *Diabetes Care* 27:1060–1065, 2004

McDonagh JE, Minnaar G, Kelly K, O'Connor D, Shaw KL: Unmet education and training needs in adolescent health of health professionals in a UK children's hospital. *Acta Paediatrica* 95:715–719, 2006

McDonagh JE, Southwood TR, Shaw KL, British Paediatric Rheumatology Group: Unmet education and training needs of rheumatology health professionals in adolescent health and transitional care. *Rheumatology* 43:737–743, 2004

McLean N, Griffin S, Toney K, Hardeman W: Family involvement in weight control, weight maintenance and weight-loss interventions: a systematic review of randomised trials. *International Journal of Obesity and Related Metabolic Disorders* 27:987–1005, 2003

McMahon BT, West SL, Mansouri M, Belongia L: Workplace discrimination and diabetes: the EEOC Americans with Disabilities Act research project. *Work* 25:9–18, 2005

Michel B, Charron-Prochownik D: Diabetes nurse educators and preconception counseling. *Diabetes Educ* 32:108–116, 2006

Mollenkopf J, Waters MC, Holdaway J, Kasinitz P: The ever-winding path: ethnic and racial diversity in the transition to adulthood. In *On the Frontier of Adulthood: Theory, Research, and Public Policy.* Settersten RA Jr, Furstenberg FF Jr, Rumbaut RG, Eds. Chicago, University of Chicago Press, 2005, p. 454–497

Munir F, Leka S, Griffiths A: Dealing with self-management of chronic illness at work: predictors for self-disclosure. *Social Science & Medicine* 60:1397–1407, 2005

Newman B, Newman P: *Development Through Life: A Psychosocial Approach.* Belmont, CA, Wadsworth Publishing, 1999

Osgood DW, Ruth G, Eccles JS, Jacobs JE, Barber BL: Six paths to adulthood: fast starters, parents without careers, educated partners, educated singles, working singles, and slow starters. In *On the Frontier of Adulthood: Theory, Research and Public Policy.* Settersten RA Jr, Furstenberg FF Jr, Rumbaut RG, Eds. Chicago, University of Chicago Press, 2005, p. 320–355

Pacaud D, Crawford S, Stephure DK, Dean HJ, Couch R, Dewey D: Effect of type 1 diabetes on psychosocial maturation in young adults. *Journal of Adolescent Health* 40:29–35, 2007

Palmer CA, Baucom DH, McBride CM: Couple approaches to smoking cessation. In *The Psychology of Couples and Illness.* Schmaling T, Sher TG, Eds. Washington, DC, American Psychological Association, 2000, p. 311–336

Peveler RC, Bryden KS, Neil HA, Fairburn CG, Mayou RA, Dunger DB, et al.: The relationship of disordered eating habits and attitudes to clinical outcomes in young adult females with type 1 diabetes. *Diabetes Care* 28:84–88, 2005

Peyrot M, McMurry JF, Hedges R: Marital adjustment to adult diabetes: interpersonal congruence and spouse satisfaction. *Journal of Marriage & the Family* 50:363–376, 1988

Polonsky WH, Anderson BJ, Lohrer PA, Aponte JE, Jacobson AM, Cole CF: Insulin omission in women with IDDM. *Diabetes Care* 17:1178–1185, 1994

Poston L, Harthoorn LF, Van Der Beek EM: Obesity in pregnancy: implications for the mother and lifelong health of the child. A consensus statement. *Pediatric Research* 69:175–180, 2011

Ramsey S, Summers KH, Leong SA, Birnbaum HG, Kemner JE, Greenberg P: Productivity and medical costs of diabetes in a large employer population. *Diabetes Care* 25:23–29, 2002

Rasmussen K, Yaktine A: *Weight Gain During Pregnancy: Reexamining the Guidelines.* Washington, DC, National Academies Press, 2008

Revenson RA: Social support and marital coping with chronic illness. *Annals of Behavioral Medicine* 16:122–130, 1994

Revenson TA, Majerovitz SD: The effects of chronic illness on the spouse. Social resources as stress buffers. *Arthritis Care Res* 4:63–72, 1991

Roberts SE, Goldacre MJ, Neil HA: Mortality in young people admitted to hospital for diabetes: database study. *BMJ* 328:741–742, 2004

Rydall AC, Rodin GM, Olmsted MP, Devenyi RG, Daneman D: Disordered eating behavior and microvascular complications in young women with insulin-dependent diabetes mellitus. *N Engl J Med* 336:1849–1854, 1997

Saarni C, Crowley M: The development of emotion regulation: effects on emotional state and expression. In *Emotions and the Family: For Better or For Worse.* Blechman E, Ed. Hillsdale, NJ, Lawrence Erlbaum Associates, 1990, p. 53–74

Schafer LC, McKaul KD, Glasgow RE: Supportive and non-supportive family behaviors: relationship to adherence and metabolic control in persons with type 1 diabetes. *Diabetes Care* 9:179–185, 1986

Schmaling KB, Sher TB: *The Psychology of Couples and Illness: Theory, Research, and Practice.* Washington, DC, American Psychological Association, 2000

Temple RC, Aldridge VJ, Murphy HR:. Prepregnancy care and pregnancy outcomes in women with type 1 diabetes. *Diabetes Care* 29:1744–1749, 2006

Testa MA, Simonson DC: Health economic benefits and quality of life during improved glycemic control in patients with type 2 diabetes mellitus: a randomized, controlled, double-blind trial. *JAMA* 280:1490–1496, 1998

TODAY Study Group, Zeitler P, Epstein L, Grey M, Hirst K, Kaufman F, Tamborlane W, Wilfley D: Treatment options for type 2 diabetes in adolescents and youth: a study of the comparative efficacy of metformin alone or in combination with rosiglitazone or lifestyle intervention in adolescents with type 2 diabetes. *Pediatric Diabetes* 8:74–87, 2007

Trief PM, Sandberg JG, Fisher L, Dimmock JA, Scales K, Hessler D, Weinstock RS: Challenges and lessons learned in the development and implementation of a couples-focused telephone intervention for adults with type 2 diabetes: the Diabetes Support Project. *Translational Behavioral Medicine* 2011a, doi: 10.1007/s13142-011-0057-8.

Trief PM, Sandberg JG, Ploutz-Snyder R, Brittain R, Cibula D, Scales K, Weinstock RS: Promoting couples collaboration in type 2 diabetes: the diabetes support project pilot data. *Families, Systems & Health* 29:253–261, 2011b, doi: 10.1037/a0024564.

Trief PM, Morin PC, Izquierdo R, Teresi J, Starren J, Shea S, et al.: Marital quality and diabetes outcomes: the IDEATel project. *Families, Systems & Health* 24:318–331, 2006

Trief PM, Wade MJ, Brittain KD, Weinstock RS: A prospective analysis of marital relationship factors and quality of life in diabetes. *Diabetes Care* 25:1154–1158, 2005

Trief PM, Ploutz-Snyder R, Brittain KD, Weinstock RS: The relationship between marital quality and adherence to the diabetes care regimen. *Annals of Behavioral Medicine* 27:148–154, 2004

Trief PM, Sandberg J, Greenberg RP, Graff K, Castranova N, Yoon M, et al.: Describing support: a qualitative study of couples living with diabetes. *Families, Systems & Health* 21:57–67, 2003

Trief PM, Himes CL, Orendorff R, Weinstock RS: The marital relationship and psychosocial adaptation and glycemic control of individuals with diabetes. *Diabetes Care* 24:1384–1389, 2001

Trief PM, Aquilino C, Paradies K, Weinstock RS: Impact of the work environment on glycemic control and adaptation to diabetes. *Diabetes Care* 22:569–574, 1999

Trief PM, Grant W, Elbert K, Weinstock RS: Family environment, glycemic control and the psychosocial adaptation of adults with diabetes. *Diabetes Care* 21:241–245, 1998

Troxel WM, Matthews KA, Gallo LC, Kuller LH: Marital quality and occurrence of the metabolic syndrome in women. *Archives of Internal Medicine* 165:1022–1027, 2005

Tunceli K, Bradley CJ, Lafata JE, Pladevall M, Divine GW, Goodman AC, et al.: Glycemic control and absenteeism among individuals with diabetes. *Diabetes Care* 30:1283–1285, 2007

Uchino BN, Cacioppo JT, Kiecolt-Glaser JK: The relationship between social support and psychological processes: a review with emphasis on underlying mechanisms and implications for health. *Psychological Bulletin* 119:488–531, 1996

Valdmanis V, Smith DW, Page MR: Productivity and economic burden associated with diabetes. *American Journal of Public Health* 91:129–130, 2001

Van Walleghem N, MacDonald CA, Dean HJ: Building connections for young adults with type 1 diabetes mellitus in Manitoba: feasibility and acceptability of a transition initiative. *Chronic Diseases in Canada* 27:130–134, 2006

Vijan S, Hayward RA, Langa KM: The impact of diabetes on workforce participation: results from a national household sample. *Health Services Research* 39 (6 Pt 1):1653–1669, 2004

Von Korff M, Katon W, Lin EH, Simon G, Ciechanowski P, Ludman E, et al.: Work disability among individuals with diabetes. *Diabetes Care* 28:1326–1332, 2005

Weissberg-Benchell J, Wolpert H, Anderson BJ: Transitioning from pediatric to adult care: a new approach to the post-adolescent young persons with type 1 diabetes. *Diabetes Care* 30:2441–2446, 2007

Whittaker C: Transfer of young adults with type 1 diabetes from pediatric to adult diabetes care. *Diabetes Quarterly* (Spring):10–14, 2004

Wing RR, Marcus MD, Epstein LH, Jawad A: A family based approach to the treatment of obese type II diabetic patients. *Journal of Consulting & Clinical Psychology* 59:156–162, 1991

Wolff S, Legarth J, Vansgaard K, Toubro S, Astrup A: A randomized trial of the effects of dietary counseling on gestational weight gain and glucose metabolism in obese pregnant women. *International Journal of Obesity* 32:495–501, 2008

Wrightsman LS: *Adult Personality Development: Theories and Concepts.* Thousand Oaks, CA, Sage Publications, 1994

Wysocki T, Nansel TR, Holmbeck GN, Chen R, Laffel L, Anderson BJ, et al.: Collaborative involvement of primary and secondary caregivers: associations with youths' diabetes outcomes. *Journal of Pediatric Psychology* 34:869–881, 2009

Paula M. Trief, PhD, is a Professor in the departments of Psychiatry and Medicine at SUNY Upstate Medical University in Syracuse, NY, where she also serves as Senior Associate Dean for Faculty Affairs and Faculty Development.

Chapter 16
Diabetes-Related Functional Impairment and Disability

Felicia Hill-Briggs, PhD

ASSESSMENT AND DIAGNOSIS OF FUNCTION AND DISABILITY

The World Health Organization (WHO) *International Classification of Functioning, Disability and Health* (ICF) serves as an overarching diagnostic and classification framework for health and disability, used for clinical, social, policy, economic, and research purposes (WHO 2001). ICF was designed to classify health and function at three levels of human functioning: the body or body part, the whole person, and the whole person in a social context (WHO 2002). Disability is described as dysfunction in one or more of the following domains (WHO 2002):

Impairments (problems in body function or structure such as a significant deviation or loss)

- Body Functions—physiological functions of body systems (including psychological and cognitive functions)
- Body Structure—anatomical parts of the body such as organs, limbs, and their components

Activity and Participation (execution of a task or action and involvement in life situations)

- Activity Limitations—difficulties an individual may have in executing activities
- Participation Restrictions—problems an individual may experience in involvement in life situations

Life activities that are encompassed in the domains of Activity Limitations and Participation Restrictions are each relevant to psychosocial areas of function and include: learning and applying knowledge, carrying out daily routines, communication, mobility, self-care (including looking after and maintaining one's health), domestic life activities, interpersonal interactions and relationships, major life areas (including education, work, economic life), and community, social, and civic life. In addition, the ICF disability framework recognizes the role of Environmental Factors, and encourages consideration of the impact of products and technology; natural environment support; relationships; attitudes; and services, systems, and policies on impairment, activity, and participation (WHO 2002).

DIABETES AS A DISEASE OF DISABILITY

Within the ICF framework, disability is something that affects a majority of people affected with diabetes. To the extent that all people experience impact of the disease in one or more life area, each person with diabetes experiences some degree of disability (WHO 2001). Diabetes is among the chronic conditions for which people are protected under the Americans with Disabilities Act Amendments Act (http://www.diabetes.org/living-with-diabetes/know-your-rights/ discrimination/employment-discrimination/americans-with-disabilities-act- amendments-act/). People with diabetes have twice the prevalence of physical disability and twice the incidence rate of new-onset disability as compared with their counterparts without diabetes (Gregg 2002, Reyerson 2003). This excess disability burden has been found even independent of diabetes complications and comorbidities (Gregg 2002, Maty 2004). Caring for diabetes can impact life areas including self-care, major life activities such as work or recreation, and interpersonal relationships. Within the ICF framework, Environmental Factors such as attitudes, technologies, and support of others are recognized as having the potential to decrease or to increase the disabling impact of a disease such as diabetes on the life activities of people living with the disease.

In addition to the impact of diabetes as a disease of disability itself, diabetes complications confer excess impairment, activity limitation, and participation restriction (Wray 2005, Von Korff 2005). People living with diabetes complications may be considered a special subgroup with regard to impact of diabetes- related disability on mood, quality of life, psychosocial and interpersonal functioning, and diabetes self-care.

DIABETIC FOOT ULCERS AND AMPUTATION

Diabetes accounts for >60% of nontraumatic lower-limb amputations in the U.S., and >65,000 lower-extremity amputations are performed on people with diabetes annually (Centers for Disease Control and Prevention [CDC] 2011). The prevalence of peripheral neuropathy, a major contributor to foot wounds and lower- extremity amputations, is 30% among adults with diabetes (CDC 2011). People with type 1 and type 2 diabetes who have any type of foot complication (i.e., foot ulceration, healed ulcers without amputation, or amputation) experience lower health-related quality of life as compared with people with diabetes who do not have foot problems (Carrington 1996, Price 2000, Ragnarson 2000, Valensi 2005, Goodridge 2006). Psychosocial symptoms and distress in people with foot ulcers or amputation include mild to severe depressive symptoms; anxiety symptoms related to worry about wounds and feet; negative affect, attitudes, and self-percep- tions about their feet; feelings of unpredictability regarding symptoms and treat- ment; and experience of pain and phantom pain (Carrington 1996, Price 2000, Ragnarson 2000, Price 2004, Valensi 2005, Vileikyte 2005, Goodridge 2006). Foot ulceration may cause more emotional distress than amputation, due to fears of recurrent infection or ulceration, and greater restriction on mobility during ulcer- ation as compared with postamputation (Price 2000, Price 2004). Patients with either foot ulceration or amputation experience reduced physical functioning, reduced ability to carry out daily activities, poorer self-care, lower medication compliance, and disrupted social-family roles (Ragnarson 2000, Valensi 2005). Prior to amputation, preoperative individuals have psychosocial concerns about life following amputation, including fears and concerns about impending financial status and inability to participate in both social activities and functional activities (e.g., walking, driving) following amputation. Some diabetic patients, when faced with the prospect of impending amputation, may experience severe depression with death wish or suicidality (Walsh 2002, Price 2004). The caregivers and spouses of people with diabetic foot ulcers also experience psychosocial distress. Concerns are associated with the poor daily functioning and impaired mobility in the person with foot ulcer, the caretaking tasks and responsibilities faced by the caregiver, and the impact of the foot ulcers on work loss and family life (Brod 1998).

Peripheral neuropathy, the leading cause of diabetic foot ulcers and subsequent lower-extremity amputation, also results in functional impairment and limits on activity and participation. Physical impairments from peripheral neuropathy lead to inability to work (Gore 2006, Candrilli 2007). Chronic neuropathic pain, which occurs in an estimated 11 to 32% of diabetic people with neuropathy, is an additional source of psychological distress, depression, sleep disturbance, and poor quality of life (Vinik 2000, Argoff 2006).

With regard to treatment, rehabilitation practice guidelines are available for managing patients following lower-limb amputation, including recommendations for addressing mood, impairments in function, and problems with activity and participation that lead to lower quality of life (Candrilli 2007). For addressing the limitations resulting from living with chronic pain, there is evidence that cognitive-behavioral therapy may have limited effectiveness for adults experiencing chronic, nonheadache pain (Eccleston 2009). However, research is needed to determine effectiveness of psychological interventions on chronic pain, coping, subsequent self-care, and quality of life specifically in diabetic people with foot ulcers and limb loss.

Evidence from one randomized controlled trial demonstrates effectiveness of a structured peer self-management intervention, but not a peer support group intervention, on multiple psychosocial outcomes in people with limb loss. The Promoting Amputee Life Skills (PALS) study (Wegener 2009), in which 37% of the sample of 500 amputees had limb loss due to diabetes, found that a nine-session (90 min in duration each) structured self-management intervention delivered by trained peer amputees resulted in decreased likelihood of depression and functional limitations, and improved self-efficacy.

DIABETES-RELATED VISION IMPAIRMENT AND BLINDNESS

Diabetic retinopathy results in 12,000 to 24,000 new cases of blindness annually in the U.S., and diabetes is the primary cause of new cases of blindness among adults 20–74 years of age (CDC 2011). People with diabetes who develop diabetes-related vision impairment or blindness are at risk for significant psychosocial distress, including anxiety, apprehension, depressive symptoms, somatization, feelings of vulnerability, poor health-related quality of life, and family stress resulting from the vision impairment (Bernbaum 1988b, Cox 1998, Coyne 2004). Even prior to vision loss, people with diabetic retinopathy may report anxiety about current and future vision loss (Sharma 2005). Factors that contribute to reduced quality of life include decreased independence, low sense of control/power, limited participation in leisure and social activities, and impaired ability to perform daily activities due to mobility restrictions (Williams 2002, Coyne 2004, Leksell 2005b). In families, vision impairment due to diabetes is a significant stressor in the marital relationship and is associated with higher rates of spousal separation (Bernbaum 1993).

People with vision impairment and blindness experience participation restriction in diabetes self-care. Barriers to participation in their self-management include perceived poor understanding on the part of health care professionals; mobility and transportation difficulties prohibiting reliable attendance at medical appointments, educational events, or support groups; lack of accessible diabetes-related health information; and lack of diabetes equipment in accessible formats (Williams 2002, Leksell 2005a). These barriers result in a reduced sense of control and engagement in the patients' health care (Williams 2002).

Treatment for psychological adjustment following new-onset vision impairment or blindness is a neglected area of research in diabetes. Studies examining prevalence of mood or adjustment disorders and both individual and marital/family intervention approaches are needed. Studies have addressed educational needs of people with diabetes and vision impairment, and diabetes self-management programs specifically designed for people with vision impairment have demonstrated effectiveness in improving quality of life, self-reliance, and diabetes self-management skills (Bernbaum 1988a, Bernbaum 1989, Bernbaum 2000).

PSYCHOSOCIAL SEQUELAE OF STROKE AND MYOCARDIAL INFARCTION (MI)

Prevalence of cardiovascular disease in people with diabetes is ~30% (http://www.cdc.gov/diabetes/pubs/estimates11.htm#12), and people with diabetes have a 200–400% higher risk of stroke (CDC 2011). Following stroke or MI, common psychosocial complications include depression, cognitive impairment, reduced quality of life, and functional impairment impacting performance of activities of daily living (Antman 2004, Bogey 2004, Duncan 2005, Thombs 2006). Depression following stroke or MI is associated with higher mortality (Frasure-Smith 1995, House 2001).

Family members and caregivers also experience significant fears, concerns, and depressive symptoms associated with caregiver burden and with the impact of impairment and disability on role functioning, interpersonal relationships, and quality of life (Moser 2004, McCullagh 2005, Cameron 2006). Caregiver distress is associated with poorer patient recovery following MI (Moser 2004). Psychosocial interventions for caregivers that address caregiver stress and well-being, role reversal, relationship concerns, and financial issues have reported effectiveness in improving quality of life for caregivers following stroke (Mant 2000) or MI (Nelson 1998, Van Horn 2002).

There is emerging evidence that poststroke rehabilitation may result in similar overall functional gains (including mobility, cognition, communication, and personal care activities of daily living) in people with and without diabetes (Mizrahi 2007, Ripley 2007). However, research is needed to determine the impact of functional impairments in language (aphasia), vision, cognition, and mobility specifically on ability to perform diabetes self-management behaviors and to participate in one's diabetes care (Golden 2005).

In people with poststroke paresis (weakness) and plegia (paralysis) affecting ability to use the hands, self-injecting insulin and self-monitoring of blood glucose are adversely impacted, resulting in loss of independence in self-care, and significantly reduced quality of life and functional health status (Kleinbeck 2004). Case studies have addressed activity limitation in self-care in patients with poststroke hemiparesis or hemiplegia. These cases demonstrate that independence in the self-care activity of insulin injecting can be restored by designing devices that compensate for functional impairment, allowing for execution of tasks using preserved function (Keon 1980, Harvey 1992, Sohmiya 2004).

COGNITIVE IMPAIRMENT AND DEMENTIA IN DIABETES

Cognitive impairment and dementia contribute to the excess burden of disability associated with diabetes (Engelgau 2004). Older adults with diabetes have a 50–100% increased risk of Alzheimer's disease and a 100–150% increased risk of vascular dementia (Biessels 2006, van Harten 2006). Diabetes is also associated with higher risk of mild cognitive impairment (Luchsinger 2007, Whitmer 2007) and structural and functional abnormalities on neuroimaging (van Harten 2006, Christman 2010). Executive functions, processing speed, and memory are the domains in which performance decrements or deficits, relative to nondiabetic control subjects, have been observed most commonly (Biessels 2006, Luchsinger 2007, Christman 2010).

Onset of symptoms of cognitive impairment, and course of decline in progressive dementia can have a devastating emotional and psychosocial impact on families and caregivers (Etters 2008). The extent to which living with diabetes may compound the impact is not known. Similarly, research is needed on the reciprocal impact of diabetes and its care on caregiver stress, burden, and behavior.

Cognitive impairment in nondemented adults with diabetes has been associated with need for assistance performing instrumental activities of daily living (e.g., using a telephone; traveling outside of walking distance; shopping; cooking; doing housework, handyman work, and laundry; taking medications; and managing money) and with poorer awareness of this functional impairment (Christman 2010). However, research is needed to determine impact of mild, moderate, and severe cognitive impairment on performance of diabetes self-management activities of medication taking, self-monitoring of blood glucose, healthy eating, physical activity, and managing acute hyper- and hypoglycemia.

There is evidence from one study that adults with type 2 diabetes who have mild to moderate cognitive impairment can exhibit learning following diabetes self-management education that uses print and oral presentation methods designed for accessibility and usability (Hill-Briggs 2008). Moreover, a follow-up randomized controlled trial testing a problem-solving–based diabetes self-management training in this patient population with impairments demonstrated that a nine-session structured program, using materials adapted for accessibility and usability, improved diabetes knowledge, problem-solving skills, self-care, and disease control (Hill-Briggs 2011).

Impact of cognitive impairment on mood, coping, and quality of life of people with diabetes requires investigation. Moreover, studies are needed to determine timing and effect of cognitive interventions (e.g., cognitive rehabilitation, medications) on ability to perform diabetes self-management activities in diabetic people with cognitive impairment. Finally, research is needed on effective training approaches for diabetes self-management assistance and effective performance of diabetes care assistance by caregivers of people with diabetes and cognitive impairment or dementia.

INTELLECTUAL DISABILITY

People with intellectual disability (ID) have significant limitations in both intellectual functioning (generally an IQ <70–75) and in adaptive behaviors, and have the onset of disability before 18 years of age (http://www.aamr.org/content_100.cfm?navID=21). Studies have reported prevalence of diabetes among people with ID ranging from 11 to 24%, in part due to the number of overweight and obese individuals in the ID population (Butler 2002, Straetmans 2007, Reichard 2011). Despite high prevalence of diabetes, there is a paucity of research regarding diabetes in people with ID. Qualitative studies have found that people with ID and diabetes may experience feelings of loss, lack of control, and poor access to understandable information to facilitate diabetes self-care (Cardol 2012), whereas professional caregivers may struggle with lack of knowledge of diabetes and dilemmas regarding autonomy vs. assistance in self-management (Cardol 2011). Future research is needed to identify psychosocial needs present in this population and to design and test effectiveness of interventions targeting needs of both the people with ID and diabetes, and of their caregivers.

RECOMMENDATIONS FOR CLINICAL CARE

Foot Ulcers and Amputations
1. Rehabilitation psychologists and counselors, and health psychologists who are trained in assessment and interventions for adjusting to functional impairment and disability, may be especially appropriate for evaluation and treatment planning for psychosocial distress and adaptation related to foot ulcers and wounds, chronic pain, and lower-extremity amputation (Wegener 2007, Renosky 2008).
2. As a part of ongoing care, use standardized questionnaires or interview formats to assess degree of function or impairment, and cognitive capacity, including mental health.
3. For coping with chronic pain, cognitive-behavioral therapy is recommended. This modality may improve mood and be effective in bringing about some pain reduction (Eccleston 2009).
4. People with diabetes who are at risk for foot ulcers should be screened for depression due to increased risk for depression and higher likelihood of poor foot care when depression is present (Vileikyte 2004).
5. Participation in rehabilitation programs that provide community integration (strategies for emotional equilibrium and healthy coping, resumption

of roles in family and community activities, and recreational activities) and vocational rehabilitation (assessment and planning of vocational abilities and opportunities, educational needs) is recommended.

6. Following lower-limb amputations, ongoing assessment of psychosocial needs and mental health services is indicated in addition to continued rehabilitation efforts targeting activity and participation in activities of daily living and diabetes self-management (Esquenazi 1996). In addition, structured peer self-management interventions can be effective for improving multiple psychosocial outcomes following amputation (Limb Loss Task Force 2011).

Vision Impairment and Blindness

1. Initiation of programs for diabetes self-management education (DSME) and rehabilitation that have been developed specifically for people who have vision impairment or blindness are recommended. Effective interventions focus on coping, updating diabetes knowledge, assisting in selection of appropriate self-management devices, and training people in use of adaptive equipment (e.g., syringe magnifiers, syringe loading devices, and blood glucose monitoring devices with speech capability and tactile aids) and low-vision strategies (Bernbaum 1988a, Bernbaum 1989, Cate 1995, Bernbaum 2000).

2. Strategies for improving participation in diabetes self-care among people with vision impairment and blindness should be followed, including:
   a) recommendation of test strips and blood glucose monitoring devices that address specific features such as speech output, size, instruction format, operating procedures, test strip use procedures, and tactual cues (Williams 1994);
   b) accessible diabetes education materials that provide materials in formats that do not require eyesight or that are easily adaptable to audio-only formats and meet low-vision guidelines for print materials including specifications regarding font, size, color of background, and paper stock for nonglare (Williams 1999);
   c) use of insulin administration mechanisms/tools that enhance ease of dose-setting adjustments, are durable, and have easily accessible instructions and procedures for operating and trouble-shooting (Williams 1994, Uslan 2005);
   d) when using insulin pumps, including a speech output capability, high-contrast displays, and consistently large print (Coyne 2004);
   e) ensuring that print materials, blood glucose monitoring devices, and insulin pumps carry all features deemed necessary for optimal accessibility for blind and visually impaired people with diabetes; to date, diabetes self-management tools carry some but not all features (Williams 1994, Uslan 2003, Uslan 2004, Uslan 2005).

3. Referral for evidence-based psychotherapies, including cognitive-behavioral therapy and interpersonal therapies is suggested when depression, anxiety, difficulty adjusting to impairment or disability, and family/spousal

stress associated with diabetes-related vision impairment or blindness are identified (Kendall 1998, Chambless 2005).
4. Identification of interpersonal support for the visually impaired individual is suggested for monitoring of or assistance with performance of regimen behaviors as needed.

Stroke and MI

1. Because disability does not inherently preclude individuals from self-managing diabetes, it is recommended that all people with poststroke or post-MI disability receive assessment of their functional limitations and capabilities related to performing diabetes self-management (e.g., manual dexterity, visual and cognitive function), and be provided with reasonable accommodations, including adapted education tools and diabetes equipment (Kleinbeck 2004, AADE 2002). Emphasis should be placed on whether the patient can perform diabetes self-management behaviors independently or with assistance or supervision.
2. Cognitive rehabilitation, which uses both remediation strategies for cognitive deficits and compensatory training, is recommended for cognitive impairment following stroke. Current evidence-based strategies with demonstrated effectiveness for specific domains should be implemented according to practice recommendations and guidelines (Lincoln 2000, Cicerone 2005, Bowen 2007, Nair 2007). In addition, general practice recommendations regarding treatment of poststroke impairments by increasing mobility and personal care, facilitating instrumental activities of daily living, and maintaining communication should be followed. The need to maintain self-care and communication is key to the well-being of poststroke patients with diabetes (Bogey 2004, Duncan 2005).
3. For people with diabetes who are unable to self-inject insulin or self-monitor blood glucose due to hemiparesis or hemiplegia following stroke, adaptive devices can be used to facilitate independence in performing these diabetes self-care activities using one hand (Keon 1980, Harvey 1992, Sohmiya 2004).
4. Screening for depression and other psychological manifestations of poor adjustment to illness following stroke or MI is recommended. Poorer functional recovery and higher rates of mortality are associated with presence of depression/significant psychopathology (Antman 2004, Duncan 2005, Thombs 2006). Health care professionals conducting psychological and cognitive screening or neuropsychological evaluation should follow practice standards and guidelines regarding test selection, use, and modification when functional impairment or disability impacts standard test administration procedures (American Educational Research Association 1999, Hill-Briggs 2007).
5. Evidence-based psychotherapies including cognitive-behavioral therapy and interpersonal therapies are recommended for treatment of depression, anxiety, difficulty adjusting to impairment or disability, and psychosocial stressors in people with diabetes following stroke (Kendall 1998, Chambless 2005, Duncan 2005). When providing psychotherapy or counseling to

people who have functional or cognitive impairments such as those following stroke, special attention must be given to the impact of sensory deficits and information-processing difficulties on ability to engage fully in treatment. Structured therapy techniques and accommodations for functional impairments are recommended (Kortte 2005).

6. After careful assessment of body systems, functional status, and psychological state poststroke or post-MI, if impairment is significant, indicating the potential for poor adjustment and adverse sequelae, medication evaluation should be considered. Antidepressants have been studied for treatment of depression following stroke. Fluoxetine is well tolerated and effective in reducing poststroke depressive symptoms, although it does not speed cognitive or functional recovery (Robinson 2000, Wiart 2000, Fruehwald 2003). Nortriptyline is effective in reducing depression following stroke, and it may also improve anxiety symptoms and functional recovery of activities of daily living (Robinson 2000). Nortriptyline and fluoxetine may be effective in reducing mortality several years following stroke (Jorge 2003).

7. Poststroke or post-MI stress/crisis management and counseling interventions are recommended for family members and caregivers of people with diabetes-related disability to address impact of impairment or disability and to improve quality of life of the caregiver (Mant 2000).

Cognitive Impairment

1. Diabetes self-management education designed for accessibility and usability using clear and simplified presentation of information (CDC 1999, Williams 1999, Kortte 2005) should be used to facilitate learning in people with mild to moderate cognitive impairment (Hill-Briggs 2008).

2. If cognitive impairment is suspected, degree and type of cognitive impairment(s) need to be established using standardized neuropsychological measures and procedures. Available practice recommendations for evaluation and intervention for cognitive impairment and dementia should be followed for people with diabetes with possible or confirmed cognitive impairment (Knopman 2001, Petersen 2001, NAN 2002, Clare 2003).

3. Assessment and treatment of mood states in the context of cognitive impairment or dementia should follow standardized and generally accepted criteria (American Geriatrics Society Clinical Practice Committee 2003) using standardized diagnostic instruments or formal psychiatric interviewing tools, such as the SCID (First 1996).

4. The diabetes management team should give education and training to the caregivers who assist people with cognitive impairment, dementia, or intellectual disability in performing diabetes self-management behaviors.

BIBLIOGRAPHY

American Association of Diabetes Educators (AADE): Diabetes education for people with disabilities. *Diabetes Educ* 28:916-921, 2002

American Association on Intellectual and Developmental Disabilities: Definition of Intellectual Disability. Available at http://www.aamr.org/content_100. cfm?navID=21. Accessed 20 July 2012

American Diabetes Association: Americans with Disabilities Act Amendments Act. Available at http://www.diabetes.org/living-with-diabetes/know-your-rights/ discrimination/employment-discrimination/americans-with-disabilities-act- amendments-act/. Accessed 2 July 2012

American Educational Research Association, American Psychological Association, National Council on Measurement in Education: Testing individuals with dis- abilities. In *Standards for Educational and Psychological Testing*. Washington, DC, American Educational Research Association, 1999, p. 101–108

American Geriatrics Society Clinical Practice Committee: Guidelines Abstracted from the American Academy of Neurology's Dementia Guidelines for Early Detection, Diagnosis, and Management of Dementia. *J Am Geriatr Soc* 51:869–873, 2003

Antman EM, Anbe DT, Armstrong PW, Bates ER, Green LA, et al.: ACC/AHA guidelines for the management of patients with ST-elevation myocardial infarction: a report of the American College of Cardiology/American Heart Association Task Force on Practice Guidelines (Committee to Revise the 1999 Guidelines for the Management of Patients with Acute Myocardial Infarc- tion). *Circulation* 110:e82–e292, 2004

Argoff CE, Cole BE, Fishbain DA, Irving GA: Diabetic peripheral neuropathic pain: clinical and quality-of-life issues. *Mayo Clin Proc* 81 (4 Suppl.):S3–S11, 2006

Bernbaum M, Wittry S, Stich T, Brusca S, Albert SG: Effectiveness of a diabetes education program adapted for people with vision impairment. *Diabetes Care* 23:1430–1432, 2000

Bernbaum M, Albert SG, Duckro PN, Merkel W: Personal and family stress in individuals with diabetes and vision loss. *J Clin Psychol* 49:670–677, 1993

Bernbaum M, Albert SG, Brusca SR, Drimmer A, Duckro PN, et al.: A model clinical program for patients with diabetes and vision impairment. *Diabetes Educ* 15:325–330, 1989

Bernbaum M, Albert SG, Brusca SR, Drimmer A, Duckro PN: Promoting diabe- tes self-management and independence in the visually impaired: a model clin- ical program. *Diabetes Educ* 14:51–54, 1988a

Bernbaum M, Albert SG, Duckro PN: Psychosocial profiles in patients with visual impairment due to diabetic retinopathy. *Diabetes Care* 11:551–557, 1988b

Biessels GJ, Staekenborg S, Brunner E, Brayne C, Scheltens P: Risk of dementia in diabetes mellitus: a systematic review. *Lancet Neurology* 5:64–74, 2006

Bogey RA, Geis CC, Bryant PR, Moroz A, O'Neill BJ: Stroke and neurodegenerative disorders. 3. stroke: rehabilitation management. *Archives of Physical Medicine and Rehabilitation* 85 (3 Suppl. 1):S15–S20, 2004

Bowen A, Lincoln NB, Dewey M: Cognitive rehabilitation for spatial neglect following stroke. *Cochrane Database Syst Rev* CD003586, 2007

Brod M: Quality of life issues in patients with diabetes and lower extremity ulcers: patients and care givers. *Qual Life Res* 7:365–372, 1998

Butler JV, Whittington JE, Holland AJ, Boer H, Clarke D, Webb T: Prevalence of, and risk factors for, physical ill-health in people with Prader-Willi syndrome: a population based study. *Developmental Medicine and Child Neurology* 44:248–255, 2002

Cameron JI, Cheung AM, Streiner DL, Coyte PC, Stewart DE: Stroke survivors' behavioral and psychologic symptoms are associated with informal caregivers' experiences of depression. *Archives of Physical Medicine and Rehabilitation* 87:177–183, 2006

Candrilli SD, Davis KL, Kan HJ, Lucero MA, Rousculp MD: Prevalence and the associated burden of illness of symptoms of diabetic peripheral neuropathy and diabetic retinopathy. *J Diabetes Complications* 21:306–314, 2007

Cardol M, Rijken M, van Schrojenstein Lantman-de Valk H: People with mild to moderate intellectual disability talking about their diabetes and how they manage. *Journal of Intellectual Disability Research* 56:351–360, 2012

Cardol M, Rijken M, van Schrojenstein Lantman-de Valk H: Attitudes and dilemmas of caregivers supporting people with intellectual disabilities who have diabetes. *Patient Educ Couns* 87:383–388, 2011, doi:10.1016/j.pec.2011.11.010

Carrington AL, Mawdsley SK, Morley M, Kincey J, Boulton AJ: Psychological status of diabetic people with or without lower limb disability. *Diabetes Res Clin Pract* 32:19–25, 1996

Cate Y, Baker SS, Gilbert MP: Occupational therapy and the person with diabetes and vision impairment. *Am J Occup Ther* 49:905–911, 1995

Centers for Disease Control and Prevention. National diabetes fact sheet: national estimates and general information on diabetes and prediabetes in the United States, 2011. Atlanta, U.S. Department of Health and Human Services, Centers for Disease Control and Prevention, 2011. Available from http://www.cdc.gov/diabetes/pubs/factsheet11.htm. Accessed 19 September 2012

Centers for Disease Control and Prevention: *Scientific and Technical Information Simply Put.* 2nd ed. Atlanta, Centers for Disease Control and Prevention, 1999

Chambless DL: Compendium of empirically supported therapies. In *Psychologists' Desk Reference.* 2nd ed. Koocher GP, Norcross JC, Hill SS, Eds. Oxford, Oxford University Press, 2005

Christman A, Vannorsdall T, Hill-Briggs F, Schretlen D: Cranial volume, mild cognitive deficits and functional limitations associated with diabetes in a community sample. *Arch Clin Neuropsychol* 25:49–59, 2010

Cicerone KD, Dahlberg C, Malec JF, Langenbahn DM, Felicetti T, et al.: Evidence-based cognitive rehabilitation: updated review of the literature from 1998 through 2002. *Archives of Physical Medicine and Rehabilitation* 86:1681–1692, 2005

Clare L, Woods RT, Moniz Cook ED, Orrell M, Spector A: Cognitive rehabilitation and cognitive training for early-stage Alzheimer's disease and vascular dementia. *Cochrane Database Syst Rev* CD003260, 2003

Cox DJ, Kiernan BD, Schroeder DB, Cowley M: Psychosocial sequelae of visual loss in diabetes. *Diabetes Educ* 24:481–484, 1998

Coyne KS, Margolis MK, Kennedy-Martin T, Baker TM, Klein R, Paul MD, Revicki DA: The impact of diabetic retinopathy: perspectives from patient focus groups. *Fam Pract* 21:447–453, 2004

Duncan PW, Zorowitz R, Bates B, Choi JY, Glasberg JJ, et al.: Management of adult stroke rehabilitation care: a clinical practice guideline. *Stroke* 36:e100–e143, 2005

Eccleston C, Williams AC, Morley S: Psychological therapies for the management of chronic pain (excluding headache) in adults. *Cochrane Database Syst Rev* CD007407, 2009. doi: 10.1002/14651858.CD007407.pub2

Engelgau MM, Geiss LS, Saaddine JB, Boyle JP, Benjamin SM, et al.: The evolving diabetes burden in the United States. *Ann Intern Med* 140:945–950, 2004

Esquenazi A, Meier RH 3rd: Rehabilitation in limb deficiency. 4. Limb amputation. *Archives of Physical Medicine and Rehabilitation* 77 (3 Suppl.):S18–S28, 1996

Etters L, Goodall D, Harrison BE: Caregiver burden among dementia patient caregivers: a review of the literature. *J Am Acad Nurse Pract* 20:423–428, 2008

First MB, Spitzer RL, Gibbon M, Williams JBW: *Structured Clinical Interview for DSM-IV Axis I Disorders, Clinician Version (SCID-CV)*. Washington, DC, American Psychiatric Press, 1996

Frasure-Smith N, Lesperance F, Talajic M: Depression and 18-month prognosis after myocardial infarction. *Circulation* 91:999–1005, 1995

Fruehwald S, Gatterbauer E, Rehak P, Baumhackl U: Early fluoxetine treatment of post-stroke depression. *Journal of Neurology* 250:347–351, 2003

Golden SH, Hill-Briggs F, Williams K, Stolka K, Mayer RS: Management of diabetes during acute stroke and inpatient stroke rehabilitation. *Archives of Physical Medicine and Rehabilitation* 86:2377–2384, 2005

Goodridge D, Trepman E, Sloan J, Guse L, Strain LA, McIntyre J, Embil JM: Quality of life of adults with unhealed and healed diabetic foot ulcers. *Foot Ankle Int* 27:274–280, 2006

Gore M, Brandenburg NA, Hoffman DL, Tai KS, Stacey B: Burden of illness in painful diabetic peripheral neuropathy: the patients' perspectives. *J Pain* 7:892–900, 2006

Gregg EW, Mangione CM, Cauley JA, Thompson TJ, Schwartz AV, et al.: Diabetes and incidence of functional disability in older women. *Diabetes Care* 25:61–67, 2002

Hackett ML, Anderson CS: Predictors of depression after stroke: a systematic review of observational studies. *Stroke* 36:2296–2301, 2005

Harvey RL, Stachowski KM, Dewulf SK: Independent insulin administration by the hemiplegic patient: stabilization of an insulin pen with a new device. *Arch Phys Med Rehabil* 73:779–781, 1992

Hill-Briggs F, Lazo M, Peyrot M, Chang Y, Doswell A, Hill M, Levine D, Wang N, Brancati F: Effect of problem-solving-based diabetes self-management training on diabetes control in a low income patient sample. *J Gen Intern Med* 26:972–978, 2011

Hill-Briggs F, Lazo M, Renosky R, Ewing C: Usability of a diabetes and cardiovascular disease education module in an African-American, diabetic sample with physical, visual, and cognitive impairment. *Rehabilitation Psychology* 53:1–8, 2008

Hill-Briggs F, Dial J, Morere D: Neuropsychological assessment of persons with physical disability, visual impairment or blindness, and hearing impairment or deafness. *Arch Clin Neuropsychol* 22:389–404, 2007

House A, Knapp P, Bamford J, Vail A: Mortality at 12 and 24 months after stroke may be associated with depressive symptoms at 1 month. *Stroke* 32:696–701, 2001

Jorge RE, Robinson RG, Arndt S, Starkstein S: Mortality and poststroke depression: a placebo-controlled trial of antidepressants. *Am J Psychiatry* 160:1823–1829, 2003

Kendall PC, Chambless DL: Empirically supported psychological therapies. *J Consult Clin Psychol* 66:3–6, 1998

Keon HM, Hanna AK: Self-administration of insulin by a hemiplegic individual. *Diabetes Care* 3:705, 1980

Kleinbeck C, Williams AS: Disabilities, diabetes, and devices. *Home Healthc Nurse* 22:469–475, 2004

Knopman DS, DeKosky ST, Cummings JL, Chui H, Corey-Bloom J, et al.: Practice parameter: diagnosis of dementia (an evidence-based review). Report of the Quality Standards Subcommittee of the American Academy of Neurology. *Neurology* 56:1143–1153, 2001

Kortte KB, Hill-Briggs F: Psychotherapy with cognitively impaired adults. In *Psychologists' Desk Reference*. 2nd ed. Koocher GP, Norcross JC, Hill SS, Eds. Oxford, Oxford University Press, 2005, p. 342–349

Leksell JK, Sandberg GE, Wikblad KF. Self-perceived health and self-care among diabetic subjects with defective vision: a comparison between subjects with threat of blindness and blind subjects. *J Diabetes Complications* 19:54–59, 2005a

Leksell JK, Wikblad KF, Sandberg GE: Sense of coherence and power among people with blindness caused by diabetes. *Diabetes Res Clin Pract* 67:124–129, 2005b

Limb Loss Task Force/Amputee Coalition: *Roadmap for Limb Loss Prevention and Amputee Care Improvement*. Knoxville, TN, Amputee Coalition, 2011. Available from http://www.amputee-coalition.org/WhitePapers/Roadmap-for-Limb-Loss-Prevention-and-Amputee-Care-Improvement.pdf. Accessed 20 July 2012

Lincoln NB, Majid MJ, Weyman N: Cognitive rehabilitation for attention deficits following stroke. *Cochrane Database Syst Rev* CD002842, 2000

Luchsinger JA, Reitz C, Patel B, Tang MX, Manly JJ, Mayeux R: Relation of diabetes to mild cognitive impairment. *Archives of Neurology* 64:570–575, 2007

Mant J, Carter J, Wade DT, Winner S: Family support for stroke: a randomised controlled trial. *Lancet* 356:808–813, 2000

Maty SC, Fried LP, Volpato S, Williamson J, Brancati FL, Blaum CS: Patterns of disability related to diabetes mellitus in older women. *Journal of Gerontology: Medical Sciences* 59:148–153, 2004

McCullagh E, Brigstocke G, Donaldson N, Kalra L: Determinants of caregiving burden and quality of life in caregivers of stroke patients. *Stroke* 36:2181–2186, 2005

Mizrahi EH, Fleissig Y, Arad M, Kaplan A, Adunsky A: Functional outcome of ischemic stroke: a comparative study of diabetic and non-diabetic patients. *Disabil Rehabil* 29:1091–1095, 2007

Moser DK, Dracup K: Role of spousal anxiety and depression in patients' psychosocial recovery after a cardiac event. *Psychosom Med* 66:527–532, 2004

Nair RD, Lincoln NB: Cognitive rehabilitation for memory deficits following stroke. *Cochrane Database Syst Rev* CD002293, 2007

National Academy of Neuropsychology (NAN): Cognitive rehabilitation: official statement of the National Academy of Neuropsychology: NAN position papers. Denver, CO, NAN, May 2002. Available at https://www.nanonline.org/docs/PAIC/PDFs/NANPositionCogRehab.pdf. Accessed 20 July 2012

Nelson DV, Baer PE, Cleveland SE: Family stress management following acute myocardial infarction: an educational and skills training intervention program. *Patient Education and Counseling* 34:135–145, 1998

Petersen RC, Stevens JC, Ganguli M, Tangalos EG, Cummings JL, DeKosky ST: Practice parameter: early detection of dementia: mild cognitive impairment (an evidence-based review). Report of the Quality Standards Subcommittee of the American Academy of Neurology. *Neurology* 56:1133–1142, 2001

Price P: The diabetic foot: quality of life. *Clin Infect Dis* 39 (Suppl. 2):S129–S131, 2004

Price P, Harding K: The impact of foot complications on health-related quality of life in patients with diabetes. *J Cutan Med Surg* 4:45–50, 2000

Ragnarson Tennvall G, Apelqvist J: Health-related quality of life in patients with diabetes mellitus and foot ulcers. *J Diabetes Complications* 14:235–241, 2000

Reichard A, Stolzle H: Diabetes among adults with cognitive limitations compared to individuals with no cognitive disabilities. *Intellect Dev Disabil* 49:141–154, 2011

Renosky R, Hunt B, Hill-Briggs F, Wray L, Ulbrecht JS: Counseling people living with diabetes. *Journal of Rehabilitation* 74:31–40, 2008

Reyerson B, Tieney EF, Thompson TJ, Engelgau MM, Wang J, Gregg EW, et al.: Excess physical limitations among adults with diabetes in the U.S. population, 1997–1999. *Diabetes Care* 26:206–210, 2003

Ripley DL, Seel RT, Macciocchi SN, Schara SL, Raziano K, Ericksen JJ: The impact of diabetes mellitus on stroke acute rehabilitation outcomes. *Am J Phys Med Rehabil* 86:754–761, 2007

Robinson RG, Schultz SK, Castillo C, Kopel T, Kosier JT, et al.: Nortriptyline versus fluoxetine in the treatment of depression and in short-term recovery after stroke: a placebo-controlled, double-blind study. *Am J Psychiatry* 157:351–359, 2000

Sharma S, Oliver-Fernandez A, Liu W, Buchholz P, Walt J: The impact of diabetic retinopathy on health-related quality of life. *Curr Opin Ophthalmol* 16:155–159, 2005

Sohmiya M, Kanazawa I, Inomata N, Yonehara S, Sumigawa M, et al.: A new device to introduce self-injection of insulin by his non-dominant hand in a patient with hemiplegia. *Diabetes Technol Ther* 6:505–509, 2004

Straetmans JM, van Schrojenstein Lantman-DeValk HM, Schellevis FG, Dinant GJ: Health problems of people with intellectual disabilities: the impact for general practice. *British Journal of General Practice* 57:64–66, 2007

Thombs BD, Bass EB, Ford DE, Stewart KJ, Tsilidis KK, et al.: Prevalence of depression in survivors of acute myocardial infarction. *Journal of General Internal Medicine* 21:30–38, 2006

Uslan MM: Analysis: beyond the "clicks" of dose setting in insulin pens. *Diabetes Technol Ther* 7:627–628, 2005

Uslan MM, Burton DM, Chertow BS, Collins R: Accessibility of insulin pumps for blind and visually impaired people. *Diabetes Technol Ther* 6:621–634, 2004

Uslan MM, Eghtesadi K, Burton D: Accessibility of blood glucose monitoring systems for blind and visually impaired people. *Diabetes Technol Ther* 5:439–448, 2003

Valensi P, Girod I, Baron F, Moreau-Defarges T, Guillon P: Quality of life and clinical correlates in patients with diabetic foot ulcers. *Diabetes Metab* 31:263–271, 2005

van Harten B, de Leeuw FE, Weinstein HC, Scheltens P, Biessels J G: Brain imaging in patients with diabetes. *Diabetes Care* 29:2539–2548, 2006

Van Horn E, Fleury J, Moore S: Family interventions during the trajectory of recovery from cardiac event: An integrative literature review. *Heart & Lung: The Journal of Acute and Critical Care* 31:186–198, 2002

Vileikyte L, Leventhal H, Gonzalez JS, Peyrot M, Rubin RR, et al.: Diabetic peripheral neuropathy and depressive symptoms: the association revisited. *Diabetes Care* 28:2378–2383, 2005

Vileikyte L, Rubin RR, Leventhal H: Psychological aspects of diabetic neuropathic foot complications: an overview. *Diabetes Metab Res Rev* 20 (Suppl. 1):S13–S18, 2004

Vinik AI, Park TS, Stansberry KB, Pitteneger GL: Diabetic neuropathies. *Diabetologia* 43:957–973, 2000

Von Korff M, Katon W, Lin EHB, Simon G, Ciechanowski P, Ludman E, Oliver M, Ruttter C, Young B: Work disability among individuals with diabetes. *Diabetes Care* 28:1326–1332, 2005

Walsh SM, Sage RA: Depression and chronic diabetic foot disability. A case report of suicide. *Clin Podiatr Med Surg* 19:493–508, 2002

Wegener ST, Mackenzie EJ, Ephraim P, Ehde D, Williams R: Self-management improves outcomes in persons with limb loss. *Arch Phys Med Rehabil* 90:373–378, 2009

Wegener ST, Kortte KB, Hill-Briggs F, Johnson-Greene D, Palmer S, Salorio C: Psychologic assessment and intervention in rehabilitation. In *Physical Medicine and Rehabilitation*. 3rd ed. Braddom RL, Ed. Philadelphia, Elsevier, 2007, p. 63–92

Whitmer RA: Type 2 diabetes and risk of cognitive impairment and dementia. *Current Neurology and Neuroscience Reports* 7:373–380, 2007

Wiart L, Petit H, Joseph PA, Mazaux JM, Barat M: Fluoxetine in early poststroke depression: a double-blind placebo-controlled study. *Stroke* 31:1829–1832, 2000

Williams AS: A focus group study of accessibility and related psychosocial issues in diabetes education for people with visual impairment. *Diabetes Educ* 28:999–1008, 2002

Williams AS: Accessible diabetes education materials in low-vision format. *Diabetes Educ* 25:695–698, 700, 702, 1999

Williams AS: Recommendations for desirable features of adaptive diabetes self-care equipment for visually impaired persons. Task Force on Adaptive Diabetes for Visually Impaired Persons. *Diabetes Care* 17:451–452, 1994

World Health Organization: *Towards a Common Language for Functioning, Disability and Health: The International Classification of Functioning, Disability and Health (ICF)*. Geneva, World Health Organization, 2002

World Health Organization: *International Classification of Function, Disability and Health (ICF)*. Geneva, World Health Organization, 2001

Wray LA, Ofstedal MB, Langa KM, Blaum CS: The effect of diabetes on disability in middle-aged and older adults. *J Gerontol A Biol Sci Med Sci* 60:1206–1211, 2005

Felicia Hill-Briggs, PhD, is Associate Professor in the Department of Medicine and Department of Physical Medicine and Rehabilitation, Johns Hopkins School of Medicine; Associate Professor in the Department of Health, Behavior, and Society, Johns Hopkins Bloomberg School of Public Health; and a member of the Core Faculty at the Welch Center for Prevention, Epidemiology & Clinical Research, Johns Hopkins Medical Institutions, in Baltimore, MD.

List of Contributors

Barbara J. Anderson, PhD, is Professor of Pediatrics and Associate Head of the Psychology Section at Baylor College of Medicine in Houston, TX.

Brooke A. Bailer, PhD, is a Postdoctoral Fellow at the Center for Weight and Eating Disorders in the Department of Psychiatry at the Perelman School of Medicine of the University of Pennsylvania in Philadelphia, PA.

Daniel J. Cox, PhD, ABPP, is a clinical psychologist and professor in the Department of Psychiatry and Neurobehavioral Sciences and the Department of Internal Medicine at the University of Virginia in Charlottesville, VA.

Mary de Groot, PhD, is an Associate Professor of Medicine at the Indiana University School of Medicine in Indianapolis, IN.

Linda M. Delahanty, MSRD, is Chief Dietitian and Director of Nutrition and Behavioral Research at Massachusetts General Hospital Diabetes Center in Boston, MA.

Lucy F. Faulconbridge, PhD, is the Director of Research at the Center for Weight and Eating Disorders in the Department of Psychiatry at the Perelman School of Medicine of the University of Pennsylvania in Philadelphia, PA.

Linda Gonder-Frederick, PhD, is an Associate Professor in the Department of Psychiatry and Neurobehavioral Sciences at the University of Virginia School of Medicine in Charlottesville, VA.

Felicia Hill-Briggs, PhD, is Associate Professor in the Department of Medicine and Department of Physical Medicine and Rehabilitation, Johns Hopkins School of Medicine; Associate Professor in the Department of Health, Behavior, and Society, Johns Hopkins Bloomberg School of Public Health; and a member of the Core Faculty at the Welch Center for Prevention, Epidemiology & Clinical Research, Johns Hopkins Medical Institutions, in Baltimore, MD.

Clarissa S. Holmes, PhD, is a Professor of Psychology, Pediatrics and Psychiatry at Virginia Commonwealth University in Richmond, VA. She also has an appointment as an Adjunct Professor of Psychiatry at Georgetown University in Washington, DC.

Suzanne Bennett Johnson, PhD, is Distinguished Research Professor at Florida State University College of Medicine in Tallahassee, FL, and President of the American Psychological Association.

Lori Laffel, MD, MPH, is Chief of the Pediatric, Adolescent and Young Adult Section and an Investigator in the Section on Genetics and Epidemiology at the Joslin Diabetes Center, and an Associate Professor of Pediatrics at Harvard Medical School in Boston, MA.

David G. Marrero, PhD, is the J.O. Ritchey Professor of Medicine and Director, Diabetes Translational Research Center at the Indiana University School of Medicine in Indianapolis, IN.

Mark Peyrot, PhD, is Professor in the Department of Sociology, Loyola University Maryland in Baltimore, MD.

Richard R. Rubin, PhD, is Professor in the Departments of Medicine and Pediatrics at The Johns Hopkins University School of Medicine in Baltimore, MD.

Christopher M. Ryan, PhD, is Professor of Psychiatry at the University of Pittsburgh School of Medicine in Pittsburgh, PA.

David B. Sarwer, PhD, is the Director of Clinical Services at the Center for Weight and Eating Disorders in the Department of Psychiatry at the Perelman School of Medicine of the University of Pennsylvania in Philadelphia, PA.

Jaclyn A. Shepard, PsyD, is an Assistant Professor in the Department of Psychiatry and Neurobehavioral Sciences at the University of Virginia School of Medicine in Charlottesville, VA.

Harsimran Singh, PhD, is a Research Scientist in the Department of Psychiatry and Neurobehavioral Sciences at the University of Virginia School of Medicine in Charlottesville, VA.

Paula M. Trief, PhD, is a Professor in the departments of Psychiatry and Medicine at SUNY Upstate Medical University in Syracuse, NY, where she also serves as Senior Associate Dean for Faculty Affairs and Faculty Development.

Thomas A. Wadden, PhD, is the Director of the Center for Weight and Eating Disorders in the Department of Psychiatry at the Perelman School of Medicine of the University of Pennsylvania in Philadelphia, PA.

Jill Weissberg-Benchell, PhD, CDE, is an Associate Professor of Psychiatry at Northwestern University's Feinberg School of Medicine at the Ann and Robert H. Lurie Children's Hospital of Chicago in Chicago, IL.

Garry Welch, PhD, is Director of Behavioral Medicine Research at Baystate Medical Center in Springfield, MA, and Research Associate Professor at Tufts University School of Medicine in Boston, MA.

Judith Wylie-Rosett, EdD, RD, is Professor and Head of the Division of Health Promotion and Nutrition Research in the Department of Epidemiology and Population Health at Albert Einstein College of Medicine of Yeshiva University in Bronx, NY.

Tim Wysocki, PhD, is Principal Research Scientist and Director of the Center for Pediatric Psychology Research in the Department of Biomedical Research at Nemours Children's Clinic in Jacksonville, FL.

Deborah Young-Hyman, PhD, CDE, is a diabetes/obesity expert at the Georgia Prevention Center, Institute for Public and Preventive Health, Medical College of Georgia, in Augusta, GA.

Sofija E. Zagarins, PhD, is a Postdoctoral Research Fellow in the Department of Behavioral Medicine Research at Baystate Medical Center in Springfield, MA, and a Visiting Assistant Professor in the Department of Public Health at the University of Massachusetts in Amherst, MA.

Index

Note: Page numbers followed by *f* refer to figures. Page numbers followed by *t* refer to tables. Page numbers in **bold** indicate an in-depth discussion.

A1C value. *See also* glycosylated hemoglobin A1C levels
  adherence intervention, 118, 120
  biomedical risk factors, 75
  Blood Glucose Awareness Training (BGAT), 40
  blood glucose monitoring (BGM), 172
  brain structure anomalies, 73, 82
  cerebral blood flow (CBF), 81
  cognitive behavioral therapy (CBT), 6
  continuous glucose monitoring (CGM), 177
  continuous subcutaneous insulin infusion (CSII), 159, 162–163
  Diabetes Self-Care Profile (DSCP), 109–110
  eating disorders (ED), 18
  electrophysiological characteristics, 80
  hypoglycemia, 37
  Juvenile Diabetes Research Foundation (JDRF) 6-month CGM Trial, 177
  medical nutrition therapy (MNT), 134, 137
  neurochemical abnormalities, 74
  Sensor-Augmented Pump Therapy for A1C Reduction (STAR3) clinical study, 177

  STeP (Structured Testing Program), 174–175
  technology-based assessments, 107–108
  work-related issues, 253
ability test, 57
academic achievement, 63–64
academic assistance, 61
Academy of Nutrition and Dietetics, 131, 134, 136
accelerometer, 152
Accountable Care Organization (ACO) model, 101–102
Accu-Chek Interview, 109–110. *See also* Diabetes Self-Care Profile (DSCP)
active medication therapy, 253
activity, 1, 2t. *See also* lifestyle modification; physical, activity
activity limitation, 273–275
Adami, G. F., 200
Adams, T. D., 201–202
adaptive behavior, 278
adaptive equipment, 278–279
adherence
  assessment tools, 122–124
  clinical care recommendations, 122–124
  defining, 117
  glycemic control and, 118–119
  inadvertent nonadherence, 117, 122–123
  medical regimen, **117–130**
  nonadherence, 117–118, 122–123
  patient, assessing and improving, 119–121
  provider, 119, 121–122

treatment, 233
willful nonadherence, 117
adiposity, 236
adjustment disorder, 1, 219, 237
adjustment-related psychiatric
disorders, 220
adolescent
behavioral characteristics, 234
behavioral intervention, 235
blood glucose monitoring (BGM),
174–175
clinical care recommendations,
236–237
collaborative teamwork, 234
continuous glucose monitoring
(CGM), 177
continuous subcutaneous insulin
infusion (CSII), 159, 161–163
depressive symptoms in, 4
disordered eating behavior (DEB),
19–20
hospitalization, 4
hypoglycemia, 39
insulin omission, 20
internet-based studies, 182–183
medical regimen nonadherence, 118
neurocognitive dysfunction, 70
psychological characteristics, 234
psychological intervention, 235
severe hypoglycemia (SH), 38
special issues, **233–250**
type 2 diabetes risk, 80
web-based intervention, 182–183
Wechsler Adult Intelligence Scale
(WAIS-IV), 57
AdultCarbQuiz, 105
adults
adult care, transition to, 251–252,
259
blood glucose monitoring (BGM),
172
childbearing/parenthood, 257–258
clinical care recommendations,
259–261
cognitive characteristics, 71*t*
cognitive domain studies, 78*t*
continuous glucose monitoring
(CGM), 176–177, 184

continuous subcutaneous insulin
infusion (CSII), 159, 161–163
diagnosis, 220
hypoglycemia, 34–35
late middle-age, 259
life course evaluation, 258–259
lifespan development issues, **251–
271**
marriage/partnering, 254–256
middle adulthood, 259
neurocognitive dysfunction, **69–99**
old-old, 259
sensor-augmented pump (SAP)
therapy, 40
sertraline treatment, 6
type 1 diabetes (T1D), 70–77
type 2 diabetes (T2D), 77–86
work/employment, 252–254
young adult, 251, 259
young-old, 259
Aerobic and Fitness Association of
America (AFFA), 150
aerobic exercise, 148, 153
affective disorders, 194, 200–201
African American, 121, 132
aging process, 77
agoraphobia, 2
AHEAD (Assessing Health and Eating
among Adolescents with Diabetes)
survey, 22
alcohol consumption, 37, 105, 109,
194
ALIVE! (A Lifestyle Intervention Via
Email), 182
Allison, D. B., 197
Alzheimer's disease, 79, 83, 277
ambulatory care, 5
American Association of Clinical
Endocrinologists (AACE), 205
American Association of Diabetes
Educators' AADE7™ Self-Care
Behaviors tool, 101, 108–109
American College of Sports Medicine
(ASCM), 150
American Council on Exercise (ACE),
150
American Diabetes Association (ADA)
adult care, transition to, 251

Clinical Practice Recommendations , vii
employment discrimination, 253, 260
Individuals with Disabilities Education Act (IDEA), 59
nutrition recommendations, 131–132, 136–137
practice guidelines, 109
self-monitoring of blood glucose (SMBG), 172
standards of care, 119, 122, 134
American Diabetes Association Interest Group on Behavioral Medicine & Psychology, 103
American Dietetic Association. *See* Academy of Nutrition and Dietetics
American Psychiatric Association [APA] manual of mental health diagnoses (DSM-IV-TR 2000). *See* DSM-IV-TR (APA)
American Society for Metabolic & Bariatric Surgery (ASMBS), 205
Americans with Disabilities Act, 253, 260–261
Americans with Disabilities Act Amendments Act, 273
amputation / amputee, 221, 278–279
amylin secretion, 21, 83–84
amyloid metabolism, 79
anhedonia, 1
anisotropic diffusion, 73
anorexia, 17. *See also* eating disorders (ED)
antianxiety medication, 196
antidepressant medication, 6–8, 196, 281
antihyperglycemic therapies, 171
antipsychotic medication, 196
anxiety
adolescent, 234
bariatric surgery, 200–202
binge eating disorder (BED), 196
cognitive impairment and, 87
continuous subcutaneous insulin infusion (CSII), 161
diabetes complications, 221
diabetes-related vision impairment or blindness, 275–276

disorders, 194–195, 198, 201, 237
exercise, 151
foot ulcer/amputation, 274
pump therapy, 164
Self-Care Inventory-Revised (SCI-R), 107
treatment regimen transitions, 222
anxiety spectrum disorders, 2
APOE ε4 allele, 83
appetite, 1
apprehension, 275
Arnett, J. J., 251
artificial pancreas, 39
assessment
of achievement, 64
function and disability, 273
methods, 101–102
technology based, 107–110
tools, 101–107, 122, 195. *see also* *specific type*
assistive learning device, 63, 65
assistive memory device, 65
atherosclerotic risk factors, 82
attention, 231
attention deficit hyperactivity disorder (ADHD), 61
Audit of Diabetes (ADKnowl), 104
Audit of Diabetes-Dependent Quality of Life (ADDQoL), 164
authoritative parenting, 233
autonomic failure, 37, 42
autonomic neuropathy, 148
avoidant coping behaviors, 219–220
avoidant disorder, 195
Axis I disorder, 193, 195, 198
Axis II disorder, 195

β-amyloid accumulation, 85*t*
Bandura, A., 106
bariatric surgery, **193–217**
affective disorders, 194, 200–201
anxiety disorders, 194
binge eating disorder (BED), 196–197, 202–203
body image, 198, 200, 204–205
clinical care recommendations, 206–207
dietary adherence, 203

eating behavior, postoperative changes in, 202–203
eating behavior, preoperative, 196
health-related quality of life (HRQoL), 204
methodological variability in assessment, 195
night eating syndrome, 196–197, 202–203
personality disorders, 195–196
psychiatric status, postoperative, 200–201
psychiatric status, preoperative, 193–194
quality of life, postoperative, 204–206
quality of life, preoperative, 197–198
sexual functioning, 198, 200, 205
substance use, 194
suicide risk, 201–202
basal ganglia, 75–76
Beck Depression Inventory (BDI), 198, 200–201
Beck Depression Inventory-II (BDI-II), 2–3
behavioral
  characteristics, 234
  evaluation, 205
  family systems therapy, 235
  goals, 137
  health, viii
  intervention, 121, 123, 147–148, 151, 258
  modification techniques, 234
  recommendations, 138
behavioral-psychosocial assessment, 193
Behavioral Research In Diabetes Group Exchange [BRIDGE], 103
Behavioral Risk Factor Surveillance System (BRFSS), 172
bereavement, 2t
beta cell function, 222
BGATHome, 40, 43
BG Monitoring Owner's Manual, 173
binge eating disorder (BED), 109, 196–197, 200, 202–203

bipolar disorder, 2
black persons, 148. *See also* African American
blindness, 275–276, 279–280. *See also* retinopathy
blood-brain-barrier permeability, 85t
blood glucose (BG). *See also* blood glucose monitoring (BGM)
  awareness training, 181–182
  control, 6, 20, 107
  estimation and accuracy evaluation, 40
  levels, 33, 35–36, 39–40, 85t, 105, 109, 149–150
  meters, 119, 123
  self-monitoring tool, 175
  symptom diary, 40
  testing, 107, 123
Blood Glucose Awareness Training (BGAT), 40, 43
blood glucose monitoring (BGM), 119, 171–175, 177, 182–183, 279
blood lipid control, 109
blood pressure, 105, 109, 135, 147. *See also* hypertension
BMI (body mass index), 6, 19, 82, 135, 159–160, 193–194, 198, 199f, 204, 236
body
  fat, 147
  function, 273
  image, 198, 200, 204–205
  pain, 198, 199f
  structure, 273
  weight, 159–160
Body Attitude Questionnaire, 200
body dysmorphic disorder, 200
body image–related quality of life (BIQoL), 205
Body Shape Questionnaire, 200, 204
Bond, D. S., 200, 205
borderline disorder, 195
brain. *See also* neurocognitive, dysfunction
  alpha activity, 80
  basal ganglia, 75–76
  cerebral blood flow (CBF), 72
  cognitive function and severe hypoglycemia, 34

cortex, 75, 83
cortical atrophy, 81–82
cortical gray matter, 72–73
delta power, 80
density measures, 73
dysfunction in T2D, 85
fast wave activity, 72
frontal region, 81
function, viii, 60, 69, 75
glucose level, 74–75
glucose transport, 83
gray matter, 72–73, 75, 80–81
gray matter choline (Cho), 84
metabolite, 75, 83
neurochemical abnormalities, 75
neurometabolite, 84
optic radiations, 73
parietal-occipital region, 81
posterior corona radiata, 73
resistance arterioles, 72
slow wave activity, 72, 80
structural abnormalities, 80
structure, 75
subcortical atrophy, 81
temporal region, 81
theta power, 80
volumes, 81–83
wave activity, 71
white matter, 74–76, 80–84
white matter microstructural
abnormalities, 73
brain-behavior relationship, 73
brainstem, 75
bulimia, 17, 19, 21, 196. *See also* eating
disorders (ED)
Bulimia Test - Revised (BULIT-R), 22
bupropion, 6

Caesarean section (c-section), 257
caloric consumption, 151
caloric restraint, 21
cancer, 193, 220
carbohydrate counting, 21, 105, 237
carbohydrate intake, 132, 150
cardiac-rehabilitation specialist, 150
cardiovascular disease (CVD), 105,
149, 193, 221, 254, 276
cardiovascular health, 121

cardiovascular morbidity, 134
cardiovascular risk, 107, 147–148
caregiver burden, 276
carotid intima media thickening, 76
case management intervention, 6, 40
Caucasian, 162, 259
cell phone, 181–182, 184
Center for Epidemiologic Studies
Depression Scale (CES-D), 3
Centers for Disease Control and
Prevention (CDC), 172
central nervous system (CNS), 69,
82–83, 85*t*
central neuropathy, 72
cerebral
amyloid angiopathy, 83
atrophy, 76
glucose utilization, 72
hypoperfusion, 77, 84
infarction, 76
metabolism rate, 72
microangiopathy, 77
microcirculation, 77
microvasculature, 72, 77
perfusion, 72, 81
cerebral blood flow (CBF), 72, 75,
80–81
cerebrospinal fluid (CSF) volumes, 81,
83
cerebrovascular reactivity studies, 72
Cerebrovascular Risk Factor Scale, 83
certified exercise specialist / trainer,
150
childbearing, 257–258, 261. *See also*
pregnancy
Child Behavior Checklist (CBCL),
230
children
academic achievement, 57–58
acute disease-related cognitive
disruption, 61
assessment of achievement, 58
autonomy, 229–230
blood glucose monitoring (BGM),
172, 178–179
chronic disease-related skill
disruption, 60–61
chronic hypoglycemia, 60–61

classroom assistance, 58–59
clinical care recommendations,
   236–237
cognitive impairment, 63
continuous glucose monitoring
   (CGM), 176–179, 184
continuous subcutaneous insulin
   infusion (CSII), 159, 161–162
depressive symptoms in, 4
diagnosis, 219–220
diagnosis-associated psychological
   problems, 219
disease duration, 60
fear of hypoglycemia (FOH), 35, 41
hospitalization, 5
hyperglycemia, 61
hyperglycemia and depressive
   symptoms, 4
hypoglycemia, 34–35, 37–39, 41,
   60–61
infancy, 229
intellectual performance, 57
internet-based studies, 183
learning disorders, 57–62
mealtime behavior, 230
metabolic control, 40, 60–61
neurocognitive dysfunction, 70
neuropsychological skills, 60–61
neuropsychological status,
   assessment of, 61–62
parent-child conflict, 233
parent-child relationship, 230
physical environment, 229–230
preschool, 229–232
remedial services, 58–59
school-aged, 232–233
self-management competence, 64
severe hypoglycemia (SH), 34,
   37–38, 60–61
skill assessment, 122–123
skill deficits, 118
social environment, 229–230
special issues in, **229–250**
toddlers, 229–232
type 1 diabetes and cognitive
   impairment, **57–68**
type 2 diabetes risk, 7, 79–80
Children's Memory Scale (CMS), 58

Children With Diabetes, Joslin.org, 181
cholesterol, 105, 147
choline, 84
choline-containing compounds (Cho),
   74
chronic neuropathic pain, 275
chronic pain, 278
chronic social dysfunction, 195
clinical
   assessment tools, 102–107
   care regimen, 8. *see also specific area*
   expenditures, 101
   management, 109
   recommendations, vii–viii. *see also
      specific area*
   research protocol, 3
   trials, 39. *see also specific trial*; studies
Clinical Practice Recommendations
   (ADA), vii
clinic-based intervention, 235
closed-loop control system, 39
Cochrane Database Systematic
   Review, 136
Cochrane review, 118
cognition, 277
cognitive
   behavioral strategies, 137
   behavioral treatment, 197
   dysfunction, 76–79, 84
   flexibility, 71*t*
   function, viii, 231
   impairment, 1, 38, **57–68**, 234,
      276–278, 281
   limitation, 5
   performance, 74, 81–82
   rehabilitation, 280
   remediation services, 87
   screening, 280
   testing, 70, 73, 75, 78, 85
cognitive behavioral therapy (CBT), 6,
   24, 275, 278–280
Cohen's d, 71*t*, 77, 78*t*
collaborative care approach, 8, 261
collaborative problem-solving, 256
Colles, S. L., 203
communication, 236, 280
community-based diabetes
   interventions, 133, 237

community integration program, 278
compensation strategies, 62
compensatory training, 280
Composite International Diagnostic
  Interview (CIDI), 3
Comprehensive Diabetes Management
  Program (CDMP), 109
comprehensive individual assessment,
  260
computerized assessment tools, 101
computerized tracking systems, 121,
  174
concentration, 1, 2*t*, 232
conceptual reasoning skills, 231
conflict, 233
conflict resolution, 236
confusion, 5
congenital malformations, 257
Consumer Price Index (CPI), 133
continuous arterial spin labeling MRI
  techniques, 81
continuous glucose monitoring
  (CGM), 39, 42–43, 171, 175–179,
  184, 237
continuous subcutaneous insulin
  infusion (CSII), **159–170**
    anxiety, 161
    body weight, 160
    children, 231–232
    clinical care recommendations,
      163–164
    depression, 161, 163
    diabetic ketoacidosis (DKA), 161
    discontinuation, 162
    eating disorders (ED), 163
    flexibility, 162, 164
    glycemic control, 159
    health-related quality of life
      (HRQoL), 222
    hypoglycemia, 160, 163
    insulin requirements, 160
    literature, summary of, 162–163
    medical nutrition therapy (MNT),
      134
    pregnancy, 258
    psychosocial outcomes, 162–163
    psychosocial risks, 164
    quality of life (QOL), 161

regimen, responsibility for, 161–162
severe hypoglycemia (SH), 38
socioeconomic characteristics, 162
treatment satisfaction, 161, 163
coping skills, 234
cortex, 75, 83
cortical atrophy, 83–84
cortical gray matter, 72–73
cost expenditures, 117–118, 120, 173
counseling interventions, 281
counterregulatory hormones, 33–34
couples-based intervention, 255, 261
Cramer, J., 118
C-reactive protein, 79
crisis management, 281

"dead in bed" phenomenon, 33
death, 2*t*. *See also* mortality
decision making, 5
delusional disorders, 2
dementia, 35, 38, 79, 85, 277–278, 281
depressed mood, 1, 2*t*
depression. *See also specific type*
    adjustment disorder, 1
    amputation, 274
    assessment and diagnosis of, 1, 3–4
    bariatric surgery candidates, mean
      symptoms of, 199*f*
    binge eating disorder (BED), 196
    BMI (body mass index), relation to,
      198
    cognitive effects of, 78
    comorbid, prevalence of, 3–4
    continuous subcutaneous insulin
      infusion (CSII), 161, 163–164
    curricula, 8
    diabetes and, viii, **1–16**
    diabetes complications, 5, 221
    diabetes predictor, as a, 5
    Diabetes Self-Care Profile (DSCP),
      109–110
    diabetes-specific emotional distress,
      136
    diagnosis, 219
    differential diagnoses, 2
    disordered eating behavior (DEB),
      21
    dysthymia, 1

early detection, 237
eating disorders (ED), 21
exercise, relation to, 147, 151, 153
family intervention, 255
foot ulcer, 274, 278
health-related quality of life
  (HRQoL), relation to, 198
insulin therapy, 222
measurement of, 2–3
medical regimen nonadherence,
  118
mixed episode, 2*t*
myocardial infarction following,
  276, 280
obesity and, 194
postdiagnosis, 5
preoperative, 202
prevention, 8
remission, 6
research, recommendations for
  future, 7–8
screening and care,
  recommendations for, 8
Self-Care Inventory-Revised
  (SCI-R), 107
severe hypoglycemia (SH), 38
sexual dysfunction, 221
spectrum disorder, 1–2
stroke following, 276, 280
subsyndromal depression, 1
suicide, 202
symptoms, 1, 175
treatment, 6–8
weight loss, 195, 201, 206
depressive disorder, 1
depressive symptoms, 3–5, 7, 275
Developmental Neuropsychological
  Assessment–Second Edition
  (NEPSY-II), 58
diabetes. *See also specific type*
  assessment tools, 101–110
  care regimen, 19–24, 42, 101, 105
  clinical care recommendations,
    222–223, 278–281
  complications, 5, 221–223, 253
  control, 220. *see also* glycemic
    control
  conventional treatment, 159

depression and, **1–16**
diagnosis, 219–220, 222–223
disease of disability, 274
distress, 175
duration, 76, 84
early disease onset, 64
eating disorders (ED), 17–18
education, 6–8, 38, 40–41, 101, 109,
  173, 255, 261, 279
educational accommodations, 59
history, 150
hybrid, 235
knowledge, assessment of, 104–111,
  124
long-term complications, 221
management, 1, 36, 40–41, 138,
  183*t*
management team, 24
maturity-onset, 235
medical management of, vii
micro-management, 36
morbidity, 131
vs. nondiabetic patients in case
  studies, 70–71, 73–74, 76–85
preventing and controlling, 138–
  139
problem solving, 106
psychological risk, critical periods
  of, **219–228**
psychosocial adjustments to,
  219–228
as a psychosocial issue, vii
regimen adherence, 117–118
self-care behavior, assessment of,
  107–111, 123
self-care skills, assessment of,
  106–111
self-efficacy, 106–107
self-management, 252–253, 276–
  280
skill assessment, 122, 124
social support, 1
symptoms, 5, 223
treatment planning, 102, 122
treatment regimen transitions,
  222–223
type 1.5, 235
work-related issues, 252–253

Diabetes and Cardiovascular Disease
Test (DCDT), 105
diabetes-associated cognitive
dysfunction, 70, 86–87
diabetes clinical information systems,
101
Diabetes Control and Complications
Trial (DCCT), 33, 64, 134, 161, 172,
179, 231, 257
Diabetes Control and Complications
Trial (DCCT) / Epidemiology
of Diabetes Interventions and
Complications (EDIC) Cognitive
Follow-Up Study, 75
Diabetes Control and Complications
Trial (DCCT) Research Group, 159,
222
Diabetes Distress Scale (DDS), 3
Diabetes Eating Problems Survey
(DEPS), 22
Diabetes Educator Tool (D-ET),
108–109
Diabetes HealthSense, 103
Diabetes Knowledge Scales (DKN A,
B, and C), 105
Diabetes Knowledge Test (DKT), 104
Diabetes Medical Management Plan
(DMMP), 59
diabetes.org, 181
Diabetes Prevention and Control
Program, 133
Diabetes Prevention Program, 134, 151
Diabetes Problem-Solving Inventory,
106
Diabetes Problem Solving Scale, 106
Diabetes Quality-of-Life Measure
(DQOL), 164
diabetes-related
complications, 147, 149
distress, 1, 3, 107, 221
functional impairment and
disability, 273–289
psychological distress, 219–220
Diabetes Self-Care Profile (DSCP),
101, 109
Diabetes Self-Management
Assessment Report Tool
(D-SMART), 108–109

diabetes self-management behaviors,
235
diabetes self-management education
(DSME), 38, 102–103, 106, 110–111,
117, 119, 183, 278–279, 281
diabetes-specific distress, 136, 223
Diabetes-Specific Quality-of-Life
Scale (DSQOLS), 164
Diabetes Support and Education
(DSE), 135
Diabetes Treatment and Satiety Scale
(DTSS-20), 22
diabetic encephalopathy, 69
diabetic ketoacidosis (DKA), 18, 24,
161, 163–164, 172, 232, 251
diagnosis-associated psychological
problems, 219
*Diagnostic and Statistical Manual of
Mental Disorders IV* (DSM IV), 58
Diagnostic Interview Schedule (DIS),
3
diet, 5, 107, 119, 133, 203
dietary assessment methods, 131
Dietary Guidelines for Americans, 2010,
132
Differential Ability Scales–Second
Edition (DAS-II), 57
diffusion tensor imaging (DTI), 73
digitized fundus photography, 77
disability, 273, 278
discrimination, 59, 260
disordered eating behavior (DEB),
17–32
adolescent, 19–20
bariatric surgery, 206
BMI (body mass index), 20
definition of, 17
diabetes care regimen, 20–21
diabetes-specific measurement
tools, 23
diabetic patients, viii, 17–18
diagnosis, 17
Eating Disorder Examination, 19
etiology of, 20–21
evaluation tools, 21–23
formal evaluation and care, 24
hypoglycemia, 23, 36
insulin dosing, 23

intervention efforts, 24
measurement of, 21–22
medication dosing, 23
nondiabetic population, 20
physiologic dysregulation, 20–21
psychiatric morbidity, 23
psychiatric symptoms, 20–21
psychological/psychiatric
evaluation, 24
regimen compliance /
noncompliance, 20–21
research findings, limitations of
current, 22–23
Restraint scale, 19
risk factors, 20
screening and care,
recommendations for, 23–24
subclinical, prevalence of, 18–20
type 1 diabetes (T1D), 17–19
type 2 diabetes (T2D), 21
Western culture, 19
Dixon, J. B., 201
DLife.com, 181
Dose Adjustment for Normal Eating
(DAFNE) randomized clinical trial,
134
Dose Adjustment for Normal Eating
[DAFNE] Study Group 2002, 104
driving, 34
drug(s), 2*t*, 194
DSM-III (APA), 20
DSM-IV (APA), 2*t*, 196
DSM-IV-TR (APA), 17, 21
Dumont, R. H., 232
dyad level model, 256
dysphoria, 87
dysthymia, 1, 6
dysthymic disorder, 194

EAT-26, 21
Eating Attitudes Test (EAT) 40, 21
Eating Disorder Examination (EDE),
19, 22
Eating Disorder Inventory (EDI-3),
21–22
eating disorders (ED), **17–32**
adolescent, 20, 237
BMI (body mass index), 20

continuous subcutaneous insulin
infusion (CSII), 163
definition of, 17
diabetic patients, viii, 17–18
diagnosable, prevalence of, 18–20
diagnosis, 17
etiology of, 20–21
evaluation tools, 21–22
measurement of, 21–22
nondiabetic population, 20
physiologic dysregulation, 20–21
psychiatric symptoms, 20–21
regimen compliance /
noncompliance, 20–21
research findings, limitations of
current, 22–23
risk factors, 20
screening and care,
recommendations for, 23–24
type 2 diabetes (T2D), 21
Eating Disorders Inventory body
dissatisfaction subscale, 200
eating patterns, 206
ecological model, 122
economic impact, 5
education, 6–8, 59, 63, 105, 173, 183*t*,
237, 255, 279, 281
educational level, 133
Education of All Handicapped
Children Act of 1974, 59
Education Rehabilitation Act of 1973,
59, 61
effort-reward imbalance, 254
8-week self-management training
program, 235
Eiser, C., 230
elderly persons, 6, 34–35, 38, 77–78,
82–83, 118, 122, 200, 255
electroencephalogram (EEG), 71–72,
80
electronic medical record (EMR)
systems, 102, 111
email, 181–182
emotional
disorders, 21. *see also specific type*
distress, 109–110
response, 106, 220, 222
support, 254, 260

employment, 251, 260
employment discrimination, 253
endothelial dysfunction, 85*t*
end-stage renal disease (ESRD), 221
energy loss, 2*t*
environmental factors, 273–274
environmental strategies, 62, 137–138
Epidemiology of Diabetes
  Interventions and Complications
  (EDIC), 64
epinephrine, 37, 39
Equal Employment Opportunity
  Commission (EEOC), 261
erectile dysfunction, 221
ethnicity, 5, 7, 148, 235–236
euglycemia, 39
evaluation tools, 21–22
event-related evoked-potential, 71
event-related potentials, 80
Evidence Analysis Library (EAL), 134
evidence-based policies, 138
evidence-based psychotherapies,
  279–280
executive function, 61, 74, 77, 78*t*,
  79–80, 277
executive skills, 231
exercise
  aerobic, 148, 153
  assessment, 150–151
  behavioral intervention, 5, 147–148,
    151, 153
  caloric consumption, 151
  care setting, 152
  clinical care recommendations,
    152–153
  depression, as a treatment for, 8
  diabetes self-management, 119
  fear of hypoglycemia (FOH), 35
  flexibility training, 148
  goal, 148
  hypertension, 149
  hypoglycemia, 35–37, 39
  indications, 148–149
  interventions, target of, 149–150
  lifestyle modification, **147–158**
  non-weight-bearing, 148
  outcomes, 152
  physical examination prior to, 149

physiologist, 150
program, 150–152
psychosocial factors in treatment,
  151–152
racial/ethnic differences in, 148
resistance training, 148, 153
resources, 151
safety procedures, 150
self-care behavior, 107
self-efficacy, 151–152
severe hypoglycemia (SH), 36
statistics, 148
swimming, 149
treatment methods, 149–150
type 2 diabetes, 121, 123, 147
walking, 150, 152
weight lifting, 149
women and, 148
exercise electrocardiogram (ECG)
  stress tests, 149
eye exam, 121

Fabricatore, A. N., 198
Facebook, 181
family. *See also* parenting; social,
  support
  communication, 234
  environment, 232
  functioning, 162, 175
  history, 235
  intervention, 235, 255–256, 261
  stress, 219–220, 255, 275, 277, 279
  structure, 219
  support, 255
  teamwork, 236
  therapy modalities, 235
family-systems perspective of diabetes
  management, 255
fasting plasma glucose (FPG) values,
  85, 105
fatigue, 1, 2*t*
fear of hypoglycemia (FOH), 35, 38,
  40–41
feedback, 121
female gender, 219–220. *See also*
  women
female sexual dysfunction (FSD), 200,
  205

fetal growth, 257
Fisher, E. B., 122
504 Plan, 59
flexibility training, 148
fluoxetine, 6, 281
food. *See also* binge eating disorder
  (BED); diet; disordered eating
  behavior (DEB); eating disorders
  (ED)
    choices, 137
    groups, 105
    insecurity, 133
    intake, 36
    records, 131
foot care, 105, 107
foot exam, 121
foot ulcer, 221, 274–275, 278–279
free appropriate public education
  (FAPE), 59
Frei, A., 107
frontal gliosis, 83
frothing, 203
functional abnormalities, 277
functional impairment, 5, 273, 278,
  281

Galatzer, A., 220
gamification, 183
γ-aminobutyric acid [Glx], 74
Garrison, W. T., 230
gastric dumping, 203
gastroparesis, 21, 221
gender, 256
generalized anxiety disorder, 2
genetic characteristics, 78
gestational diabetes (GDM), 7, 257,
  261
gestational weight gain (GWG), 258
glargine, 232
glial proliferation, 74
gliosis, 83–84
glipizide GITS, 253
glucose. *See also* blood glucose (BG)
    brain transport, 83
    dysregulation, 83
    metabolism, 80
    toxicity, 79. *see also* hyperglycemia
glutamate, 74, 84

glutamine, 74, 84
glyburide, 85
glycemia, viii
glycemic control. *See also* blood
  glucose (BG); blood glucose
  monitoring (BGM)
    adherence, 118–119, 233
    adherence assessments, 123
    cognitive remediation services,
      86–87
    depressive symptoms, 4–5
    exercise and, 148
    gestational diabetes, 257
    insulin pump therapy, 159
    insulin sensitivity, diminished, 233
    internet-based insulin pump
      monitoring system, 183
    intervention efforts, 121
    patient expectations, 24
    physical activity and, 147
    pregnancy, 257
    school, 62, 232
    technology, 171
    treatment methods, 6
    weight control *vs.*, 20
    weight loss, 135
    work-related issues, 253
    young adult, 252
glycemic patterns, 175
glycohemoglobin levels, 159, 221
glycosuria, 19
glycosylated hemoglobin A1C levels,
  118, 120–121, 123. *See also* A1C value
gray matter, 72–73, 75, 80–81
gray matter choline (Cho), 84
Grey, M., 219–220
Grilo, C. M., 200
guilt, 1, 2*t*

Hamburg, B. A., 219
Haynes, R., 117, 119
HDL cholesterol, 105
health care expenditures, 5, 35, 120,
  122, 254
health care system, 252
health care team. *See* medical, team;
  specific type of provider
Health Problem Solving Scale, 106

health profession training, 138
health-related quality of life
  (HRQoL), 136, 197–198, 199*f*, 204,
  206, 221–222, 275–276
Healthy People 2010, 172
hemiparesis, 277, 280
hemiplegia, 277, 280
Herpertz, S., 195
Higa, K. D., 201
high-density lipoprotein (HDL)
  cholesterol, 105
hippocampal atrophy, 82–83
hippocampus, 75
Hispanic, 4, 148
Honolulu-Asia Aging Study, 83
hormonal counterregulation, 37, 42
hormonal dysregulation, 21–23
hormone replacement, 23
hospitalization, 18, 24
Hsu, L. K., 201
hypercholesterolemia, 82, 86
hyperglycemia
  blood glucose monitoring (BGM),
    175
  cerebral blood flow (CBF), 81
  children and adolescents, 61, 64
  cognitive dysfunction, 84
  cognitive function, viii
  cognitive impairment, 277
  dementia, risk of, 35
  depressive symptoms and, 4
  exercise and, 149–150
  medical nutrition therapy (MNT),
    134
  microvascular disease, 74, 77
  overtreatment of, 36, 42
  pregnancy, 257
  Sensor-augmented pump (SAP)
    therapy, 39–40
hyperglycemia-associated
  neurotoxicity, 79
hyperinsulinemia, 78
hyperperfusion, 72, 75
hypersomnia, 1, 2*t*
hypertension, 78–79, 81–83, 86, 196
hypoglycemia, **33–55**
  acute transient, 61
  adrenergic symptom, 37

asymptomatic, 231
behavioral intervention, 40
biological definition, 33
biopsychobehavioral model, 37
blood glucose monitoring (BGM),
  175
children, 60–61, 230
chronic, 60–61, 234
CNS damage in T2D, 85*t*
cognitive dysfunction, 86
cognitive impairment, 84, 277
comprehensive interview, 41
continuous glucose monitoring
  (CGM), 39, 177–179
continuous subcutaneous insulin
  infusion (CSII), 160, 163
"dead in bed" phenomenon, 33
definition of, 33–34
depression remission treatment, 6
Diabetes Self-Care Profile (DSCP),
  109
disordered eating behavior (DEB),
  viii, 21, 23
diurnal, 38
emotional well-being, impact on,
  34–35
exercise and, 149–150
hippocampus sensitivity to, 82
management, 105
mild, 33, 37, 42, 61–62, 231
moderate, 33, 37, 62
mortality, 33
neurocognitive outcomes and, 75
neuroglycopenic symptom, 37
nocturnal, 33, 38, 42, 232
overtreatment of, 40, 134
patient belief, 42
patient cognition, 36
physical well-being, impact on,
  34–35
physiological factors, 35
precursor to, 36
prevalence of, 33–34
profound, consequences of, 75
psychotherapy treatment, 41
recommendations for care, 41–43
risk factors, 35–38
seizure, 231

severe, 33–41, 60–62, 75, 160, 231–232, 234, 253
  studies, 160
  symptomatic definition, 33
  type 2 diabetes (T2D), 84–85
  work-related issues, 253, 260
hypoglycemic agent, 222
hypoglycemic-associated autonomic failure (HAAF), 37, 42
hypoglycemic awareness (HA), 37, 39, 42
hypoglycemic symptomatology, 38
hypoglycemic unawareness, 42
hypomanic periods, 2
hypoperfusion, 72, 75
hyposomnia, 1

impairment, 273–274
impotence, 221
inactivity, 235
inadvertent nonadherence, 117
income level, 133, 254
incretin production, 21
indecisiveness, 2t
Individual Education Plan (IEP), 59
Individualized Health Plan (IHP), 59
Individuals with Disabilities Education Act (IDEA), 59
infancy, 229
infant-parent attachment, 229
inflammation, 85t
information processing, 71, 281
Inoff, G. E., 219
insomnia, 2t
Institute of Medicine (IOM), 258
instrumental support, 260
insulin
  abnormalities, 80
  action, 105
  administration, 36, 134, 279
  appetite regulation, 21
  basal, 38–39, 180
  bolus, 180
  care regimen, 38
  disordered eating behavior (DEB), 17–20, 22–23
  dose adjustment skills training, 104
  dysregulation, 84
  endogenous, 21
  excessive administration, 36
  flexible regimen, 237
  gestational diabetes, 257
  glargine, 232
  injection-based basal bolus insulin programs, 180
  intensive insulin therapy, 33, 35, 37–38, 40, 159, **171–195**, 222, 231
  long-acting insulin analog, 180, 232
  manipulation, 17–20, 22, 38
  metabolism, 79
  pen use, 222
  physical activity effect on, 147
  pump therapy, **159–170**, 279
  quality of life (QOL), 222
  rapid-acting, 180
  requirement, 163
  resistance, 78, 83, 135
  sensitivity, 233
  stacking, 36
  syringe, 222
  therapy, 109
insulin pen, 171, 184
insulin pump therapy, 38, 119, 171, 177, 183, 231, 237, 258. *See also* continuous subcutaneous insulin infusion (CSII)
insulin resistance, 85t, 148
insurance coverage, 172–173
integrative cognitive therapy, 24
intellectual disability (ID), 278
intellectual performance, 57–58
intelligence, 71t, 231
intensive diabetes management training, 184
intensive diabetes therapy, 134
intensive insulin therapy, **171–195**
  blood glucose monitoring (BGM), 172–175
  clinical care recommendations, 183–185
  continuous glucose monitoring (CGM), 175–179
  hypoglycemia, 33, 35, 37–38, 40
  internet programs, 181–183
  pen use, 179–181
  psychosocial considerations, **171–195**

technology, 171, 181–183
intensive lifestyle intervention (ILI),
  236
intensive lifestyle intervention (ILI)
  behavioral weight loss treatment, 135
interactive technologies, 184
interactive voice recognition systems,
  103
interleukin-6, 79
internalizing behavior, 230
*International Classification of
  Functioning, Disability and Health*
  (ICF), 273–274
International Fitness Professionals
  Association (IFPA), 150
internet, 185
internet-based diabetes self-
  management program, 181
internet coping skills training
  program, 183
internet programs, 171, 181–184
interpersonal interactions, 276
interpersonal support, 279
interpersonal therapies, 24, 279–280
intervention efforts, ix, 220, 234
interview assessment, 3
interview format, 278
interview protocols, 3–4
IQ score, 57–59, 64, 80
ischemic cerebrovascular disease, 79
islet cell transplant, 39
iTunes®, 182

Jacobson, A. M., 233
Jette, A. M., 152
job strain, 254
Joslin, E. P., 147
Juvenile Diabetes Research
  Foundation (JDRF) 6-month CGM
  Trial, 176–179
Juvenile Diabetes Research
  Foundation (JDRF) trial, 39

Kalarchian, M. A., 193–194, 198, 202
Kaufman Assessment Battery for
  Children–Second Edition (K-ABC–
  II), 57
knee pain, 136

Kodl study, 73
Kovacs, M., 219–220, 233
Kruseman, M., 203

language, 71*t*, 277
laparoscopic adjustable gastric banding
  (LAGB), 193, 201, 204
Laron, Z., 220
lateral ventricles, 83
Latino, 121
LDL cholesterol, 105
learning cognition, 71*t*
learning disorders, 57–63, 234, 237
learning skills, 70, 77, 78*t*, 79, 84, 231
legacy affect, 179
life. *See* health-related quality of life
  (HRQoL); quality of life (QOL)
life activities, 273–275
life course issues, viii, ix
lifestyle intervention program, 136
lifestyle modification, 109, **131–145,
  147–158**, 204, 258
lipid, 147
lipid abnormalities, 18
lipid assays, 121
lipid metabolism, 80, 135
Liss, D. S., 232
locus of control, 162
Look AHEAD (Action for Health in
  Diabetes) study, 134, 136, 147, 151
low-calorie diet, 203
low-density lipoprotein (LDL)
  cholesterol, 105
lungs, 257

macrosomia, 257
macrovascular complications, 76, 82,
  84, 149
macrovascular disease, 5, 85*t*
magnetic resonance imaging (MRI),
  73, 81–82
magnetic resonance spectroscopy, 74
major depressive disorder (MDD),
  1–3, 5–6, 194–195, 202, 206
management strategies, 8, 121–122
manic periods, 2
marital/family intervention, 276
marriage, 254–256, 261

maturity-onset diabetes, 235
McQuiston, S., 230
meal plan, 110, 134
mealtime behavior, 230
measurement tools. *See* assessment,
  tools
medical
  advice, 119, 123–124
  care, 7, 110
  condition, 2t
  equipment, 122
  insurance coverage, 58, 62
  morbidity, 252
  record audits, 121
  regimen, 64
  regimen adherence, 117–130
  team, 8, 24, 87, 101–102, 119, 150,
    183, 206, 237, 260, 280
medical nutrition therapy (MNT),
  20–21, 24, 42, 131–139, 257
Medicare, 136
medication. *See also specific type*
  adherence, 118–119, 123, 183t,
    274–275
  antidepressant, 6, 8
  cost expenditures, 123
  delivery system, 223
  disordered eating behavior (DEB),
    23–24
  evaluation, 281
  major depressive disorder (MDD),
    2t
  metformin, 85, 139, 236
  oral, 119, 123
  oral hypoglycemic agents, 5, 222
  prescription expenditures, 5, 118,
    122
  psychotropic, 87, 196
  severe hypoglycemia (SH), 38
  treatment regimen transitions, 222
  tricyclic antidepressant, 6
Medication Event Monitoring
  Systems (MEMS caps), 119, 123
memory, 71t, 74, 77
memory loss, 5
memory skills, 70, 78t, 79, 82, 84,
  231–232, 277
MEMS caps, 119, 123

men, 4, 205, 221, 256
Mendelson, M., 198
menopause, 200
mental health disorders, 252. *See also*
  specific type
mental health services, 8, 58, 164, 175,
  184, 206, 279
mental illness, 7–8. *See also specific type*
mental performance, 77, 198
metabolic
  control, 18, 40, 60–61, 82, 84–86,
    131, 159, 163, 231
  derangement, 24
  memory, 179
  syndrome, 7, 255
metformin, 85, 139, 236
method of assessment, 195
Mexican-American, 148
Michigan and Vanderbilt Diabetes
  Research Training Centers, 103
microangiopathic disease, 149
microstructural abnormalities, 84
microvascular complications, 72,
  75–77, 82, 84, 86, 149, 252
microvascular disease, 5, 85t
Miller-Johnson, S., 233
minority population, 19, 123
miscarriage, 257
mixed-methods assessment, 133
mobility, 204, 275–277
Monitoring of Individual Needs in
  Diabetes (MIND) program, 103
mood, 86, 164, 175, 200
mood disorders, 194–195, 198, 202
morbidity, 18, 20–21, 23, 130, 134,
  148, 257
mortality, 5, 33, 148, 193, 201, 255,
  276, 281
motivation, 151
motivational interviewing, 137, 235
Motivational Interviewing Network of
  Trainers (MINT), 132
motivation enhancement, 138
multicomponent intervention, 121, 123
multilevel assessment, 133
multilevel framework, 138
multiple daily injections (MDI), 134,
  159–160, 177, 222, 232, 258

multisystemic therapy, 235
muscle-skeletal injuries, 149
myelin metabolism, 74
myocardial infarction (MI), 276–277, 280–281
Myo-inositol (mI), 74, 83–84

N-acetyl-aspartate (NAA), 74, 84
National Committee for Quality Assurance (NCQA) certification program, 111
National Diabetes Education Outcomes System (NDEOS), 108
National Diabetes Education Program, 181
National Diabetes Information Clearinghouse, 137
National Health and Nutrition Examination Survey (NHANES), 133, 194
National Institutes of Health Consensus Development Conference on Gastrointestinal Surgery for Severe Obesity, 193, 205
National Standards for Diabetes Self-Management Education, 117
Native American, 121
nature, 133
neonatal morbidity, 257
nephropathy, 5, 221
neural slowing, 84
neural transmission, 75
neuritic plaques, 83
neurobehavioral tests, 230
neurochemical abnormalities, 75
neurocognitive
    complications, 84–85
    dysfunction
        in adults with diabetes, **69–99**
        recommendations for clinical practice, 86–87
        type 1 diabetes (T1D), 70–77
        type 2 diabetes (T2D), 77–86
    functioning, viii, 231
    phenotype, 74–75
neuroendocrine effects of stress, 222
neurofibrillary tangles, 83
neuroglycopenia, 33, 37

neuroimaging techniques, 57, 73
neurometabolite, 84
neuronal calcium homeostasis, 85*t*
neuronal demyelination, 74
neuronal necrosis, 74
neurons, 74–75
neuropathy, 5, 18, 72, 80, 84, 148, 221, 275
neuropsychological
    assessments, 61–62, 231
    evaluation, 280
    screening and evaluation, 86
    skills, 60
    tests, 58
neuropsychologist, 61, 87
neurotransmitter, 74
neurovegetative symptoms, 1
Nguyen, N. T., 204
night eating syndrome, 197
nocturnal counterregulation, 37
nocturnal hypoglycemia, 33, 38, 42, 232
nonadherence, prevalence of, 117–118
Northam, E. A., 230–231
nortriptyline, 6, 281
nurture, 133
nutrition
    assessment, 131
    counseling, 137
    Diabetes and Cardiovascular Disease Test (DCDT), 105
    goals, 137
    lifestyle modification, **131–145**
    medical nutrition therapy (MNT), 131
    psychosocial assessment, 131
    social ecological model, 138*f*
    strategies, 134

obesity
    bariatric surgery, 193, 196–198, 206
    children and adolescents, 235–236
    community and environment factor, 133
    health-related quality of life (HRQoL), 135
    medical nutrition therapy (MNT), 131, 139

neurocognitive dysfunction, 78, 80, 86
pregnancy risk, 258, 261
O'Brien, P. E., 204
obsessive-compulsive disorder, 2, 195
Omalu, B., 201–202, 206
Onyike, C. U., 194
optic radiations, 73
oral hypoglycemic agents, 5, 222
oral medication, 119, 123
organic pathology, 221
organizational adherence systems, 122
organizational interventions, 121
osteoarthritis, 198
oxidative stress, 79, 85*t*

pain, 198, 199*f*, 255, 274–275, 278
panic disorder, 2, 194
Pankowska, E., 160
paralysis, 277
paranoid disorder, 195
parental involvement, 233–234
parent-child conflict, 233
parent-child relationship, 230
parenting, 219–220, 229, 257–258, 261
parenting stress, 162, 230
paroxetine, 6
participation limitation, 273–275
partnering, 261
partner stress, 256, 261
Pathways study, 6
patient-centered medical home (PCMH), 101–102
patient education, 38, 40–41, 181
Patient Health Questionnaire (PHQ-9), 2–3, 153, 206
patient-provider approaches, 121
patient self-report assessments, 101–110
patient self-report measures, 102
PCMH/ACO model, 101–102, 110–111
pediatric diabetes management, 163
Pediatric Quality of Life Inventory™ (PedsQL) Diabetes Module, 164
pedometer-based interventions, 152
peer influence, 234
peer self-management intervention, 275, 278–279

pen use, 179–181
perfectionism, 200
performance accomplishments, 106
peripheral nerve conduction velocity, 72
peripheral neuropathy, 72, 80, 84, 274–275
personality disorders, 195
personally controlled health records (PCHRs), 102
personal relationships, 251
phantom pain, 274
pharmacotherapy, 24, 204
phospholipid cell membrane, 74
physical
    activity, 36, 105, 135, 137–138, 147, 235. *see also* exercise
    function, 204
    functioning impairment, 199*f*
    performance, 198
physiological responses, 106
physiologic effects of stress, 222
physiology, basic, 105
Pickup, J. C., 160
plegia (paralysis), 277
plugging, 203
Polonsky, W. H., 221
positron emission tomography (PET), 72
postbariatric surgery patients, 201
posterior corona radiata, 73
poststroke paresis (weakness), 277
poststroke rehabilitation, 276, 279
postsurgical counseling, 206
post-traumatic stress disorder (PTSD), 194
Powers, S. W., 230
preconception counseling (PC), 258, 261
pregnancy, 257, 261. *See also* childbearing
pregnancy planning, 258, 261
premature delivery, 257
preoperative depression, 202
preoperative psychopathology, 195, 206
prepregnancy diabetes-related complications, 257
preschooler, 229–232

preterm delivery, 257
primary care provider, 101–102
primary care setting, 6, 8
private school, 59
Problem Areas in Diabetes (PAID), 3
Problem Areas In Diabetes (PAID-
  Revised), 223
problem-solving, 77, 234
problem solving–based diabetes self-
  management training, 277
problem solving interventions studies,
  106
problem-solving skills, 234
problem-solving therapy (PST), 6
processing speed, 78*t*, 79, 231, 277
Project Implicit, 139
proliferative diabetic retinopathy
  (PDR), 221. *See also* retinopathy
Promoting Amputee Life Skills
  (PALS) study, 275
protein glycation, 85*t*
proton magnetic resonance
  spectroscopy (1H-MRS), 74, 83
psychiatric
  complications, 202, 206
  disorders, 38, 193, 196, 232
  illness, 221
  interview protocols, 3–4
  status, 193, 200–201
  symptoms, 195
  treatment, 24, 237
psychoeducation, 40
psychoeducational assessment, 58, 62
psycho-educational strategies, 234
psychological
  characteristics, 234
  distress, 222
  intervention, 121
  morbidity, 252
  screening, 280
  testing, 62
  treatment, 24, 63, 237
  well-being, 148
psychologist, 61–62
psychomotor agitation, 1, 2*t*
psychomotor efficiency, 63
psychomotor speed, 71*t*, 74–77, 80
psychopathology, 3, 202

psychosocial
  assessment, 153, 223
  complications, 276
  crisis intervention clinic, 220
  distress, 275, 278
  evaluation, 195
  functioning, 138
  group counseling, 220
  health, 109
  intervention, 220, 276
  issues, vii, 151, 162, **171–195**
  needs, 279
  status, 200
  symptoms, 274
psychotic disorders, 2
psychotic symptoms, 2*t*
psychotropic medication, 87, 196
pump therapy. *See* continuous
  subcutaneous insulin infusion (CSII);
  insulin pump therapy

qualitative methods, 133
quality of life (QOL), 161, 163, 175,
  177–178, 193, 204, 220–221, 232,
  255, 276
Quality of Life Instruments Database
  [QOLID], 103
quality-of-life scales, 222
quantitative surveys, 133
questionnaires, 21–22, 101–115, 119,
  131, 152–153, 206, 278

racial minorities, 235–236
Rand, C. S. W., 202
randomized controlled trials (RCTs),
  134, 159–161, 163, 235, 253, 255,
  257–258, 275
reasonable accommodation, 253,
  260–261, 280
rebelliousness, 234
rehabilitation program, 278–279
remediation strategies, 62, 280
renal complications, 76
renal function, 38
resistance training, 148, 153
Reske-Nielsen case studies, 69
Resource Centers for Minority Aging
  Research, 103

resources, 103–104, 131
respiratory system, 149
Restraint scale, 19
retardation, 1, 2t
retinal detachment, 148
retinal microvascular abnormalities, 76–77
retinopathy, 4–5, 18, 72–74, 76, 81, 148–149, 221, 275
retirement, 259
risk-taking, 234
Robert Wood Johnson Diabetes Initiative, 103, 133
role functioning, 276
Rosenberger, P. H., 200
rosiglitazone, 85, 236
Rotterdam Study, 83
Roux-en-Y gastric bypass (RYGB), 193, 203
Rovet, J. F., 230–231
Ryan, C., 230

safety assessments, 260
Sarwer, D. B., 198, 200, 203–204
Schedule for Affective Disorders and Schizophrenia-Lifetime Version (SADS-L), 3
schizoaffective disorder, 2
schizophrenia, 2
school, 232
school-age developmental period, 232–233
school assessments, 58
school assistive services, 62
school-based medical care plans, 59
school-based multicomponent intervention, 236–237
SCID. *See* Structured Clinical Interview for the DSM-IV-TR (SCID)
seizure, 61
self-appraisal, 106
self-care behavior, 5, 64, 107–111, 119, 123, 276
Self-Care Inventory and the Diabetes Regimen Adherence Questionnaire, 119, 123
Self-Care Inventory-Revised (SCI-R), 107, 109

self-efficacy, 162, 175
self-esteem, 63, 107, 162, 200, 232
self-management, 117
self-management behavior, viii, ix, 65
self-management devices, 278–279
self-monitoring of blood glucose (SMBG), 39, 105, 132, 134, 172, 257
self-perception, 223
self-report
    depression, 200–201
    depression questionnaires, 3
    diet behaviors, 134
    health status, 5
    instruments, 120, 196
    measures, 195, 197
    regimen adherence, 220
    symptom inventories, 2–3
semistructured clinical interview, 196–197
Sensing With Insulin Pump Therapy to Control HbA1c [SWITCH], 39–40
Sensor-augmented pump (SAP) therapy, 39–40, 42–43
Sensor-Augmented Pump Therapy for A1C Depression and Diabetes 39 Reduction [STAR 3], 39–40
Sensor-Augmented Pump Therapy for A1C Reduction (STAR3) clinical study, 177
sensory deficits, 281
sensory-evoked potentials, 80
sensory measurement, 71
serotonin and norepinephrine reuptake inhibitor (SNRI), 7
serotonin reuptake inhibitor (SSRI), 6–7
sertraline, 6
severe hypoglycemia (SH), 33–41, 60–62, 75, 160, 231–232, 234, 253
sexual dysfunction, 221, 223
sexual functioning, 198, 200, 205
SF-36® Health Survey scales, 204
sick day management, 105
single photon emission computerized tomography (SPECT), 72
skill deficits, 117–118
sleep, 35, 86

sleep apnea, 196, 198
sleep-related eating disorder (SRED), 197
smartphone apps, 183
smoking, 37, 105, 107, 255
social
 class status, 64
 dysfunction, 195
 ecological model, 137, 138*f*
 media, 181
 network, 220
 performance, 198
 phobia, 2, 194
 self-perception, 221
 skills, 234
 support
  adolescent diabetes, 234
  continuous glucose monitoring (CGM), 184
  dementia, 277
  depression, 5
  Diabetes Self-Care Profile (DSCP), 109–110
  diagnosis of diabetes, 220
  eating disorders (ED), 24
  exercise, 152–153
  family, 255
  infant diabetes, 229
  insulin pump therapy, 164
  internet and interactive technologies, 183*t*
  marriage/partnering, 254, 261
  medical regime adherence, 122–123
  weight loss, 135
social cognitive theory (SCT), 106–107
social-emotional adjustment, 232
Society of Behavioral Medicine Diabetes Special Interest Group, 103
socioecological assessment, 133
socioeconomic status (SES) groups, 38, 64, 235–236
somatization, 275
specific phobia, 2, 194
spectrum disorder, 1–2
SPECT techniques, 80–81
spousal stress, 279

spouse participation, 255–256
standardized assessment methods, 101–102
standardized neuropsychological measures and procedures, 281
standardized patient-care flow sheets, 121
STeP (Structured Testing Program), 122, 174–175
stepped-care approach, 8
stigmatization, 63
stress, 151, 222, 229
stress-management techniques, 234
stress test, 149, 153
stroke, 276–277, 280–281
structural abnormalities, 277
Structured Clinical Interview for the DSM-IV-TR (SCID), 3, 22, 193, 195, 281
structured clinical interviews, 195–196
Structured Testing Program (STeP), 122, 174–175
structured therapy techniques, 281
studies. *See also specific study*
 continuous subcutaneous insulin infusion (CSII), 159–163
 depression, treatment of, 6–7
 depression and diabetes, risk factors, 5
 depressive symptoms, 4
 diabetic ketoacidosis (DKA), 161
 diabetic *vs.* nondiabetic patients in, 70–71, 73–74, 76–85
 Honolulu-Asia Aging Study, 83
 hypoglycemia, 39, 160
 internet-based, 182–183
 Juvenile Diabetes Research Foundation (JDRF) 6-month CGM Trial, 176–177
 medical nutrition therapy (MNT), 134
 neurocognitive dysfunction, 70–72
 problem solving interventions, 106
 research, 102
 Rotterdam Study, 83
 Sensor-Augmented Pump Therapy for A1C Reduction (STAR3) clinical study, 177

STeP (Structured Testing Program), 122, 174–175

Studies to Treat Or Prevent Pediatric Type 2 Diabetes (STOPP-T2D), 236

Sweet Talk, 174

Trials of the National Institutes of Health, 236

web-based intervention, 182

Studies to Treat Or Prevent Pediatric Type 2 Diabetes (STOPP-T2D), 236

Stunkard, A. J., 198, 200

subsyndromal depression, 1

suicide, 1, 2*t*, 3, 201–202, 206, 251, 275

sulfonylurea, 34, 85

Summary of Diabetes Self Care Activities (SDSCA), 107, 109

support, 6–7. *See also* social, support

surgical intervention, 193. *See also* bariatric surgery; *specific type*

surveys, 21–22

Swedish Obese Subjects (SOS) study, 200, 204

Sweet Talk, 174

swimming, 149

systematic assessment methods, 101–102

systolic blood pressure, 76

Tau phosphorylation, 85*t*

technology, 171, 174, 181–184, 273

telemedicine approach, 235

testing guidelines, 61–62

text messaging, 181–182, 184–185

The Obesity Society (TOS), 205

therapy, 8

thiazolidinedione insulin sensitizer, 85

Third National Health and Nutrition Examination Survey (NHANES III), 5

tissue water diffusion, 73

tobacco, 37

TODAY study (Treatment Options for Type 2 Diabetes in Adolescents and Youth), 236

toddlers, 229–232

transient lipid abnormalities, 18

transition programs, 252

transition to adult care, 260

transplantation, 39

treatment. *See also specific treatment*

complexity, 118

goals, 121–122

racial disparities, 7

resources, 42

technology, implementation of, viii, ix

Trials of the National Institutes of Health, 236

tricyclic antidepressant medication, 6–7

triglycerides, 82

Tukey's honestly significant difference comparison, 199*f*

tumor-necrosis factor-α, 79

12-Item Short Form Health Survey (SF12), 177

24-hour recall interviews, 120, 123, 131

2010 Dietary Guidelines from the U.S. Department of Health and Human Services and the U.S. Department of Agriculture, 137–138

type 1 diabetes (T1D)

adherence interventions, 121

adolescent, 4, 34, 235

Beck Depression Inventory-II (BDI-II), 3

blood glucose monitoring (BGM), 172

BMI (body mass index), 19

brain structure anomalies, 82

children, 4–5, 34–35, **57–68**

cognitive characteristics, 71*t*

cognitive impairment, 34

depression, rates of, 3–4

Diagnostic Interview Schedule (DIS), 3

disordered eating behavior (DEB), 17–20

eating disorders (ED), 18–19

glycemic control adherence, 118–119

hypoglycemia, 33

hypoglycemic awareness (HA), 37

men, depressive symptoms in, 4

neurochemical abnormalities, 83–84
neurocognitive dysfunction in adults with, 70–77
severe hypoglycemia (SH), 34
weight, 17–18
young adult, 251
type 1.5 diabetes, 235
type 2 diabetes (T2D)
    Beck Depression Inventory-II (BDI-II), 3
    blood glucose monitoring (BGM), 172
    BMI (body mass index), 19
    brain structure anomalies, 82
    CNS damage, potential routes of, 85t
    cognitive impairment, 277
    depression, 3–5
    Diagnostic Interview Schedule (DIS), 3
    disordered eating behavior (DEB), 19, 21
    eating disorders (ED), 21
    ethnicity, 235
    fear of hypoglycemia (FOH), 35
    glycemic control adherence, 118
    hypoglycemia, 34
    medication adherence, 121
    men, depressive symptoms in, 4
    minority population, 19
    neurocognitive dysfunction in adults with, 77–86
    obesity, 193, 198
    pediatric age-group, 235
    psychiatric morbidity, 21
    psychological insulin resistance, 18
    racial minorities, 235
    regimen adherence, 255

unconsciousness, 61
unemployment, 5, 253–254
United Kingdom Prospective Diabetes Study (UKPDS), 179
United Kingdom Prospective Diabetes Study (UKPDS) Group, 159
unstructured practitioner-based assessment, 195
urine protein, 121

U.S. health care delivery system, 110
usual care (UC), 6

valsalva activity, 149
vascular alterations, 80
vascular dementia, 79, 83, 277
vascular disease, 78, 85t
vascular risk factors, 84
vasopressin, 85t
verbal ability, 231
verbal fluency, 60–61
verbal memory, 80
verbal persuasion, 106
vertical banded gastroplasty, 201
Veteran Survey of Weight Management, 132
vicarious learning, 106
vision, 277
vision impairment, 221, 275–276, 279–280
visual evoked potential latencies, 80
visual learning, 60
visual perception, 71t
visual-spatial orientation, 230
vitreous hemorrhage, 148
vocational rehabilitation, 278–279
vomiting, 203
voxel-based morphometry (VBM), 73
vulnerability, 275

walking, 150, 152
Waller, D. A., 232
Waters, G. S., 201–202
web-based educational discussion boards, 181–182
web-based emotional support discussion boards, 181–182
web-based interventions, 181
Wechsler Adult Intelligence Scale (WAIS-IV), 57
Wechsler Individual Achievement Test–Third Edition (WIAT-III), 58
Wechsler Intelligence Scale for Children–IV (WISC-IV), 57
Wechsler Intelligence Scale for Preschoolers (WPPSI-III), 57
Wechsler Memory Scale–Third Edition (WMS-III), 58

Wechsler scales, 57–58
weight. *See also* obesity
  cognitive effects of excess, 78
  control, 235
  depression, as a symptom of, 1
  gain, 20, 163–164
  lifting, 149
  loss, 2*t*, 151, 204
  loss intervention, 134–136, 147–
    148, 193, 195, 197, 201, 254–255.
    see also bariatric surgery; exercise
  management behaviors. *see*
    disordered eating behavior (DEB);
    eating disorders (ED)
  management strategies, 21
  medical nutrition therapy (MNT)
    goals, 131
weight-related pain, 204
weight-related postural abnormalities,
  204
Weight Watchers, 151
Weissberg-Benchell, J., 161–162
white matter, 74–76, 80–84
white matter microstructural
  abnormalities, 73
white persons, 148. *See also* Caucasian
Wide Range Achievement Test–
  Fourth Edition (WRAT-4), 58
Wide Range Assessment of Memory
  and Learning–Second Edition
  (WRAML-II), 58
willful nonadherence, 117
women
    body image, 200
    brain structure anomalies, 81

childbearing, 257
coping skills, 256
depressive symptoms in, 4
diabetes-specific emotional distress,
  136
disordered eating behavior (DEB),
  17–19, 23
eating disorders (ED), 17–19
exercise and, 148
female sexual dysfunction (FSD),
  200, 205
gestational diabetes, 7
insulin omission, 20
metabolic syndrome, 5
mood disorders, 194
motivational interviewing, 135
nutrition management, 132
postmenopausal, 4
Woodcock Johnson Tests of
  Achievement (WJ-III-ACH), 58
work disability, 5
work/employment, 251–254, 260
working memory test, 85–86
workplace-sponsored programs, 254,
  260
work-related issues, 252–253
worksite interventions, 254
World Health Organization (WHO),
  273
worthlessness, feelings of, 1, 2*t*
Wysocki, T., 230

YMCA, 150
young adult (YA), 251, 257, 259–260
YouTube, 181